MW01528125

LIBRARY

College of Physicians and Surgeons
of British Columbia

Psychosurgery

Marc Lévêque

Psychosurgery

New Techniques for Brain Disorders

Preface by Bart Nuttin
Afterword by Marwan Hariz

Springer

Marc Lévêque
Service de Neurochirurgie
Hôpital de la Pitié-Salpêtrière
Paris
France

ISBN 978-3-319-01143-1   ISBN 978-3-319-01144-8   (eBook)
DOI 10.1007/978-3-319-01144-8
Springer Cham Heidelberg New York Dordrecht London

Library of Congress Control Number: 2013946891

Illustration: Charlotte Porcheron (charlotte@chapodesign.com)
Translation: Noam Cochin
Translation from the French language edition 'Psychochirurgie' de Marc Lévêque,
© Springer-Verlag France, Paris, 2013; ISBN: 978-2-8178-0453-8

© Springer International Publishing Switzerland 2014
This work is subject to copyright. All rights are reserved by the Publisher, whether the whole or part of the material is concerned, specifically the rights of translation, reprinting, reuse of illustrations, recitation, broadcasting, reproduction on microfilms or in any other physical way, and transmission or information storage and retrieval, electronic adaptation, computer software, or by similar or dissimilar methodology now known or hereafter developed. Exempted from this legal reservation are brief excerpts in connection with reviews or scholarly analysis or material supplied specifically for the purpose of being entered and executed on a computer system, for exclusive use by the purchaser of the work. Duplication of this publication or parts thereof is permitted only under the provisions of the Copyright Law of the Publisher's location, in its current version, and permission for use must always be obtained from Springer. Permissions for use may be obtained through RightsLink at the Copyright Clearance Center. Violations are liable to prosecution under the respective Copyright Law. The use of general descriptive names, registered names, trademarks, service marks, etc. in this publication does not imply, even in the absence of a specific statement, that such names are exempt from the relevant protective laws and regulations and therefore free for general use.
While the advice and information in this book are believed to be true and accurate at the date of publication, neither the authors nor the editors nor the publisher can accept any legal responsibility for any errors or omissions that may be made. The publisher makes no warranty, express or implied, with respect to the material contained herein.

Printed on acid-free paper

Springer is part of Springer Science+Business Media (www.springer.com)

Preface

Neurosurgical interventions to ameliorate the suffering of desperately ill patients, suffering from a psychiatric disorder, and who cannot be helped otherwise, have caught the attention of neurosurgeons, psychiatrists, and psychologists for several decades. The title of this book, "psychosurgery," summarizes these types of interventions in one word. Everybody understands the word, and given the history, it has positive and negative connotations. In the book it is clearly explained what is really meant by psychosurgery. In fact, a surgical intervention on the brain is performed, and the wanted effect is an improvement of pathological behavior. Unfortunately, this beneficial effect is not always obtained and sometimes one encounters adverse events.

The members of the Committee of Neurosurgery for Psychiatric Disorders, which is a committee installed by the World Society for Stereotactic and Functional Neurosurgery (WSSFN), are convinced that at this moment in time, this kind of surgery can only be performed in a multidisciplinary approach, where psychiatrists work together with neurosurgeons and psychologists. It cannot at this moment be used to improve normal function (one calls this "enhancement") and not as prevention, but only to reduce important suffering.

It was interesting to observe that during the Toronto meeting of the WSSFN in 2009, more papers were presented talking about neurosurgery for psychiatric disorders than for movement disorders, which is opposite to what happened many years before.

Marc Lévêque succeeds in providing a detailed overview of the history of neurosurgery for psychiatric disorders. Furthermore, he explains many aspects of the neuroanatomy of emotions. This chapter makes it understandable why several neurosurgical techniques have been developed. These techniques are described in extenso, together with their results. He gives an overview of the psychiatric disorders for which psychosurgery is performed. The author describes ethical principles that remain relevant for this kind of surgery, and he looks into the future as well.

In summary, I like the book as it provides a very nice overview of psychosurgery in general. It is easy to understand for any (para)medical practitioner, but even specialists in the field may learn new things. They may also enjoy looking at the well-known and less-known figures which illustrate the book. The French edition of the book (which I read) seems to be a success, I presume the English version (which I did not see yet) will see an even wider readership.

Bart Nuttin
Neurosurgeon, UZ Leuven
Research Coordinator, Group of Biomedical Sciences, KU Leuven

Foreword

Acting on the brain, that intimate domain of mind and identity, can appear transgressive and hazardous. How do we justify this intrusion, and how do we guarantee appropriate professional practices when the procedure seems legitimate? What of a patient's ability to formulate clear and informed consent when what they are undergoing is so unbearable that they are willing to try any therapeutic alternative, even an uncertain one? Choosing between forgoing possible succor or attempting the medical intervention is a complex and delicate process. This choice is made even more difficult by the fact that protocols are often experimental and that surgery of the brain can lead, among other things, to altered judgement, attention, and behavior: everything that constitutes a social being. The person can be profoundly altered and his dignity and quality of life negatively impacted. Even when the purpose or objective is to improve or stimulate in order to compensate for a dysfunction or regain certain functions, the procedure is not devoid of problems and risks, notably to the mental integrity of the person.

The strength of this work by Marc Lévêque devoted to psychosurgery is that it offers an in-depth analysis of the various elements, both scientific and medical, which make up this often underestimated field. His thoughtful analysis balances between radical criticisms of psychosurgery's "inhuman or degrading treatment" and pragmatic defense of it as a "lesser evil." This approach, which informs the reader of the extent to which this specialty has in the past been tragically obsessed with correcting behavior considered socially or morally reprehensible rather than building a rigorously scientific, humane, and ethical field of research, makes a significant contribution to the literature. Indeed, it allows the reader to grasp the social, cultural and, therefore, political factors which underpin medical and scientific decisions and can lead them to being used to buttress deviant or pernicious logics. But rather than pass summary judgement, the text strives to present the context, motives, and ideologies, which can illuminate our current paradigms of caution, efficiency, efficacy, and "over-caution." Marc Lévêque's book is a shining example of a curriculum in ethics, one which supports the various types of procedures today part of a reasoned psychosurgical practice, which aims to heal those whom other therapies have failed.

This work plays a dual role. First, it surveys the field drawing on scientific rigor and extensive experience to present the current state of understanding and the latest surgical protocols. Second, it examines the criteria and conditions necessary for a justified, acceptable, and prudent practice of the specialty. One which is respectful of the patient although the context may be challenging and the therapeutic alternatives both limited and limiting. At a time when our notion of illness is shifting, our therapies are becoming more personalized and profiled, patients' rights and preferences are increasingly being factored in, and the impact of the disease on the quality of life and personal environment of the patient is ever more important. Psychosurgery examines these issues and offers a critically useful framework. Its examination of ethical dimensions of the practices is precious as well. Concepts such as autonomy, consent, assent, and responsibility are evaluated within the context of diseases which sometimes strain these principles nearly to their breaking point. What then are the safeguards which the practice can adopt in order to protect these vulnerable patients and their families? What are the pertinent ethical guidelines to draw on and who is best able to watch for the challenges specific to this type of surgery?

During preliminary debates ahead of the vote on law no. 2011—814 of 7 July 2011 regarding bioethics, it became clear that the consequences of advances being made in neuroscience today are not being sufficiently scrutinized, whether in terms of democracy, individual freedoms, or the use of biomedicine for purposes beyond simply healing patients. Consequently, the framework it implemented seems insufficient to deal with the challenges at hand. Take for example, theories aiming to lead humanity toward a transcended state, to break with our traditions and representations, to augment living systems with heretofore unimaginable abilities and capacities. Integration of the brain with other resources such as microcomputers will upend our conception of what "humans are capable of" and will radically transform our relationship to reality and those around us. What are the moral obligations and responsibilities we should strive to adopt and defend as human beings in order to preserve the common good and our identity as humans?

Marc Lévêque gives us an opportunity to share in the sometimes demanding and troubling responsibility of helping fellow human beings suffering from illness and vulnerabilities which not only alter their quality of life but also their very being as well. He expresses with great sensitivity, subtlety, and intelligence the importance of solicitude, respect, a high-degree of competency, and societal responsibility, which have always guided the practice of medicine. For this reason, we are extremely honored to be associated with his work, which I see as a rallying cry calling for solidarity and greater understanding being put in service of patients and their relatives. The notion that, "the interests and welfare of the human being shall prevail over the sole interest of society or science,"[1] is always at the forefront. Marc Lévêque gives us the possibility of learning about a scientific advance and its medical implications from its inception to the present while always

---

[1] Convention for the Protection of Human Rights and Dignity of the Human Being with regard to the Application of Biology and Medicine: Convention on Human Rights and Biomedicine Oviedo, 4.IV.1997.

remaining vigilant as to its implications. The aim is to warn us of the danger inherent in an intervention which risks affecting the consciousness and freedom of a person if it is not used responsibly and carefully. Such situations arise when, for whatever dubious reasons and objectives, we become indifferent to the plight of a patient and lose sight of the fact that not only our neglect but also our abuse of power can endanger him. This book superbly illustrates how respect of the other can lead to a truly ethical practice of medicine.

Emmanuel Hirsch
Philosopher
Professor of Biomedical Ethics
Director of AP-HP Center for Ethics
Paris, France

Preface to the French Edition

Psychosurgery is a rapidly expanding field of functional neurosurgery. This is due, on the one hand, to the considerable progress made in neurosciences, which has led to a better understanding of cerebral function; and on the other hand, to the numerous technological advances made in neurosurgery in the past few years which have enabled us to make procedures safer, more effective, and more consistent in terms of results. This is the case with deep brain stimulation. Its great therapeutic efficacy in patients undergoing treatment for neurological diseases (Parkinson's, dystonia, and essential tremors) along with low complication rates, the absence of brain lesioning, the ability to finely modulate therapeutic effects, and reverse adverse effects make the practice a logical choice for the treatment of certain neuropsychiatric diseases refractory to standard treatments. A new chapter is beginning for this fascinating field of medicine.

A reference work such as this explaining and synthesizing the latest results and looking ahead at future clinical research possibilities is absolutely necessary.

I thank Dr. Marc Lévêque for giving me the opportunity to write this Preface and having allowed me to follow the entire writing process, which has given me new appreciation for the subject. I am certain that all practitioners in this challenging and very specialized field will share my acute interest in this well written and clearly formulated book, which contains a detailed bibliography and provides a wealth of useful and pertinent information.

Patients and their families should also find this text a useful source of information. After all, the purpose of sharing this information and, consequently, improving the understanding of the neurobiology and the treatments for neuropsychiatric diseases is to improve their lives.

Philippe Cornu
Head of the Neurosurgical Department
Hôpital de la Pitié-Salpêtrière
Paris, France

Contents

Figures

Introduction

Psychosurgery, or the surgical treatment of mental pathologies, has long been one of the most controversial fields in medicine. Today, thanks to the astounding progress made in neurosciences over the past decades and the availability of new technologies, psychosurgery, now sometimes called neuromodulation, is once again at the forefront of medicine. Deep brain stimulation, a technique initially developed in the treatment of Parkinson's disease is now being offered to patients suffering from severe OCD, treatment refractory depression and addictions, very severe cases of anorexia nervosa, debilitating Gilles de la Tourette syndrome, and certain aggressive behavior disorders.

In the past 12 years, the number of indications has been steadily growing and functional imaging of the brain has revealed many new potential targets both at the surface and deep within the brain. Other techniques such as brain stimulation and vagus nerve stimulation are also being perfected. However, the greatest potential comes from convergence in the emerging fields of nanotechnology, biotechnology, information technology, and cognitive science, the so-called "great NBIC convergence," which may very well revolutionize treatment for thousands of patients currently in treatment-failure.

Curiously, even though the number of scientific articles on the subject has increased exponentially over the last decade, these advances and their implications are rarely presented in the media and remain known only to neurosurgeons, psychiatrists, and neurologists. What is the reason for this discretion? First, the very small number of patients currently concerned by these techniques and the preliminary nature of the results obtained. Second, the scientific community is apprehensive of the changing and often unpredictable nature of public opinion. Indeed, it is true that the excesses of psychosurgery in the 1950s, epitomized by the tragically widespread lobotomy, have colored the public's perception. However, current techniques have nothing in common with those of the past. The effects of deep brain stimulation are reversible, and modern lesional techniques are extremely precise with none of the deleterious effects on the brain, which lead to such serious mutilations in the personalities of patients in the 1950s. What then is the reason for the scientific community's timidity? It may stem from fears of a backlash similar to the one experienced in the field of genetics, where the public has become increasingly wary of genetically modified products and stem cell research. In spite of these fears, research continues unabated and is leading toward a paradigm shift. The neuroscientist and ethicist Nicolas Kopp wonders, "Should we feel very worried or even just pessimistic about the future of these technologies? No! We believe we should remain vigilant. We must understand, first, that the media play up people's fears; second, that the public is not given enough information about the science; third, that we must remain watchful in terms of ethics and science, in particular with regards to toxicology, as well as psychology and society. The debate surrounding GMOs illustrates these considerations well"[1].

The purpose of this volume is to summarize the findings of the hundreds of articles published in journals specializing in neurosurgery, psychiatry, neuroscience, and bioethics so that everyone may have access to the information they contain, not only specialists. The content of these pages is also drawn from material presented at scientific symposia over the past 5 years, extensive interviews with practitioners and researchers, and my experience in psychiatry, general neurosurgery, functional neurosurgery, and stereotaxy.

In order to help the reader assimilate the information contained in these pages, the volume is divided into six chapters. A certain amount of repetition, particularly with regard to descriptions of the surgical techniques and the anatomical targets, is present in order to enable readers new to the subject to understand the contents of a single chapter without having read the entire volume.

Chapter 1 retraces the history of this specialty, which by design makes no distinction between the mind and the body. From extractions of the stone of madness in the Middle Ages to the tragic epidemic of lobotomies after the close of the Second World War up to the latest developments of the twenty-first century, this retrospective will help the reader understand why this speciality, in spite of strong public opposition in the past, has continued to thrive, and how current scientific research has learned from past mistakes and successes. To understand this history and to measure the extent of the progress made over the past decades, a basic knowledge of the anatomy of the brain and of the biochemical circuitry underlying emotions and their dysfunctions is essential and can be found by reading Chap. 2.

Once the scene is set, Chap. 3 presents the technical details, indications, and complications for each type of surgery according to which anatomical structure is targeted. When presenting lesional techniques, deep brain stimulation, cortical stimulation or vagus nerve stimulation, the neurophysiological mechanisms, and remaining gaps in scientific understanding are discussed specifically.

Chapter 4 reviews the major psychiatric pathologies which have already or may in the future benefit from modern advances in psychosurgery. Clinical concepts are presented alongside epidemiological data, and wherever necessary, we have included explanations on the underlying physiopathological mechanisms for clarity. Finally, the various anatomical targets already in use or currently being explored for each of these mental illnesses are reviewed.

Chapter 5 discusses autonomy, beneficence, nonmaleficence, and justice, the principles on which modern bioethics is founded, and how research and advances in psychosurgery can deviate from these principles. The various ethical safeguards suggested or already implemented to protect an often vulnerable population are detailed as well.

Finally, Chap. 6 contains equal measures of science-fiction and science-fact. The astounding progress made in the fields of nanotechnology, information technology combined with developments in biology and cognitive science pave the way for an NBIC convergence in which every discovery leads to another. This chain of discoveries may lead us over the next 20 years to move beyond healing humans to augmenting them. Lozano's team in Toronto may have stumbled across the first instance of such possible augmentation when they accidentally increased the memory recall capacity by stimulating the hypothalamus of a patient being treated for obesity [2] [a: Similar observations have more recently been made following stimulation of the entorhinal area (Suthana…)]. This move toward an Augmented Human is discussed within the context of socio-philosophical concepts such as meliorism and transhumanism.

Psychosurgery's frightening potential for both good and evil has always made it a controversial subject. In 1954, in his book Psychochirurgie et Fonctions mentales [3], Jacques Le Beau warned that, "everything which pertains to mental functioning seems to as particularly adept at raising ire as the proverbial stick in a bees' nest." The neurosurgeon of the Salpêtrière hospital classified the "confused and often aggressive buzzing" of his detractors, including the psychiatrist Baruk [4] according to three types: the first, which proclaimed on theological grounds the impossibility of analyzing the mind, now seems antiquated. The second, which stigmatized the lack of rigor in the clinical and statistical evaluation of results and complications, now seems antiquated as well. The last, moral objections, today referred to as ethical warnings, is still relevant and must garner all our attention. In order for these ethical objections to be debated effectively, psychosurgery must be understood not just by those in the medico-technical field. The latest information about the major anatomical, surgical, and therapeutic principles must be available to everyone. This book strives to not only provide answers for psychiatrists and their patients but also to the public as a whole.

References

1. Kopp N (2007) Neuroethique et nanotechnologies. In: Hervé C (ed) La nanomedecine: Enjeux éthiques, juridiques et normatifs. Dalloz, Paris
2. Hamani C, McAndrews MP, Cohn M, et al (2008) Memory enhancement induced by hypothalamic/fornix deep brain stimulation. Ann Neurol 63:119–123
3. Le Beau JC, Gaches M, Rosier J (1954) Psycho-chirurgie et fonctions mentales: Techniques-résultats applications physiologiques. Masson, Paris
4. Baruk H (1951) [Medico-legal and moral problems of psychosurgery]. Ann Med Psychol (Paris) 109:472–474

Abbreviations

AC-PC	Anterior-Posterior Commissure
ACTH	Adrenocorticotropic Hormone
BDNF	Brain-Derived Neurotrophic Factor
BPD	Borderline Personality Disorder
CRF	Corticotropin-Releasing Factor
DBS	Deep Brain Stimulation
EEG	Electroencephalogram
FDA	Food and Drug Administration
GABA	*gamma*-Aminobutyric acid
GAF	Global Assessment of Functioning
GPe	Globus Pallidus External
GPi	Globus Pallidus Internal
HFS	High-Frequency Stimulation
HPA	Hypothalamic-Pituitary-Adrenal
HRSD	Hamilton Rating Scale for Depression
MRI	Magnetic Resonance Imaging
NBIC	Nanotechnology Biotechnology Information Technology and Cognitive Science
OCD	Obsessive Compulsive Disorder
PET	Positron Emission Tomography
PTSD	Post-traumatic Stress Disorder
STN	Subthalamic Nucleus
TRD	Treatment-Refractory Depression
VNS	Vagus Nerve Stimulation
Y-BOCS	Yale-Brown Obsessive Compulsive Scale

Chapter 1
A Controversial Past

Abstract Psychosurgery was born from the need to manage patients suffering from untreatable mental pathologies. In 1935, the Portuguese neurologist Moniz, a pioneer in the field, devised the prefrontal leucotomy, for which he received the Nobel Prize a decade and a half later. Psychosurgery reached its apex in the first half of the 1950s with over 60,000 interventions performed throughout the world. Thereafter, the evolution of frontal lobe surgery was shaped by two trends: simplification and greater selectivity of lesions. The first, simplification, was initiated by the American Walter Freeman who popularized the transorbital lobotomy as a procedure performed outside the operating room thus making it more broadly available. The second, greater selectivity of lesions, stemmed from a desire to reduce the serious negative effects, cognitive alterations, and personality changes associated with previous techniques. Some of these more targeted procedures, such as the capsulotomy and the cingulectomy, are still relevant today. After 1955, following the advent and successes of psychopharmacology, the number of interventions dropped significantly. By the end of the 1960s though, a lack of effective medication for certain patients along with improved surgical methods, notably stereotaxy, led to renewed interest in psychosurgery. This revival was short-lived: abuses, an already wary public, and fears of "psycho-enforced" authoritarianism led to strict regulations and even bans in several countries. Since 1999, the success of deep brain stimulation, a new reversible and adaptable therapy devised for the treatment of Parkinson's disease, has offered the hope of new forms of treatment for patients with severe psychiatric disorders like OCD. Today, these new neuromodulation-based treatments are reshaping the field of psychosurgery.

M. Lévêque, *Psychosurgery*, DOI: 10.1007/978-3-319-01144-8_1,
© Springer International Publishing Switzerland 2014

The Beginnings of a Surgery of the Mind

From the First Trephined Skull to Hippocrates

The first skull showing signs of trepanning dates back 5,100 years before our era to the Neolithic. Although we do not know the reason for this intervention, we do know from bone scarring around the burr hole that the "patient" survived [1, 2]. Evidence of such interventions, performed with a measure of finesse, has been found on all the continents: in Europe, Siberia, North Africa, Abyssinia, Melanesia, New Zealand, Peru, and Bolivia [3]. The first written accounts of the procedure, however, come much later. In 1500 BCE, the first surgeons of early antiquity recorded that they trepanned "to let out a spirit imprisoned in the body" and "sooth pains and melancholy or release demons" [4]. Hippocrates himself was the first to give indications for its use and detail the procedure and necessary instruments. Galen (129–201 CE), a Greek physician at the gladiatorial school in Pergamon, undertook the first rudimentary study of neuroanatomy using combatants' wounds as "windows into the body." His knowledge of anatomy encouraged him to perform numerous daring operations, including brain surgery. He considered the brain the "Prince of viscera" and the seat of reason, consciousness and the senses. This diverged from the older Aristotelian view, which held the heart as the center of thought and emotion.[1]

The "Stone of Madness" in the Middle Ages: A Pictorial Myth?

In 1170, in his work entitled *Practica Chirurgiae*, Roger of Parme professes that to remedy melancholy, a cross-shaped incision should be made at the top of the head and the skull penetrated in order to release the *"noxious humors."* Nonetheless, such written records from the Middle Ages are scarce. For the most part, we have only pictorial representations of treating mental illness with trepanning. Many painters depicted the excision of the *"stone of madness"* whose origin can be found in the imagination and symbols of that period, a time when analogy played an important role in therapy. The painting by Hieronymus Bosch appropriately titled

---

[1] Aristotle's view was long the accepted version. This ancient belief is apparent in some of our expressions: 'to learn by heart,' 'you're breaking my heart,' 'to have a heart of stone.' This concept probably originated in observations that heart rate changes, the pulse quickens, when experiencing intense emotions. The heart's reaction to emotions contrasts with the brain's placidity.

"*The Extraction of the Stone of Madness*" is the most well-known example and as such merits a few lines (Fig. 1.1) [5, 6]. In the midst of a summery landscape, a barber–surgeon can be seen extracting an object from the skull of a seated man while a monk and a nun look on. The surgeon is depicted wearing a hat shaped like a funnel suggesting he is a physician of insanity. Curiously, unlike the title of the work indicates, the surgeon is extracting not a stone but a tulip from the patient's head. The Gothic inscription above and below the scene translates to *Master, cut away the stone. My name is Lubbert das*, a Dutch name designating a simpleton. These details suggest that perhaps the painter was using allegory to denounce those who would take advantage of the ill. Lithotomy, as it is known medically, was a "psychiatric" remedy during Bosch's lifetime. Madness, symbolized by a stone, was believed to disappear with the extraction of this stone. Popular belief held that healing madness required only the removal of this mineral body. Whether therapeutic procedure, fraud, symbol, or artistic fancy, the stone of madness remains a mystery. Despite many paintings portraying this theme, especially paintings from the fifteenth- and seventeenth-century Dutch and Flemish schools,[2] we have no medical texts on the topic. Our only sources are iconographic [7]. Nonetheless, we can suppose it was a superficial intervention and not intracranial surgery. First, a vertical incision would have been made in the middle of the forehead and the scalp. Following this cut, the healer could by slight of hand have produced a small stone to show the patient as proof of the complete success of the intervention. This was of course charlatanism, but it may also hint at an intriguing early use of the placebo effect. Unknown at the time, the effect could have led to some successes and contributed to the spread of the practice. Although understanding of neurology and neuroanatomy continued to progress from the Middle Ages until the nineteenth century, records of surgical interventions with psychological objectives remain rare. Two notable exceptions are Robert Burton [8], who in his 1621 work, *Anatomy of Melancholy*, defended perforation of the skull in order to let out "*fuliginous vapors*" and Thomas Willis, a well-known anatomist at Oxford. In 1664, Willis recommended in *Cerebri Anatome* that trepanning be administered in combination with Saint John's Wort,[3] for treating severe melancholy [9]. Although often depicted in paintings, this type of surgery was not widely performed due to its high mortality rate.

---

[2] Of note are the works of Carel Allard, Jérôme Bosch, Andries Both, Pieter Brueghel, Adriaen Brouwer, Jan de Bray, Théodore de Bry, De Wael, A. Diepraem, Frans Hals, Pieter de Huys, Jan Steen, David Téniers, Jan Van Der Bruggen, Jan Van Hemessen, Franz Van Mieris, Jan Van Mieris and Nicolas Weydmans.

[3] A plant traditionally used for treating mild depression. Its efficacy is now accepted.

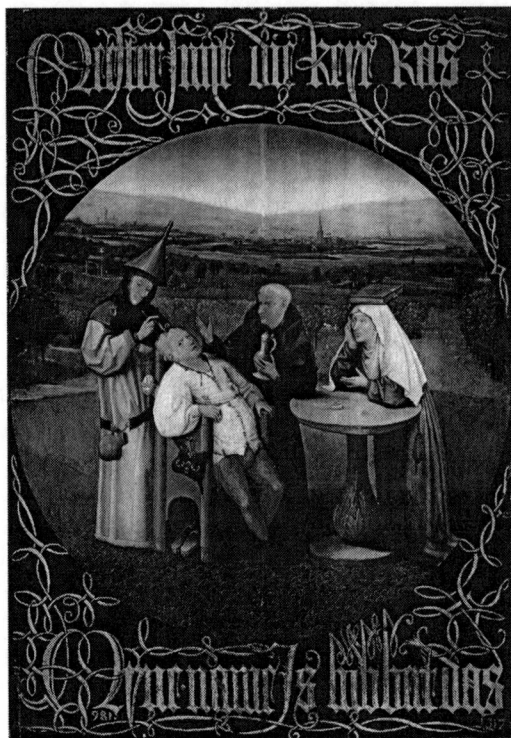

Fig. 1.1 The extraction of the stone of Madness by Hieronymus Bosch

The Nineteenth Century and the First Scientific Observations

Cranial surgery progressed little from the time of Hippocrates to the end of the nineteenth century, and we must wait until 1887[4] for the British Victor Horsley and the American Harvey Cushing and the birth of neurosurgery. It developed thanks to *the elaboration of an even more anatomically, physiologically and clinically precise medicine of the nervous system which thus enables greater understanding of why and how to affect a given region or clinical symptom of the encephalo-medular axis* [10]. The discovery of penicillin by Pasteur further stimulated the development of neurosurgery by reducing the risk of post-surgical infections when exposing the meninge. The work of Paul Broca and Carl Wernicke along with an increase in the number of clinical observations of cranial trauma and autopsy reports enabled a more precise understanding of cerebral cortex functions. The link between certain brain lesions and changes in behavior was firmly established.

---

[4] In 1887, Horsley was the first to operate on a tumor compressing the spinal chord. This prompted the famous physician William Osler to comment "With this operation, perhaps the most brilliant in all the history of surgery, victory was achieved."

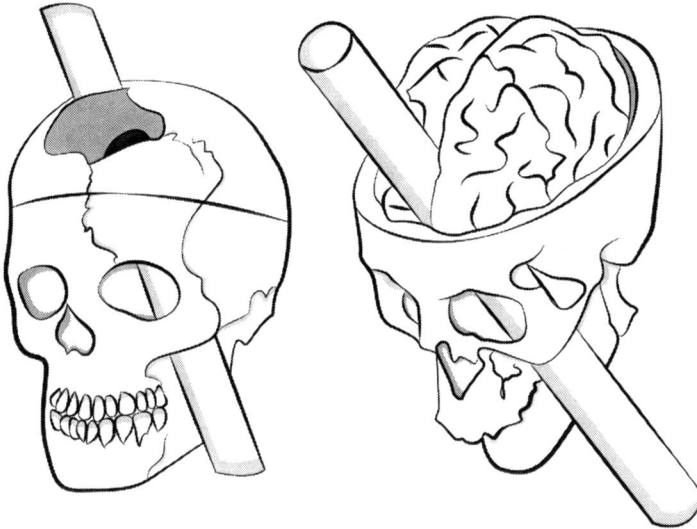

Fig. 1.2 Skull of Phineas gage and trajectory of the packing rod

Phineas Gage, the Most Famous Injury in Medicine

Though its actual impact on the nascent field of psychosurgery is debatable, the most widely cited case remains that of Phineas Gage [11]. In 1848, a young sociable and reserved man, a foreman on a railway construction site, was packing powder with a rod when the powder accidentally went off. The sudden explosion propelled the packing rod through the front part of his skull (Fig. 1.2). Miraculously, the man survived the accident and seemed to have lost none of his intellectual abilities. But afterwards, *Gage was no longer Gage* [12]. He lived out the remaining 12 years of his life in a state of behavioral disinhibition, which made him incapable of thoughtful, critical decision-making. The idea of modifying behavior through the use of brain lesions was slowing emerging from observations of this and dozens of other cases. Meanwhile, alienists were desperately searching for treatment options, but their solutions, though creative, were failing to cure patients.[5]

---

[5] This desperation and the wide array of "therapies" alienists resorted to is illustrated in an account by Quétel from his fascinating book, History of Madness. He tells the story of a 33-year-old mental patient who was "interned at the Bon Sauveur [hospital] in Caen in 1848 [...] with a diagnosis of 'very intense and continuous mania with extreme and continual agitation' [to whom] we administered local and general bloodletting, purgatives, daily baths, and 'long-term and high doses' of digitalus. Nothing calmed him. We isolated him, and then after one month, we applied a "seton" to the back of the neck [a skein of cotton is passed below the skin with the end protruding to promote drainage. In other words, an artificial ulcer is made to cause local suppuration]. Three months passed and the agitation continued so we prescribed a mercurial treatment. No improvements, and finally, cholera took the mental patient in July 1849 before we were able to try another medication… or had given up" (Quétel, C. 2009. Story of Madness. Tallandier).

Gottlieb Burckhardt, a Psychiatrist-Surgeon

The forerunner of psychosurgery is probably the daring Gottlieb Burckhardt (Fig. 1.3), an alienist at the Prefargier hospice in Switzerland who, though not a surgeon, was the first to delve into the human brain *in order to pull out the disease by the root,* and thus directly affect mental disorders [13]. His avowed goal was *to transform agitated lunatics into calm lunatics* [14]. In 1891, he published a report based on observations of six of his patients operated for psychosis [15]. Based on the physiological knowledge of his time, especially observations by Mairet [16], who had shown that patients suffering from severe auditory hallucinations possessed hypertrophied temporal lobes, he hypothesized that agitation stems from hyperactivity in a sensorial center. He posited that by excising a portion of the cerebral cortex he could disconnect the source of the perturbation. He operated on chronic patients who had not responded to prior treatments and whose psychomotor agitation made asylum life difficult. Burckhardt carried out the procedures under general anesthesia with the help of his medical assistant.

Taking between 2 and 4 h, they began by cutting a bone flap. Then, using a curette, they excised about 10 g of cortex primarily from the temporal lobe but sometimes also from the frontal lobe. We have very few details either on patients' post-surgical recovery or their very probable neurological deficits [17]. All we know is that one of those who received the operation perished 6 days later amid convulsions, and another had a seizure which was brought under control with bromides. A third patient was released a year after the procedure but committed suicide soon after. The three remaining subjects, meanwhile, seem to have exhibited reduced signs of agitation. When the Swiss psychiatrist presented his findings at the Berlin medical congress in 1889 [18], his colleagues disapproved [19]. The French psychiatrist Semelaigne indignantly asked, *Where will this surgical frenesy end? If a patient kicks is that sufficient cause to remove the motor center of his lower limbs?* [20]. Similarly, attempts made between 1906 and 1910 by an Estonian neurosurgeon working in Saint-Petersburg, Lodovicus Puusepp, to calm agitation in three maniacal or epileptic patients by sectioning the frontoparietal white matter also remained isolated undertakings [21, 22]. At a meeting of the *Hypnology and Psychology Society* in 1907, the French surgeon E. Doyen[6] defended the use of decompressive craniectomies[7] in mentally handicapped children in order, as he put it, to free the brain from its bony stockade. He alleged *rapid and astonishing* surgical results... [23].

---

[6] A surgeon from the French city of Reims known around the world for his improvements brought to surgical techniques and the development of surgical cinematography. He developed the disengageable trephine, a drill which stops spinning once the bone has been perforated and the tip reaches the meninx, for use in neurosurgery.

[7] A trepanning surgical technique involving ablation of a portion of the cranial vault.

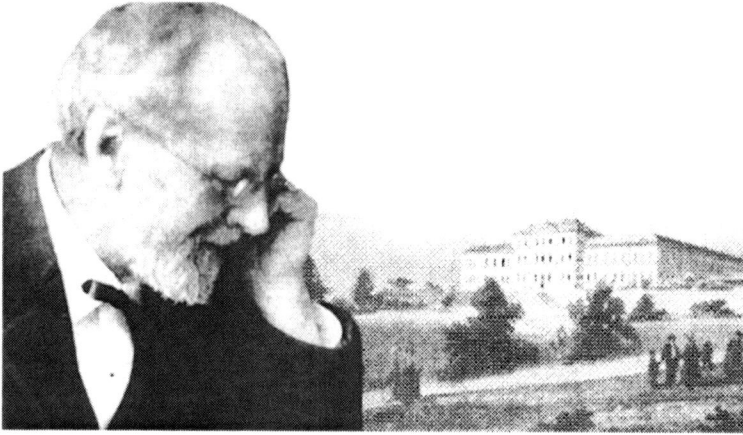

Fig. 1.3 Gottlieb Burckhardt

"Shock" Therapies in Psychiatry

For most of their history, asylums were little more than oversized holding cells: showers and bromides—made from potassium or camphor—were practically the only therapeutic tools available. For violent inmates there were straightjackets or perhaps a padded room in more luxurious establishments. Psychiatrists made creative attempts to fill this therapeutic vacuum. One such treatment, *malariatherapy*, was suggested in 1917 by J. Wagner-Jauregg for patients suffering from neuro-psychiatric disorders as a result of syphilis [24]. This Austrian neuropsychiatrist had observed that his patients improved following a febrile infectious disease. He therefore injected a group of patients with malaria, a disease chosen for its fever and because it could be controlled with quinine. This "malaria treatment" was practiced until the advent of antibiotics, and in 1927 its inventor received the Nobel Prize in medicine, the only such prize ever given to an alienist. The same year, a Polish psychiatrist by the name of M. Sackel proposed treating psychosis by inducing a coma with insulin injections [25]. In his opinion, insulin coma treatment represented the future of psychiatry [26]. Afterwards, patients were slowly woken from their hypoglycemic coma, often associated with seizures, through a progressive "resugaring" under the watchful supervision of nurses. The purpose of these "*Sackel cures,*" which were practiced in hospitals until the 1960s, was to temporarily dissolve consciousness. It was believed that during the reawakening phase the subject became calm and psychologically receptive to psychotherapy. A few years earlier, "*coloido*[8]" shocks and "*pneumoshocks*[9]" had also been tried, but experimentation was cut short because of complications and a lack of efficacy. In 1934,

---

[8] Injection of various products resulting in potentially fatal anaphylactic shock.

[9] Equivalent to pneumoencephalography, or the injection of gases into the ventricles.

the Hungarian psychiatrist L. von Meduna, hypothesizing that there was a biological antagonism between epilepsy and schizophrenia, provoked convulsions by
administering *Cardiazol®*, a tonicardiac [27]. This shock therapy led to favorable
outcomes in a small percentage of psychotic patients, but it was quickly abandoned
because the convulsions were at times extremely severe. However, the notion that
convulsions could result in clinical improvement persisted. Working at the
Salpêtrière hospital at the turn of the twentieth century, Babinski administered a
series of *voltaic electrifications of the head* to a patient suffering from melancholia
for whom all other therapies (hydrotherapy, opium, high doses of belladona) had
failed. He concluded that *in some vague way this agent altered the orientation of the
brain and triggered a process which restored balance"* [28]. In 1938, Cerletti,
working at the University of Rome and inspired by previous experiments, decided
to replace *Cardiazol* with an applied electrical current to produce the convulsions.
He performed 11 sessions of electroshock therapy on a schizophrenic patient and
obtained spectacular results. His electroconvulsive therapy (ECT) technique
quickly spread. By 1940, when it was understood that the muscle contractions held
no therapeutic benefit, curare was administered during sessions as a muscle
relaxant. Of all these various "shock" therapies, only ECT remains in use today.
Electroconvulsive therapy has been perfected and is now performed under general
anesthesia and curarization with satisfactory results in certain patients suffering
from severe depression or delirious melancholia as will later be discussed[10] [29].
Meanwhile psychiatry was evolving. It transformed from a purely philosophical
field into a medical discipline. The underlying causes of certain mental disorders
were now clearly defined, and this knowledge enabled the healing of an increasing
number of patients. Treatments for general paralysis or diffuse syphilitic menin-
goencephalitis were thus improved through the use of *malaria treatment* and
pyrotherapy. The mechanisms underpinning psychoses resulting from endocrine
problems, intoxication, deficiency, or infection were described, and Baruk was able
to cure catatonia syndromes of "colibacillary" origin. As Puech, who in 1939
founded the "neuro-psycho-surgery" department at the Saint-Anne hospital, writes
in his book, *Introduction à la psychochirurgie* [30], the discovery of *Luminal®* and
other anti-convulsives *made it possible to free many epileptics with mental disorder
from the stultifying effects of bromide*. On another level, Freud's discoveries and the
practice of psychoanalysis fundamentally reshaped classical psychotherapy and
opened up new avenues of treatment for neuroses.

The Birth of Psychosurgery

In 1910, the psychiatrist Bernard Hollander published in London a work entitled
The Mental Symptoms of Brain Diseases. In Montreal, William Penfield reported
in 1935 improvements in psychiatric symptoms following removal of tumors or

---

[10] Cf. p. 321.

cerebral abscesses from the frontal lobes [31]. Such findings revealed the important part these frontal areas play in emotional and behavioral phenomena. Neurosurgeon P. Wertheimer's account before an assembly of philosophers in 1950 described this growing awareness well: *Without neurosurgery, without the documentation it provides* [...] *psychosurgery would not have been born; it is a younger more vigorous offshoot. This knowledge gleaned through rigorous observation of operated patients, however, was complemented by findings on craniocerebral wounds and brain trauma of the frontal lobes as well as information about evolutionary atrophic processes.* The celebrated physician from Lyon then added, *This documentation enabled greater appreciation of the function of the frontal lobe and the significance of the thalamofrontal connections. The prefrontal region seems to be where the individual is projected into what lies ahead; it is the future zone; it governs the ideas of self; it is the seat of expectation and introspection. To these functions, the thalamus adds the emotional component which colors the ideas born in the prefrontal corticality. Patients without frontal lobes are euphoric, indifferent, lack initiative and social sensibility. Intelligence is little affected, but the capacity to rise to synthesis or descend to analysis is eliminated. The emotional threshold is lowered* [...]. *Functional surgery eliminates worries about the future, anxiety about tomorrow and thoughts of death. The price for this sense of security is undoubtedly a certain degree of indifference, of relative inertia. In reality, the surgery creates a regressive state. Simply put, it brings the individual back down to earth; it places him face to face with day-to-day realities. It discolors the affective tied to the self/it separates the affective from the self and places the latter back into context, the family or social surroundings. It appears to be a cure for anxiety, for worry and for painful introspection* [32]. The same clinical results had been outlined 15 years earlier at Yale University by Fulton during his pioneering studies with primates.

John Fulton and His Work on the Frontal Lobes of Monkeys

John Fulton, who was head of the physiology department, and his colleague Carlyle Jacobsen were studying the cortical functions of the frontal lobes in great apes. They studied two chimpanzees, Becky and Lucy, who had been trained to perform complex tasks and to expect a reward afterwards. They found that ablation of part of the frontal lobes did not prevent the chimpanzees from completing the tasks, but it did make them more distracted and eliminate frustration behavior when they were not rewarded [33, 34]. Their research, presented at the Second International Congress of Neurology in London in 1935, alongside the work of French neurosurgeon Clovis Vincent on the function of the frontal lobes [35], captivated the attention of one of the neurologists in attendance: Egas Moniz [34].

Fig. 1.4 Egas Moniz
(courtesy of Pr João Lobo-
Antunes)

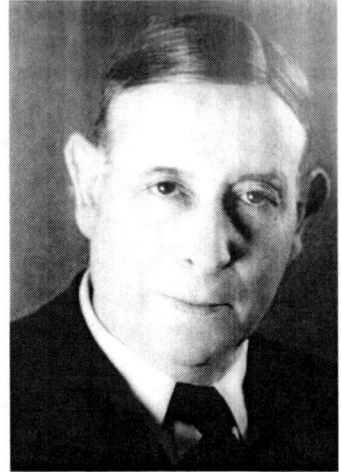

Egas Moniz, the Inventor of Psychosurgery

Egas Moniz (Fig. 1.4), was a well-known Portuguese neurologist [36]. He was an eclectic and talented individual who had been Portugal's minister of foreign affairs after WWI and then ambassador to Spain. He was highly regarded by his peers for his work developing cerebral angiography in 1927 [36–38]. Based on the findings of Fulton and Brickner [39], an American neurologist, Moniz hypothesized that *mental disorders must be related to the formation of more or less fixed cellulo-connective groupings [...]. To heal these patients we need to destroy the groupings of connections which must exist in the frontal lobes*[11] [40]. Three months after attending the London conference and without performing any preliminary experiments on animals, the Portuguese neurologist asked his colleague, the neurosurgeon Almeida Lima [41], to perform the first attempts to interrupt the afferent[12] and efferent connections of the frontal lobes. The surgical technique was elaborated on a cadaver [40].

---

[11] To support his hypothesis, Moniz also borrowed from the work of Spanish neuroanatomist Santiago Ramon y Cajal, who had been awarded the Nobel Prize in 1906 for his contributions to the "neuron doctrine." Moniz had frequented him in Madrid while serving as ambassador. His frequent references to Ramon y Cajal's research would seem to stem more from a desire to buttress his work with the name a respected scientific eminence than from actual scientific necessity (in Valenstein, E.S. 1986. Great and desperate cures: the rise and decline of psychosurgery and other radical treatments for mental illness. Basic Books, New York).

[12] Afferences: incoming nerve fibers as opposed to efferences, which are outgoing fibers.

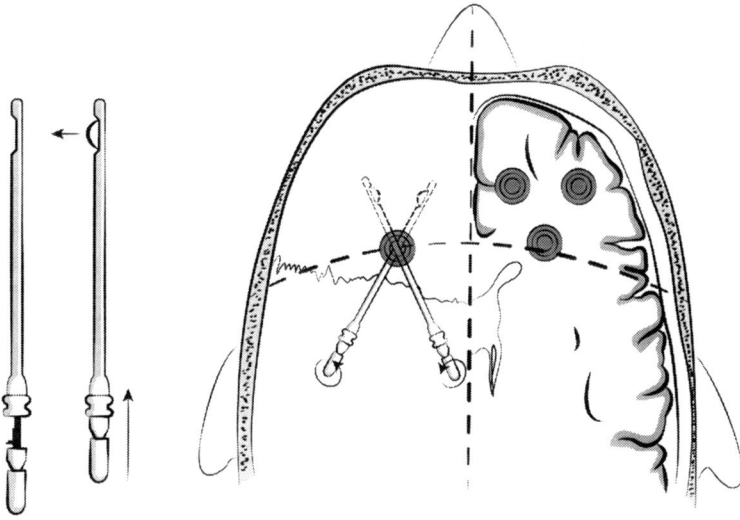

Fig. 1.5 Standard prefrontal leucotomy technique. A burr hole is made at the top of the skull and the leucotome inserted into the brain parenchyma to the desired depth. Once the instrument is in place, the cutting loop at the tip is extended by depressing the flexible plunger into the trocar. The trocar is then rotated in order to sever the white fibrous matter. The procedure is repeated from three different angles on both sides

The First Intervention: The Prefrontal Leucotomy

The operations, performed at first under local and then general anesthesia, involved making two burr holes in the upper frontal region 3 cm to each side of the median line (Fig. 1.5). A graduated syringe was inserted through these openings and absolute alcohol injected into the white matter on each side. By the eighth patient, the graduated syringe was replaced by a needle with a retractable metal loop at the tip, a leucotome, which he deemed more precise (Fig. 1.9). And so the prefrontal leucotomy was born. The Portuguese team went on to perform 100 such operations.

Premature Results

The first operation was performed on 12 November 1935, on a 63-year-old woman suffering from melancholia, anxiety and paranoid delusions. Two months later, according to a young psychiatrist who examined her, *the patient was very calm, well oriented, slightly sad and no longer exhibiting pathological ideas* [42]. In spite of this, she never left the hospital. After 4 months and a total of 20 operations Moniz quickly shared his results with the members of the Paris Neurology Society on 5 March 1936. He reported *no deaths, no aggravations,*

Table 1.1 Initial results of the prefrontal leucotomy

20 patients[a]	Anxiety/mood disorder	Schizophrenia
Cured	7	–
Improved	5	2
No change	2	5

[a] One of the patients suffered from all three pathologies

35 % of patients cured, 35 % clinically improved and 30 % without change (Table 1.1) [43]. The Portuguese neurologist added that better results were achieved in patients with mood disorders than in those suffering from schizophrenia [40].

The Skepticism of European Psychiatrists

In Paris, Moniz's work met with a mix of indifference and skepticism. It was known that any mutilation of the frontal lobe, the *majesty of the brain* according to French anatomist Gratiolet, risked undermining the intellect [44]. Despite this and his work being both methodologically and ethically suspect, his report did not receive as much criticism as it perhaps merited, especially in France, a bastion of Freudian thought. It is true that Moniz benefited from the prestige of having been Minister of Foreign Affairs and a signatory at the Paris Peace Conference in 1919, and that many thought his work on cerebral angiography deserving of a Nobel Prize (which he was destined to receive in 1949) [45]. Moniz and Lima continued practicing without any significant changes to their procedure and with minimal follow-up. They operated on nearly 100 patients and published over 100 reports and two books on their series of interventions [40]. In Europe, at first only the Italians showed any interest in their work, among them Emilio Rizatti in Turin. Later, Puusepp in Estonia also became interested [46, 47]. Both began practicing the technique and by 1939 had performed over 200 operations [21, 47]. Across the Atlantic, Walter Freeman, a neuropsychiatrist at Washington University who closely followed Fulton's research, also took an interest in the procedure. On 14 September 1936, with the assistance of James Watts, a neurosurgeon at Washington University, he performed the procedure on a 63-year-old, *agitated and depressive* woman. Some 600 similar interventions soon followed.

The Rise and Fall of Psychosurgery

To fully understand the success in the United States of the technique imported by Freeman and Watts, it is necessary to consider the crisis facing American psychiatry at the time. The only available treatments for psychotic patients were internment and various shock therapies as described above[13] [48]. In 1937, 400,000 patients were hospitalized in some 500 psychiatric institutions throughout the country. This amounted to a little over half the hospital beds in the country [49] and more than 1.5 billion dollars. At the start of WWII, over 1.8 million men were exempted for psychiatric reasons out of the 15 million who were drafted [50]. In one of his publications, Fulton estimated that *a million dollars per day could be saved if, through a more widespread use of lobotomies, 10 % of hospitalized patients could be treated on an ambulatory basis* [51]. The major American news outlets, meanwhile, were fairly casual in their coverage of the new technique [52] (Fig. 1.17). The neurophysiologist and historian of psychosurgery E.S. Valenstein concludes in his seminal work, *Great and Desperates Cures,* that *the absence of effective neuropharmacological agents, asylum overpopulation, and the high financial and social costs of psychiatric pathologies at the time contributed to the warm welcome given to frontal lobotomy* [4].

Freeman, Tireless Promoter of the Lobotomy in the United States

At first Freeman and Watts simply copied Moniz's technique, but soon they decided that modifications should be made in order to improve on the results, which they deemed disappointing. The burr holes would no longer be drilled into the top of the skull but into the sides (Fig. 1.6). The duo also began performing the surgery under

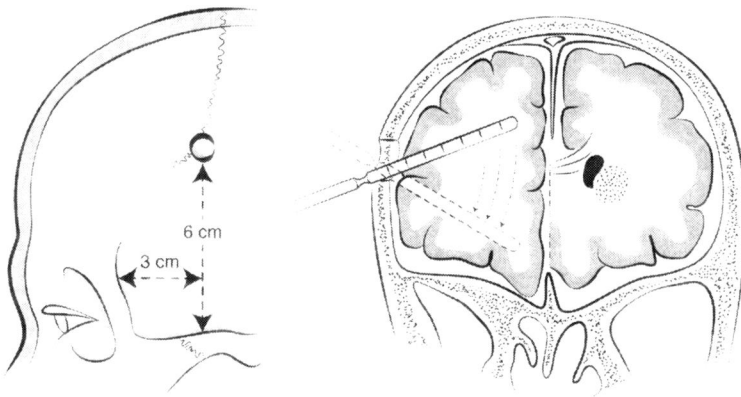

Fig. 1.6 Lateral prefrontal lobotomy *Right* Extent of prefrontal cut. The cut to the *left side* is performed slightly farther back and impacts the anterior point of the ventricle where the thalamocortical bundle (*dotted area*) remains compact and can thus more easily be avoided

---

[13] Cf. p. 28.

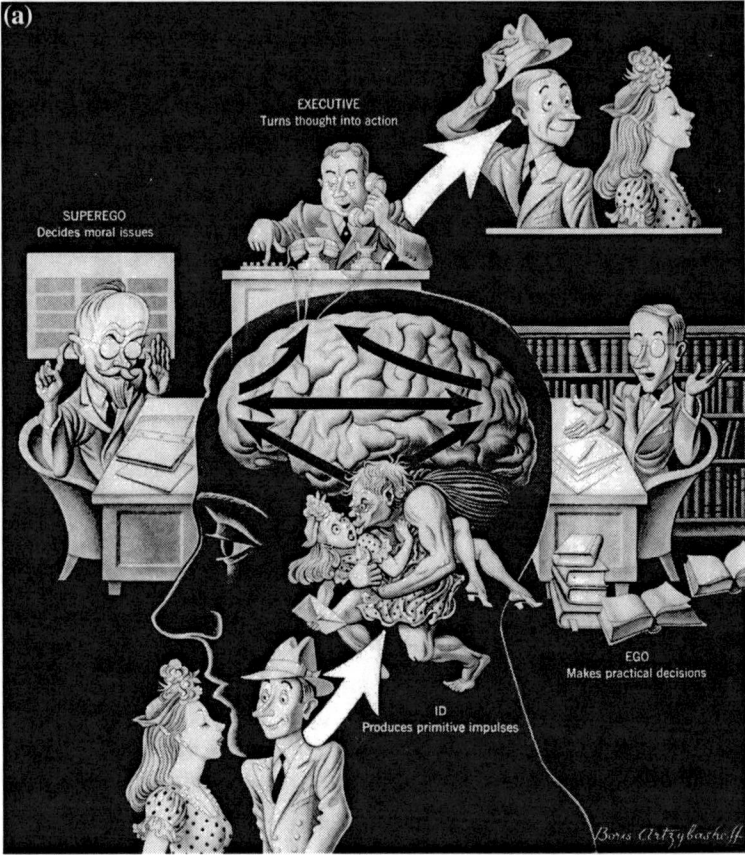

Fig. 1.7 "Psychosurgery" a drawing by Boris Artzybasheff in *Life Magazine* (17/03/1947) **a** In this artist's depiction, when the man sees the woman, the thalamus, which is the source of emotionally driven behavior, releases a primitive sexual impulse (the "id"). On the *right*, the "ego," which represents intelligence and experience, advises the man against throwing himself on the young woman as does the "superego" on the *left*, which represents moral conscience. These various impulses come together in a compromise, and by way of the executive functions, the man politely tips his hat. **b** In cases of melancholy, when the "superego" becomes excessively inhibiting, guilt, or anxiety provoking, the balance is broken and the subject lays prostrate (*top*). **c** A lobotomy, considered at the time particularly effective in this indication, allows the "superego" to be neutralized and balance to be restored (*bottom*). The author nonetheless adds that this operation must be limited to subjects who "possess sufficient intelligence to master their impulses once their moral conscience has been eliminated"

local anesthesia only so that they could put questions to the patient and monitor their perception as they performed simple mental tasks. As long as the patient did not show signs of deterioration, the leucotomy was extended. Through trial and error, Freeman formulated two *cutting strategies* according to which pathology was being treated: a limited anterior cut for *emotional psychoneuroses* and an extensive posterior cut for schizophrenia [53]. At the same time, J. Lyerly, a neurosurgeon in

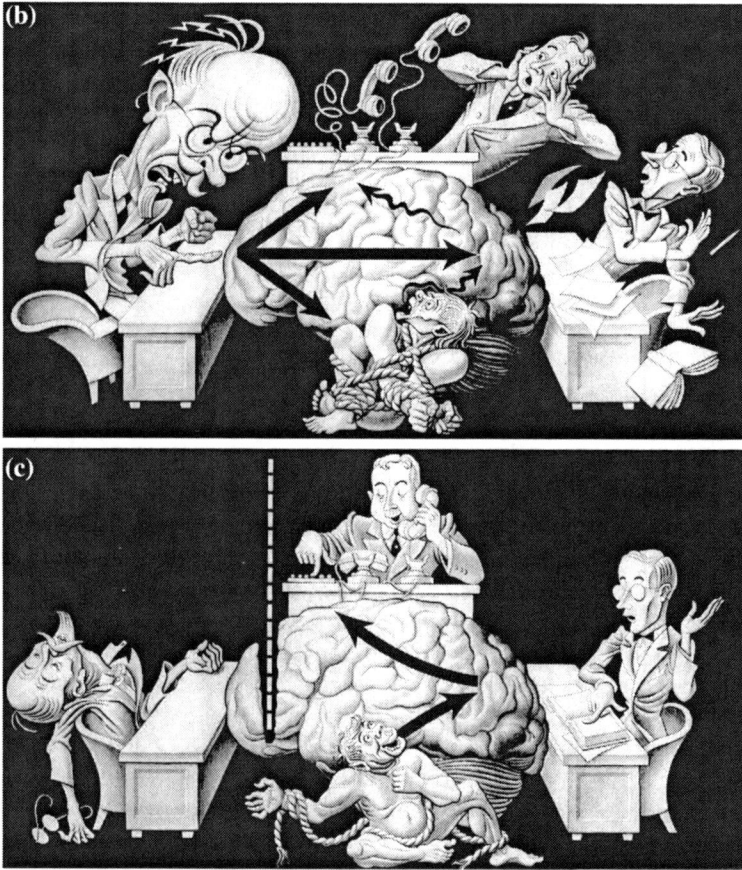

Fig. 1.7 (continued)

Florida, presented the results of a series of 21 operations and concluded that the best results were achieved in *melancholic, anxious or depressed* patients. In 1942, Freeman and Watts published *Psychosurgery,* in which they provided information gathered during the treatment of 80 patients [53]. In the preface, the authors defended the idea that the frontal lobes, which are essential to social adaptation, function improperly in the mentally ill, and that partially disconnecting the lobes from the rest of the brain allows for better social adaptation. According to Freeman, without frontal lobes there could be no emotional psychosis. The psychiatrist was echoing the then popular notion that the thalamus[14] is responsible for the emotional dimension of thought. Cutting the fronto-thalamic bundles was therefore a way of freeing the intellect from an overbearing emotional hold. Many such simplifications

---

[14] For more information on the subject, read the excerpt of Wertheimer's conference on the "justification and results of a psychosurgery."

were likewise formulated for the benefit of the public. One portrayal likened structures in the brain to Freud's *Id, Ego* and *Superego* (Fig. 1.7). Freeman's book, written in simple terms and enthusiastically promoted by *Time Magazine*, had a huge impact both on the medical world and on public opinion. Concern over conditions in asylums prompted many in the United States to turn to Freeman and Watts' lobotomy. According to *Time Magazine*, by the end of 1946, over 2,000 operations had been performed; and according to a Senate report, by June 1951 20,000 operations had been performed [50].

A Global Movement

A Timid Start in France

Although Moniz had himself studied in France under Pitre, a neurologist in Bordeaux, and then under Pierre Marie, Joseph Babinski and Jules Dejerine in Paris, he had few disciples in France. According to the neurosurgeon Puech, *his first reports along with his book published in Paris in French in 1936 were for the most part greeted with skepticism and disapproval* [30]. We do have a record of an exchange with Gaston Ferdiere [54] in 1940 concerning the treatment of a schizophrenic patient suffering from catatonic stupor using the Portuguese neurologist's leucotomy technique. But Ferdiere, head of psychiatry at the hospital in Rodez is primarily remembered for having been Antonin Artaud's[15] psychiatrist [54, 55]. Another notable exception is the small set of patients who were operated on by Puech at the Sainte-Anne hospital in 1944 [56]. Overall though, as Marcel David writes, *only after [the war] did we learn in France of the extensive use of leucotomies in Anglo-Saxon countries following the work of Freeman and Watts. Primitive techniques were improved, new surgical methods were devised and then the whole world began practicing psychosurgery with an enthusiasm that now seems ill-founded* [57]. French psychiatrists, less pressed by financial concerns and preferring shock[16] therapies, waited longer before beginning to refer their patients to neurosurgeons [58, 59]. Only several years after WWII did psychosurgery start to spread in France under the impetus of the neurosurgeons David [60], Puech [30], Talairach [61], Wertheimer [62], and Le Beau [63]. The last, influenced by Fulton's work, pioneered the topectomy[17] and the cingulectomy[18]—variant of the cingulectomy[19]—is one of the few ablative surgeries still practiced today (Fig. 1.15) [64].

---

[15] A French director, actor, and poet.

[16] Notably Cardiazol® and Insulin, cf. "shock thérapies" p. 28.

[17] Cf. p. 48.

[18] Cf. p. 49.

[19] Cf. p. 173.

Popularity in the United States

Starting in 1937, East Coast neurosurgeons like Poppen [65, 66], Grant [67] in Philadelphia, Pool [68] in New York, Lyerly [69] in Jacksonville, Florida [69], as well as Love at the *Mayo Clinic* in Minnesota, followed in Freeman's footsteps. By the end of WWII, so many were practicing the procedure that it would be impossible to name them all. In 1948, the situation in asylums had become critical. The *American Psychiatric Association* (APA) estimated a deficit of 800,000 beds, and the journalist Deutsch wrote a scathing and widely read report of poor sanitary conditions and lack of personnel in the country's psychiatric hospitals [70].

Elsewhere in Europe and the World

In England, 200 interventions had been performed by 1942. By 1947, 1,000 had been performed, almost half of them by McKissock at London's St George's Hospital. And by 1954, at the height of its popularity, over 10,000 leucotomies had been performed [71–73]. The practice spread to the rest of the British Empire, including India, after 1944. Working in Turin in 1936, Rizzati was an early Italian adopter of psychosurgery. Today however, the name Fiamberti of Varese is better remembered [74]. Indeed, in 1937, this psychiatrist simplified Moniz's technique by accessing the prefrontal part of the brain through the roof of the orbit[20] (Fig. 1.8, p. 18). This was the technique adopted by Freeman, which led to such dangerous excesses in the United States[21] [46]. In Istanbul, first Saltuk and then Berkay performed about 400 interventions between 1952 and the early 1960s, despite the opposition of Turkey's psychiatric community to the practice [75, 76]. In the USSR, the neurosurgeons Babtchin in Leningrad and Egorov performed more than 100 prefrontal leucotomies or transorbital lobotomies before a ruling by the health minister suddenly put a stop to their research. Jdanov blamed the practice on certain Jewish doctors stating that the technique was *incompatible with the basic physiological principle of Pavlov's doctrine* [77]. In an article relating the incident, Lichterman explains that the prohibition, which remained in effect until 1982, was probably the consequence of a lobotomy having been performed on the son of an *apparatchik* without his father's consent [78, 79]. This scandal foreshadowed the infamous *Doctor's Plot*, an anti-Semitic conspiracy orchestrated by Stalin's government as part of an intended purge of the Communist Party. In Japan, the first lobotomies were performed by Nakata in 1938 [80]. However, the procedure was not widely practiced in the archipelago until after Japan's surrender when Schrader, a neurosurgeon with the US army in Osaka,

---

[20] Fiamberti had himself been inspired by his compatriot A. Dogliotti, who had devised his transorbital technique in 1933 in order to inject a contrast agent for radio ventriculographies of certain brain structures.

[21] Cf. p. 42.

Fig. 1.8 Transorbital
lobotomy. Once the patient is
"anesthetized" by a series of
two electroshocks, the thin
layer of bone at the back of
the orbit is pierced by the
orbitoclast and the instrument
inserted 5 cm into the brain
parenchyma. The instrument
is then swung medially and
laterally. The procedure is
repeated on each side and
generally completed in less
than 10 min

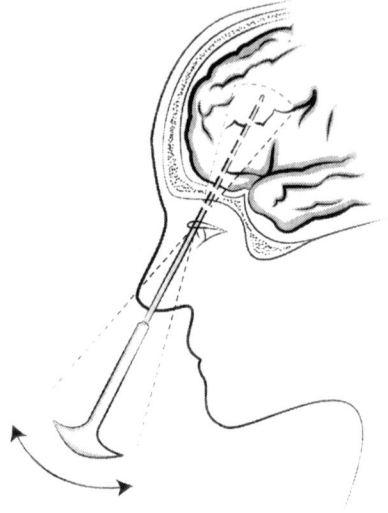

disseminated Freeman's technique. In South America, Mattos Pimenta began
working in Sao Paulo with Moniz's technique in the summer of 1936 before
switching to Freeman's method in 1942 [81].

The Transorbital or "Ice-Pick" Lobotomy

In 1945, with increasing numbers of patients being referred to him, Freeman began
to search for a way of further simplifying the technique so that it could be performed outside an operating room. He therefore adopted the method developed by
Fiamberti: rather than accessing the upper part of the frontal lobes, the lobes are
accessed just above the eye through the fornix conjunctiva in the roof of the orbit,
in other words *transorbitally* (Fig. 1.8).

The frontal lobes are thus disconnected from the rest of the brain from below
instead of from above. Rather than using a leucotome like Fiamberti, Freeman
made use of an orbitoclast, the infamous "ice-pick," whose tip located in the
frontal area of the brain he wiggled back and forth in a wagging motion in order to
sever the thalamocortical white matter (Fig. 1.9, p. 19).

In January 1946, after a few trials on cadavers Freeman began performing his
new technique in his office at Washington University. However his associate, the
neurosurgeon Watts, considered the procedure too dangerous to be performed in an
office setting [82]; and eventually, having grown increasingly critical of the patient
selection process, he decided to end their collaboration [82, 83]. Fulton, who was
also scandalized, wrote Freeman a letter in October 1947: *I hear about your are
performing lobotomies in your office with an ice pick* [...] *Why not use a shot gun?
It would be quicker!* [50]. From then on, Freeman operated alone (Fig. 1.10) [84].

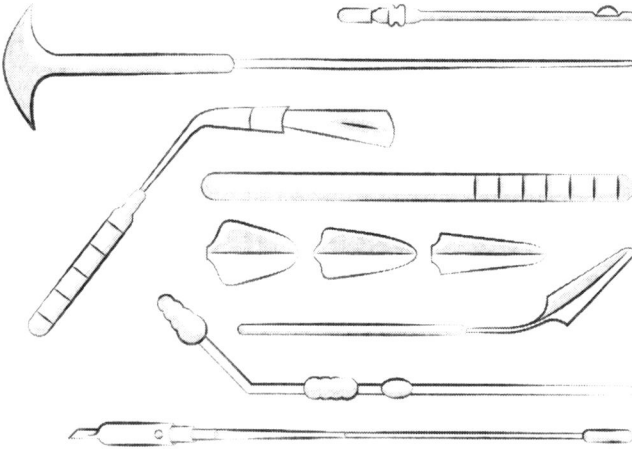

Fig. 1.9 Psychosurgical instruments formerly used in leucotomies. From *bottom* to *top* illuminating rod (Clovis Vincent), suction cannula, set of brain retractors (Clovis Vincent), graduated blade in centimeters (Walter Freeman–James Watts), bent and graduated spatula-forceps (modified from William Scoville), orbitoclast or "ice-pick" (Walter Freeman) and leucotome (Egas Moniz–Almeida Lima), found in [132]

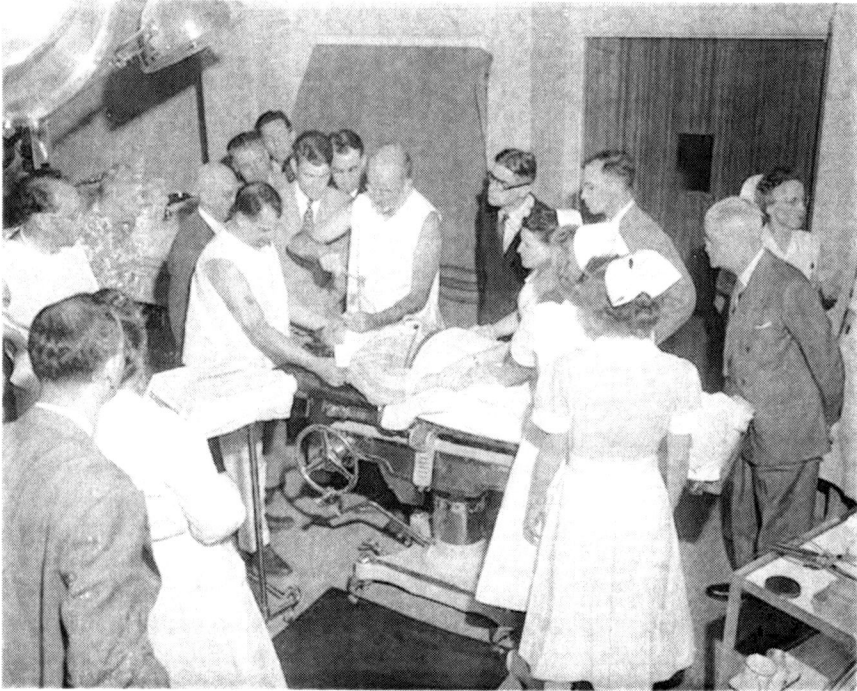

Fig. 1.10 Walter Freeman performing a transorbital lobotomy at Western State Hospital, Washington in 1949. The patient had first been "anesthetized" through a series of electroshocks. Notice the questionable aseptic conditions

He went on to perform or supervise over 4,000 interventions [84–86]. He attracted the ire of a large number of surgeons for practicing without a degree in surgery, without an operating room, and without proper sterilization.

One such detractor, Bailey, who in addition to being a surgeon was also a psychiatrist and an anatomical pathologist, declared that *this new technique, highly risky even for a neurosurgeon, is now being practiced in the offices of psychiatrists who are incapable of dealing with the possible complications of this intervention* [73, 87]. In spite of criticism, Freeman a natural salesman, managed to train many psychiatrists in the use of his technique while crisscrossing the United States in his *lobotomobile* [4]. His technique was fast and simple and allowed him to perform up to 15 interventions in a single morning [58]. Despite a high rate of complications, mostly hemorrhages but also infections from the non-sterilized equipment, Freeman's ambulatory-based technique was welcomed by his neuropsychiatrist colleagues and applauded in the media [52, 88–92] (Fig. 1.17, p. 31).

Lobotomy at Its Peak[22]

Sixty-Thousand Interventions

Over 60,000 lobotomies were performed in the United States between the years 1936 and 1956 [93]. After the end of WWII, the *Veterans Administration* went so far as to recommend it for the treatment of what we today refer to as post-traumatic stress disorder (PTSD).[23] Some well-known people were also lobotomized[24] including Rosemary Kennedy, President Kennedy's sister. She exhibited very slight signs of mental retardation and was too promiscuous according to her father. Consequently, at 23 she received a transorbital lobotomy at the hands of Freeman and Watts. The operation was a disaster which severely affected her cognitive abilities, and she remained in a psychiatric institution until her death at the age of 86. Rose Isabel Williams, the sister of writer Tennessee Williams, suffered a similar experience.[25] The famous Quebecois singer, Alys Robi, was interned and then lobotomized at the St-Michel-Archange psychiatric hospital in Quebec City in 1952 after she suffered a severe depression. She returned to music in 1960 and was knighted by Queen Elizabeth II in 1985 for her work defending the rights of the mentally ill.

---

[22] Title drawn from a chapter heading in E.S. Valenstein's Great and desperate cures: the rise and decline of psychosurgery and other radical treatments for mental illness. 1986. Basic Books, New York.

[23] Cf. p. 384.

[24] Unlike what is portrayed in the 1982 movie "Frances," the Hollywood actress Frances Farmes was never lobotomized (J. El-Hai, 2005. The lobotomist: a maverick medical genius and his tragic quest to rid the world of mental illness. John Wiley & Sons, Hoboken, N.J.).

[25] T. Williams based his play "Suddenly Last Summer" on this tragic event. cf. p. 58.

In addition to its psychiatric indications, the lobotomy was also offered to patients suffering from chronic pain in order to relieve them of the emotional component of their pain. In the final weeks of her life, Evita Perón, an icon and symbol of twentieth-century Argentina, received a lobotomy for antalgic[26] reasons in 1953. The procedure, accomplished in utmost secrecy by Poppen, was meant to relieve the Argentine leader's wife of the anxiety and unbearable pain caused by a uterine cancer which had metastasized to the bones [94]. Warner Baxter, the highest paid actor of his generation, died as a result of the procedure in 1951. The surgery had been indicated to treat his hard to chronic arthritic pain.

Crowned with a Nobel

In 1949, the Nobel Foundation in Stockholm divided the Nobel in Physiology or Medicine equally between the Swiss neurophysiologist Walter Hess and Egas Moniz (Fig. 1.11). The first was being honored for his achievements in understanding the neural mechanism involved in emotions. The second was being rewarded for his *discovery of the therapeutic value of leucotomy in certain psychoses*. Moniz's political standing and his highly regarded work on cerebral angiography were, it would seem, instrumental in the Academy's decision. Regardless, the leucotomy had been consecrated [36–38, 95, 96].

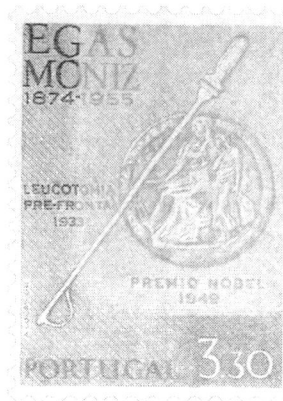

Fig. 1.11 Portuguese stamp commemorating Moniz's Nobel Prize. Notice the incorrect date, the first prefrontal leucotomy having been performed in 1935

---

[26] Some of Poppen's collaborators believed that it was in fact a hypophysectomy, excision of the pituitary gland particularly effective in the treatment of hormonal-dependant cancer pains originating in the bones. (D.E., Nijensohn, L.E. Savastano, A.D. Kaplan, and E.R. Laws, Jr. 2012. New evidence of prefrontal lobotomy in the last months of the illness of Eva Peron. World Neurosurgery 77:583–590.)

Toward More Selective Surgery

The previous year, the first *World Psychosurgery Congress* had been organized by
Freeman in Lisbon with participants from 28 countries (Fig. 1.12). This unofficial
event held in homage to Moniz and in support of his nomination for the Nobel was
an opportunity to evaluate the various lobotomy techniques being developed around
the world (p. 24). In his welcoming speech for Freeman in front of Portugal's
Academy of Sciences, Moniz admitted: *I do not know what is to become of the
cerebral leucotomy as a treatment. It is probable that sooner or later it will be
replaced by better and safer methods* [42]. Although the idea of psychosurgery had
fewer detractors, the debate shifted to those who supported the *standard* bilateral
leucotomy as practiced by Freeman and those who wished for less deleterious
techniques. Indeed, as Le Beau notes, many neurosurgeon observed *too significant
and often unpredictable a change in the subject's overall personality* following a
classic bilateral leucotomy [97]. This deterioration was identified as *post-leucotomy
syndrome* and associated *urinary incontinence, egocentrism, indifference and
puerility of the patient.* In 1939, the Swedish psychiatrist Rylander was one of the
first to become concerned by these complications and begin quantifying their extent
through psychotechnical tests [98]. Over time an increasing number of European
and American neurosurgeons directed their attention toward much more precise and
less invasive selective frontal surgery.

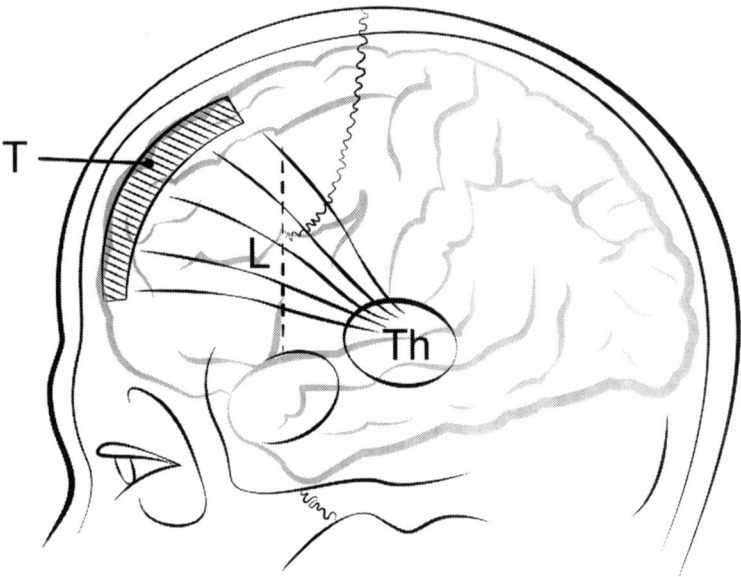

Fig. 1.12 The various psychosurgical procedures in use in 1950. *T* Prefrontal cortical excision
(topectomy), *L* Lobotomy, *Th* Thalamotomy [30]

Cortical Undercutting or the "Mini" Lobotomy

In order to prevent the occurrence of cognitive deterioration and mutilation of the personality, William Scoville of Yale promoted a more targeted procedure, a technique known as *cortical undercutting*, which targeted the connective fibers of the prefrontal cortex[27] and the cingulate gyrus[28] (Fig. 1.13) [99, 100]. The latter's role in controlling emotions, pain, and anxiety had recently been ascertained through animal experimentation [82]. This technique was popularized in France under the name *topotomy* by D. Ferey.

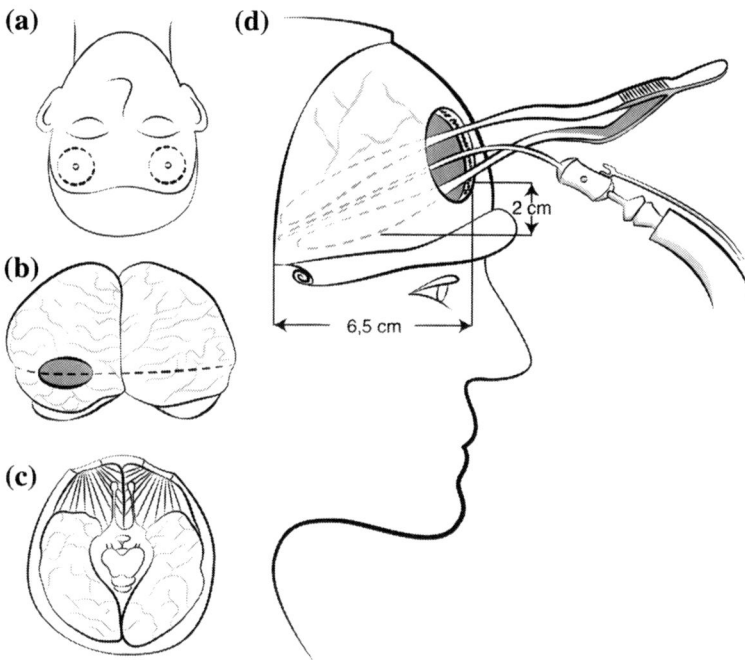

Fig. 1.13 Cortical undercutting technique. **a** Two burr holes 4 cm in diameter are made at the anterior base of the frontal lobe **b** and **c** extended toward the cingulate cortex and the fronto-thalamic connections. **d** Lesioning is then accomplished using an aspiration cannula

---

[27] Cf. p. 93.

[28] Cf. p. 95.

Topectomy: From Sectioning to Ablation

As Le Beau explains in 1949, unlike earlier techniques the topectomy involves not, *cutting projection fibers but actually eliminating cortical areas*[101]. On a functional level, *it has the same effect as a lobotomy with less drastic functional mutilation. It causes the same degeneration of the thalamus and the same impact on the hypothalamic core,* as Wertheimer [32] writes. Another advantage, this one surgical, was being able to operate directly on the uncovered surface, thus reducing the risk of hemorrhage inherent in previous techniques, which were performed *blind* (Fig. 1.14). The technique made it possible to see the gyri of the prefrontal dorsolateral cortex,[29] (Brodmann areas 9, 10 and 46), which were believed to be involved in anxiety. Pool in New York and Le Beau were the first to perform partial ablation of this region in patients suffering from severe anxiety. Patients with chronic pain involving an emotional component were also eligible. Painful anxiety, *the tension of anticipation,* associated with pain thus became one of the indications for this type of surgery [63, 68, 102, 103]. The approach was somewhat empirical as can be seen in these recommendations for topectomy of areas 9 and 10 recorded in 1949: *the weight of resected cortex varies from 25 to 30 grams on each side (Pool, for psychoses) to 10 to 12 grams on each side (Le Beau, for chronic pain)* [101]. Depending on the cortical areas concerned the procedure was either called a standard topectomy (Brodmann areas 9, 10, and 46), orbital topectomy (11, 13, and 14), polar topectomy (10 and 11) or a cingulectomy (24 and 32).

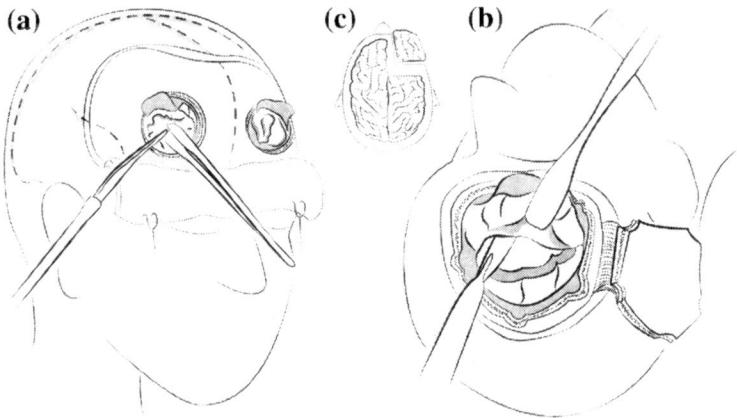

Fig. 1.14 Examples of prefrontal topectomies. **a** Bilateral orbitofrontal topectomy using a trephine, found in [181]; **b** and **c** Extended prefrontal topectomy, found in [73]

---

[29] Cf. p. 92.

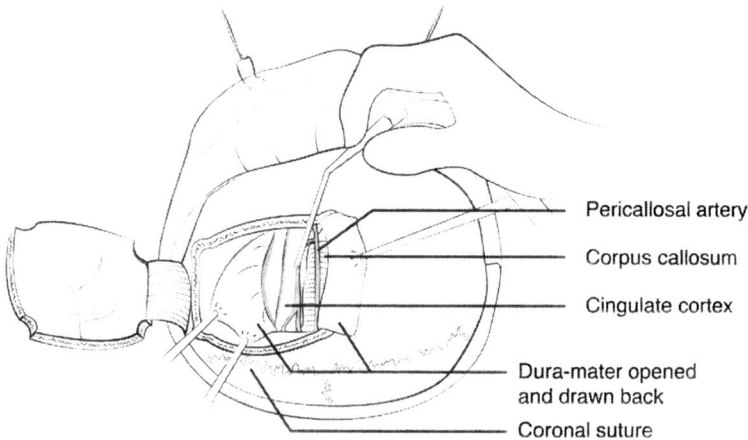

Pericallosal artery

Corpus callosum

Cingulate cortex

Dura-mater opened
and drawn back

Coronal suture

Fig. 1.15 Cingulectomy Once the scalp has been drawn back over the forehead, a frontal flap is made to allow incision into the dura mater ahead of the coronal suture. The suction cannula is then slipped between the two hemispheres just above the corpus callosum in order to aspirate the anterior part of cingulate cortex on both sides. During the intervention care must be taken to not damage the interhemispheric vessels, especially the peri-callosal artery, found in [132]

Cingulectomy: A Promising Target

The cingulectomy (Fig. 1.15), devised almost simultaneously in 1948 by the British neurosurgeon Cairns, the American Scoville and the French Le Beau, was intended for patients suffering from psychomotor agitation [104–106]. As early as 1937, research by James Papez hinted that the amygdala and the hippocampus are part of a same circuit implicated in emotion, the *limbic system.* Experiments on animals led by Paul MacLean showed that targeted lesions in one of these structures made the subject more docile [107]. The purpose of this intervention was to fight states of agitation and violence independent of anxiety through partial destruction of the cingular gyrus, especially the anterior part (area 24). A standard topectomy was still the indicated treatment when dealing with anxiety.

In Philadelphia, Wycis and Spiegel favored the thalamotomy. As the founder of neurosurgery in Marseille, Paillas, explains, *whereas leucotomies are meant to interrupt the thalamo-frontal circuit and topectomies to eliminate the cortical pole of this circuit, the purpose of thalamotomy is to destroy the other pole of this same circuit located in the mediodorsal area of the thalamus* [108]. French surgeons, especially David [109] and Talairach [60] also began targeting this area. *In this more complex procedure,* Paillas explains, *radiography, ventriculography and electroencephalography are combined to record precisely the position in the thalamus of a needle at whose tip electrocoagulation is performed.* The procedure made neurosurgery history not for its results, which were on par with previous methods, but for the technical advances it entailed. In order to reach the dorsomedial nucleus[30] with precision, Spiegel and Wycis devised a sophisticated piece of equipment, which rested on the patients' head called a *stereotactic frame* (Fig. 66). What set their procedure apart was not so much the material innovation, such a device had already been described in 1908 [110] and had remained little used, but their method. For the first time, radiological data was being used to pinpoint the target coordinates [111]. Before Spiegel and Wycis, the few neurosurgeons who used the device relied solely on surface skull features to guide their procedure. This was inherently imprecise as these ridges vary from one individual to another [112].

Anterior Capsulotomy: A Procedure Still Relevant Today

The anatomical research of Wyeis and Meyer having established that the fibers of the frontal cortex converged on the thalamus in a region known as the *anterior limb of the internal capsule*,[31] Talairach[32] and the Swede Leksell suggested in 1949 targeting the anterior limb using the new stereotactic technique [113]. Thanks to its precision and satisfactory clinical results, this intervention is the only type of *selective frontal surgery* still practiced today, as we will discuss further.[33]

Recording, Stimulation, and Frontal Electrocoagulation

Three years after developing their stereotactic frame, Spiegel and Wycis began carrying out electrical recordings and electrical stimulation of the relevant anatomical region before performing a lesion in the targeted anatomical structure. The purpose was to combine this data with observed clinical manifestations to confirm that the tip of the instrument was in contact with the target [114–116]. At the same time, one of Fulton's students at Yale, the neurophysiologist Delgado, based on experiments with cats and monkeys [117], also suggested a cerebral stimulation and recording technique to evaluate therapeutic options for psychotic patients [118]. In both methods, the electrode remained in place only temporarily, sometimes several weeks, and was used both for recording and for making lesions through an electrothermal coagulation process during removal of the electrode (Fig. 1.16). With his technique, Delgado performed lesions in the frontal lobes of a dozen patients; but curiously, he never shared the clinical results [119]. In Bristol,

---

[30] Cf. p. 124.

[31] Ibid.

[32] Before becoming a neurosurgeon at the Sainte-Anne hospital, Jean Talairach was a psychiatrist. He may have been encouraged in this pursuit by his cousin, the celebrated psychiatrist Henri Ey. His doctoral thesis was on the subject of "ovarian psychoses." Tailarach, along with Jean Bancaud, is also the father of stereo-electro-encephalography (SEEG), which involves the implanting of intracerebral electrodes in order to explore the activity of various brain structures during the diagnosis and treatment of epilepsy.

[33] Cf. p. 167 and concerning gamma-capsulotomy, p. 188.

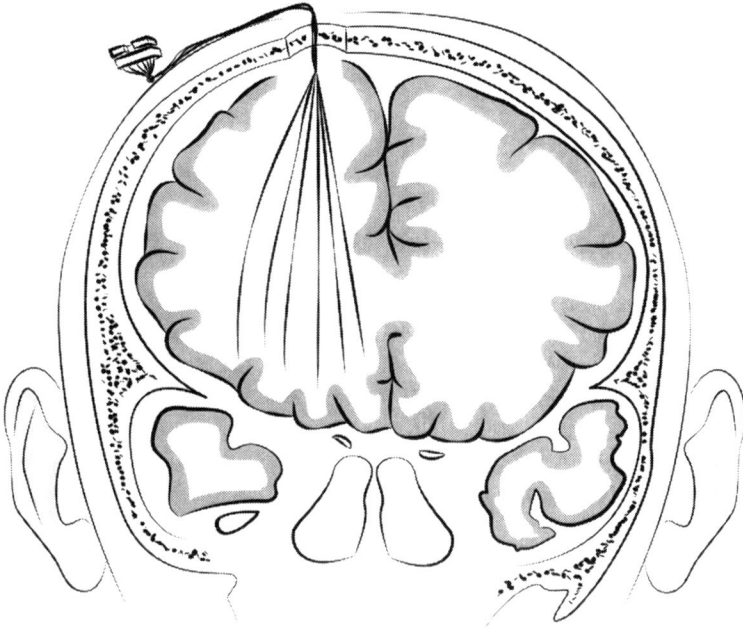

Fig. 1.16 Bundle of prefrontal stimulation and recording electrodes with a connection for attaching the external device. After a frontal burr hole is made, the electrodes are inserted along the same trajectory as in a prefrontal leucotomy and inspected radiographically (cf. Fig. 1.5, p. 11). An Electrophysiological recording and electrical stimulations are performed at the tip of each of these electrodes. Each electrode is then pulled out a few millimeters and with electrothermal coagulation used to make a lesion. Based on the clinical results of the electrical stimulation, a series of lesions can be stacked as the electrodes are progressively withdrawn, found in [120, 182]

Cooper and Crow performed the same type of intervention with the electrodes implanted in the manner of a prefrontal leucotomy[34] in patients suffering from anxiety disorders [120, 121]. On both sides of the Atlantic, about 100 patients with psychiatric pathologies as well as untreatable chronic pain were implanted, sometimes for several months, with widely varying results and levels of follow-up [122].

Condemnation

The decade spanning 1945–1955 was psychosurgery's golden age, and the Nobel attributed to Moniz its apogee. Nonetheless criticism of the first, ruinous

---

[34] Cf. p. 34.

techniques, which had already started in 1939 [98], spread in the 1950s. By 1955, criticism was widespread and the medical world and the public were paying closer attention, especially given that advances in neuropharmacology—including the discovery of neuroleptics—were finally creating effective and, significantly, reversible alternatives. Between 1955 and 1975, legislatures voted to entirely outlaw psychosurgery in Germany, Japan and many US states among others. In France, the UK, Sweden, Spain, India, Belgium, the Netherlands, and a few US states, research was allowed to discreetly continue under oversight. This first era of psychosurgery was summed up by J. Laborie, a psychiatrist from Toulouse, thusly: *With overly broad and sometimes illusory indications, more or less abandoned after the development of chemotherapies, having no strong scientific basis in neuropsychology, shocking to some because of its irreversibility, was it not inevitable that this method should meet with resistance from many physicians and face so much opposition?*[35] [77], which led a member of the Academy of Medicine, the neurosurgeon G. Lazorthes, to conclude that: *psychosurgery was hotly contested, its supporters and detractors argued over moral, religious and medical issues. As with many precursor therapies, enthusiasm was excessive and indications were sometimes abusive. After the influx came the backlash, and its abandonment too was excessive. We have seen this happen in other fields of medicine* [123]. Publications became scarcer, less enthusiastic, and more critical as more data became available.

Freeman's Excesses

Freeman was undoubtedly responsible for some of the abuses and excesses of psychosurgery during that period. After transforming the lobotomy into a fast and simple transorbital[36] procedure, he contributed to its popularization as a technique performed in a practitioner's office in under 15 min. Additionally, as seen above, the procedure was no longer being performed under general anesthesia but followed a session of electroshocks which plunged the subject into stupor or even unconsciousness for a few minutes (Figs. 1.8, p. 18 and 1.10, p. 19) [124]. The spread of this blind and complication-laden technique among practitioners without

---

[35] As an example, in 1975 a doctoral thesis showed that of the 1,100 people receiving treatment at the Marchant psychiatric hospital in Toulouse, France, 44 patients (4 %) had been treated with a lobotomy, topectomy, or prefrontal infiltration for the most part between 1950 and 1955 (60 %) or 1965 and 1970 (20 %). Eight patients received two operations and three received three operations. For nine patients, clinical results were deemed "good," for 21 "minimal," for 11 "null," and for three "worse." Best results were obtained for patients with obsessive neurosis (two patients), psychosomatic disease (two patients), maniaco-depressive psychosis (six patients), while results were disappointing for psychoses (31 patients) and hypochondria (two patients). A weakening of the intellect, often progressive, was reported in 11 cases (25 %). Of the 44 patients, half remained hospitalized while the other half was released following the procedure [44].

[36] Cf. p. 42.

surgical training only aggravated the situation. The Washington State psychiatrist was responsible for nearly 4,000 such operations, which represented about 10 % of all the lobotomies performed in the United States. The last took place in 1967 at Berkley's *Herrick Memorial Hospital* [125].[37] In response to critics, Freeman, an excellent communicator [93, 125], would often denounce the older lobotomy technique as the main source of complications and point out that his technique was the least aggressive [126, 127]. In fact, the quick and easy procedure resulting in no visible wounds or trepanning marks advocated by Freeman only offered the illusion of relative innocuity. Without systematic records or follow-ups, the full extent of tragedies due to transorbital lobotomies was realized only too late [50].

A Painful Realization

In 1949, the same year Moniz received the Nobel Prize conferring the undeniable backing of the scientific community to the frontal lobotomy, a *Newsweek* article reported on a heated argument between Freeman and Lewis which had taken place at a symposium of the *American Psychiatric Society* [128]. Lewis, the director of the *New York State Psychiatric Institute* and a respected practitioner, asked *Is the quieting of the patient a cure? Perhaps all it accomplishes is to make things more convenient for the people who have to nurse them* [...]. *It disturbs me to see the number of zombies that these operations turn out* [...]. *I think it should be stopped before we dement too large a section of the population* [73]. The following year, Jay Hoffman, chief of the *Veterans'* Affairs Neuropsychiatric Service, concluded *The evaluation of the results after prefrontal leucotomy will be greatly influenced by the frame of reference one uses. If the condition of the patient is compared with his condition prior to the onset of his psychosis, all the result must be considered failures* [...] *I think it should be re-emphasized that by psychosurgery an organic brain-defect syndrome has be substituted for the psychoses* [73, 129]. Following work by the Swede Rylander [98], two psychologists from McGill University in Montreal, Rosvold and Mishkin, confirmed a very marked reduction in Intellectual Quotient (IQ) following the procedure in a study of a group of lobotomized Canadian veterans. The comparative study, the first of its kind, relied on the results of IQ tests given to the soldiers during their initial medical visit at the time of enlistment [130]. In France, the psychiatrist Baruk, an early and vocal critic, exclaimed *these interventions are veritable mutilations which add other disorders, sometimes extremely grave ones, on top of the first disorders* at a meeting of the *French Neurological Society* on 2 July 1953. Three years before, the Portuguese psychiatrist Barahona-Fernandes, had characterized the lobotomized personality as having *a tendency towards euphoria associated with a certain degree of emotional instability, loss of initiative and infantilism* [131]. The first retrospective studies,

---

[37] The operation resulted in the death of the patient following a cerebral hemorrhage.

published in the mid-1950s, painted a grim picture of the standard lobotomy. As J.-N. Missa writes, *the results are far from positive. In 1955, tens of thousands of people (including children) received a psychosurgical treatment. These operations raise obvious ethical concerns. They are based on rather vague physiological knowledge. Surgical indications are often applied indiscriminately to almost all mental pathologies. In addition, results are often disappointing: little improvement, numerous operating room fatalities, major side effects (apathy, loss of spontaneity, amnesia, various personality changes)*[38] [58].

The Promise of Neuropharmacology

In the preface to his work published in 1954, Le Beau declares that *psychosurgery was born from the inadequacy of traditional therapy: we hope that 1 day it will be replaced by more subtle and reversible methods, pharmacodynamic for example* [132]. And indeed, the discovery 2 years earlier of a new molecule, chlorpromazine, a sedative without hypnotic properties, spelled an end to the development of psychosurgery. In 1950, the molecule, the first neuroleptic, was developed and tested at the Sainte-Anne hospital in Paris under the direction of the military surgeon Henri Laborit. In 1952, the psychiatrists Jean Delay and Pierre Deniker reported on encouraging preliminary results obtained in psychotic patients [133]. Deniker toured European asylums with samples of chlorpromazine, and it spread throughout Europe. With the support of the Canadian psychiatrist Heinz Lehmann, it quickly reached North America where it was commercialized under the name *Thorazine*®. Due to its efficacy and, in contrast to lobotomies, its reversibility, it was approved by the FDA in 1954 and quickly became popular. Soon, chlorpromazine had been prescribed to over two million patients. The widespread use of the molecule and its success encouraged research into other medications such as Haloperidol in 1959, which had the benefit of being more incisive than chlorpromazine [134].

Mounting Public Criticism

As the public increasingly began to place its hopes in neuropharmacology, awareness of psychosurgery's excesses grew. A cinema adaptation was made in 1959 of Tennessee Williams' play, *Suddenly, Last Summer* [135] in which a character persuades a young neurosurgeon to practice a lobotomy on his niece in order to prevent her from revealing a terrible secret. Ken Kesey's novel, *One Flew Over the Cuckoo's Nest* [136], met with enormous success in 1962. In it, the author

---

[38] Cf. chapter on ethical questions p. 418.

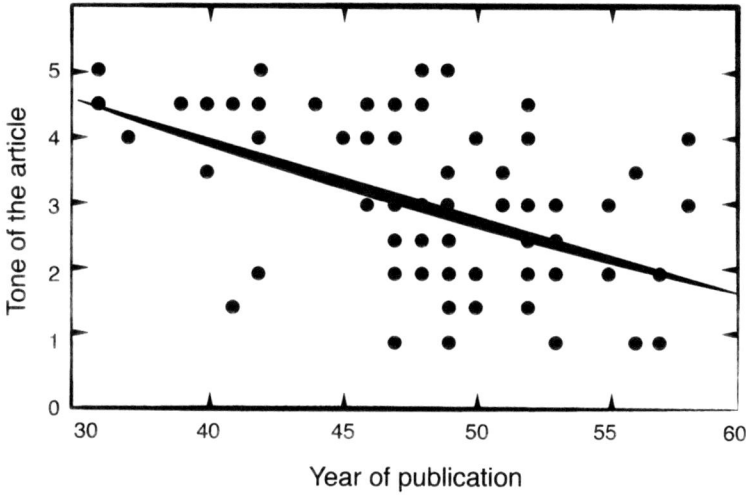

Fig. 1.17 Correlation between the tone of an article and the year of its publication. The data gathered in American newspapers and magazines published between 1935 and 1960 show the evolving tone of articles on the subject (from 5, extremely positive, to 0, extremely negative), found in [52]

recounts the trials of a rebellious and affable man wrongly interned in a psychiatric institution. The turbulent hero is rendered docile and disembodied through electroshocks and finally lobotomy. The film adaptation by Milos Forman with Jack Nicholson, was an international success and received the Oscar for best film in 1975. Over the years, articles in the press became increasingly negative (Fig. 1.17) [52].

A Timid and Much Criticized Revival

Psychopharmacology in turn flourished. After the discovery of neuroleptics, the first antidepressor molecules were developed through research into histamine derivatives in 1957. The first anxiolytics were commercialized, first *Librium*® and then *Valium*® in 1963. The efficacy of lithium salts in the treatment of bipolar disorder was also established at that time. Following these unarguable advances in pharmacology, a period of stagnation ensued at the start of the 1970s. People also became aware of some of the adverse effects and limitations of these new molecules. In 1970, Le Beau remarked: *It is also interesting to note that currently we are once again being offered cases for possible psychosurgery: indeed, failure of the new medical therapies is, naturally, more and more common as the years pass.* Functional and stereotactic neurosurgery was perfected during this time and past errors were analyzed. Still writing in the *Cahier de Médecine* journal, the neurosurgeon at the Salpêtrière hospital advocated *selective frontal psychosurgery as opposed to classical lobotomy, which is relatively blind and hence dangerous and which incapacitates too large an area of the frontal lobes and is hence mutilating* [137]. Thus, by the late 1960s the speciality was garnering renewed interest. This revival resulted in the *Second International Congress on Psychosurgery*[39] being held in Copenhagen in the summer of 1970 [138]. The congress, a follow-up to the Lisbon Congress 22 years earlier, brought together a little over 100 participants [139].

Unarguable Technical Progress

Early on, even as Moniz's was beginning his research, neurologists had learned that a targeted approach was crucial to the success of psychosurgical interventions. Experiments on animals and, it must be said, a certain amount of trial and error drew a more refined map of the brain and helped isolate the anatomical targets, notably the cingulate cortex[40] and the anterior limb of the internal capsule, relevant to the treatment of psychiatric pathologies. This period also saw a proliferation of new techniques. The need to reach cerebral targets with a maximum of precision and a minimum of damage encouraged others to continue the work of Spiegel and Wycis, to which the French Talairach [140] contributed, and perfect stereotactic surgery. With these techniques and the help of anatomical atlases compiled from dissections, it became possible to perform limited lesions in precise areas deep in the brain. The procedures developed for psychosurgery were quickly used in many other fields of neurosurgery,[41] namely in the treatment of abnormal movements. As precise as these new surgical techniques were, they did not eliminate the risk of infection or cerebral hemorrhage. As early as 1951, the Swedish neurosurgeon Lars Leksell tried to minimize these complications by replacing the metal instruments used to create targeted lesions in brain tissue with a beam of protons produced in a cyclotron [141, 142]. However radiosurgery,[42] as this method is called, truly became effective only once focused gamma rays were used. Twenty years later, Leksell performed the first *gamma-capsulotomy* on a patient suffering from severe anxiety disorder [143]. Radiosurgery found many other applications, such as the treatment of brain tumors, arteriovenous malformations, and certain forms of epilepsy.

---

[39] Freeman and Lima were honorary presidents, Scoville president, Knight vice-president, and Hitchcock secretary. The third conference was held in 1972 in Cambridge.

[40] Cf. p. 95 and Fig. 2.4.

[41] Stereotaxy is now routinely used to perform biopsies of brain tumors, in the treatment of abnormal movements (Parkinson's disease, tremors), or even pain.

[42] Cf. p. 187.

Narrower Indications and Better Monitoring of Results

During its timid revival at the start of the 1970s, psychosurgery was more closely supervised and was practiced exclusively by neurosurgeons. Interventions for psychiatric pathologies as well as indications were more limited. In addition to cases of untreatable pain, two main indications persisted: *cases of severe suicidal anxiety associated with depression* and *severe obsessive neuroses*. For the first category, the preferred treatment in France was a bilateral topectomy[43] of the prefrontal cortex (area 10). For the second, an anterior cingulectomy[44] was favored. Along with the well-known IQ test, nonstandardized neuropsychological and personality[45] tests were systematically given before and after the intervention. The procedures were less deleterious to cognition as the Parisian neuropsychiatrist Gaches explains: "*We have not observed* [...] *any post-surgical intellectual deterioration. This important point is confirmed by the resumption of professional activities in cases of success, including high-level activities (engineer, professor, business), and by the scores on baseline IQ tests being maintained.*" Gaches and his associates at the Salpêtrière observed that "*in a number of mentally ill patients, scores appear to have increased thanks to suppression of the pseudo-deterioration linked to the disease and to improvement in what psychologists call 'efficiency'* [137]. Concerning the modifications in mood and mutilations of personality observed in the past, the same team concluded, *in terms of mood, we have never observed (beyond the post-surgical phase) the disinhibition, the 'brazenness' so commonly described in the follow-up to excessive lobotomies. Nonetheless, it would seem that a number of subjects are more selfish and less docile with those around them after some interventions aimed at convexity* [topectomy of area 10, A/N]. *In terms of obsessional psychosis, we do feel that the subject is freed from his obsessions and rituals without the fundamental psychasthenic structure actually being changed. Our incomplete successes in this area in fact show how the same obsessive themes persist, in attenuated form, cut off from the stifling ritual obligation.* (Fig. 1.18) [137]. Depending on the type of procedure, post-surgical complications lasting between 3 days and 6 weeks were observed: euphoria, excitation, and sphincter problems due to topectomies of the dorsolateral cortex; inertia, apathy, and mutism due to topectomies of the orbitofrontal cortex; and reduction in spontaneous movements and speech, excessive docility, and noticeable emotional indifference following procedures on the cingulate [137]. In many

---

[43] Cf. p. 48.

[44] Cf. p. 49.

[45] The best-known and most used personality test at this time was the Minnesota Multiphasic Personality Inventory (MMPI), which comprises 550 questions to which the subject must answer "true," "I do not know," or "false." After the answers are tallied a profile is constructed from three validity scales and ten clinical scales (hypochondriasis, depression, hysteria, psychopathic deviate, masculinity–femininity, paranoia, psychasthenia, schizophrenia, hypomania, social introversion).

Table 4.2 Diagnostic Labels and Site of Brain Operation (United Kingdom)

Diagnostic Label[a]	Total Number of Patients[b]	Frontal Lobe Procedure	Cingulum[c]	Limbic Leucotomy[d]
Aggression, including self-mutilation	12		2(16.7%)	
Depression	201	169(84.1%)	2(1.0%)	28(13.9%)
Fear and anxiety	82	58(70.7%)	1(1.2%)	23(28.1%)
Obsessive-compulsive neurosis	96	50(52.1%)	5(5.2%)	41(42.7%)
Anorexia nervosa	13	11(84.6%)		2(15.4%)
Psychopathic behavior	13	7(53.8%)		6(46.2%)
Schizophrenia and other psychoses	13	6(46.2%)		7(53.8%)
Drug addiction and alcoholism	13	13(100.0%)		
Epilepsy with psychiatric disorders	36		3(8.3%)	

Fig. 1.18 Some indications given for psychosurgery

cases, scientific rigor would have required more regular and long-term follow-up of clinical results.[46] In addition, the absence of reproducible and standardized scales in some circumstances can make comparison of the results from different research teams problematic. For this reason, as we will see later, it is impossible to draw overall conclusions about interventions performed during this period.

New Lapses with Brain Stimulation

As mentioned above, recording and stimulation of deep brain structures had been carried out on a very limited number of patients suffering from mental disorders and chronic pain since the 1950s (Fig. 1.16, p. 27) [144]. The attempts, however, never left the experimental stage and produced overall only disappointing results. At the beginning of the 1970s, the *Electrical Brain Stimulation Program* at Tulane University in New Orleans started raising preoccupying ethical questions [145]. Launched in 1950 by the psychiatrist Heath, it began implanting brain electrodes in over 100 patients with a wide range of pathologies: schizophrenia, neurosis, obesity, narcolepsy, aggressive behavior disorders, epilepsy [146, 147]. A number of areas region as the cerebellum [148] and the amygdala [149] were targeted. Particular attention was paid to the septal area[47] [150]. During his research, Heath

---

[46] Cf. p. 184.

[47] Cf. p. 120.

observed that stimulation of this region provoked states of *pleasure and sexual motivation*. When he noticed that autostimulation of this zone provoked pleasant sensations [151] in some of his "patients," he began trying to modify their behavior using a so-called *positive reinforcement* technique [145]. Other dubious projects ensued including one in 1972 to transform the homosexual tendencies of a schizophrenic man into heterosexual behavior [152]. Surprisingly, few in the medical community condemned these aberrations. Notable exceptions were the American psychiatrist Breggin, who did not hesitate to denounce this program as a *crime against humanity* [153, 154], and the Scandinavian neurosurgeon Laitinen, who, as Hariz reminds us [155], would 5 years later write that *There is no doubt that in this study all standards of ethics had been ignored. The ethical responsibility of the editors who accept reports of this kind for publication should also be discussed* [156]. In contrast, media portrayal of Delgado's work was different: a few years earlier in an arena in Cordoba, the Yale neurophysiologist had made the headlines after he managed to halt a charging bull from a distance using intracerebral electrodes [157]. On the front page of the *New York Times*, Delgado's demonstration was described as *probably the most spectacular demonstration ever performed of the deliberate modification of animal behavior through external control of the brain* [158]. In 1970, with the publication of his book *Physical Control of the Mind: Toward a Psychocivilized Society* [159], whose title is abundantly clear, Delgado was once again in the press, but this time opinions were less favorable. In presenting his research on modifying behavior in monkeys through the implantation of electrodes, this former student of Fulton's called for a *psycho-controlled"* society. He believed that advances in *"neurotechnology* would lead to a *less cruel, happier and better man.* Also published in 1970, *Violence and the Brain,* by the neurosurgeon Mark and the psychiatrist Ervin stirred considerable controversy [160]. These two Harvard researchers claimed that the behavior of certain dangerous individuals could be linked to dysfunction of the limbic circuit, and that a surgical intervention could put them back on *the right track* [84]. In 1972, the *Washington Post* published a front-page article reporting that psychosurgical interventions had been performed on three recidivist delinquents in a prison in Vacaville, California [161]. At the same time, a violent legal battle surrounding the attribution by the state of Michigan of research funds for psychosurgical treatment of sexual delinquents resulted in the *G. Kaimowitz decision* [162]. The public became extremely wary of the somewhat fantastical prospect of a "psychocontrolled"[48] individual. Not only were the tragic events surrounding lobotomies in the 1960s still fresh in everyone's mind, but in that 10-year period mentalities had also changed significantly. In the West at the end of the 1960s, a rebellious and vocal movement spread denouncing the excesses of a police state wanting to control individuals considered to be deviant and among them the mad.

---

[48] This coincided in 1975 with the shocking revelation in the press of the MK-Ultra project conducted by the CIA from 1953 to 1963. The code name, MK for "Mind Control," designated a secret and illegal program to mentally manipulate certain people, notably through administration of psychotropic [77].

The *antipsychiatry* movement was also at the height of its popularity and lambasted disciplinary psychiatric power [163]. The release in cinemas around the world of two immensely popular films, Kubrick's *A Clockwork Orange* and Forman's *One Flew Over the Cuckoo's Nest*, only increased suspicion in the recently rehabilitated specialty. In the United States, the psychiatrist Breggin, soon joined by Senator Gallagher, took the lead in warning of the dangers and potential for abuse inherent in psychosurgery. In 1972, they presented Congress with two reports advocating a ban on psychosurgery in the United States.

The Unexpected Results of an American Report

In response to these two reports and the significant interest in the issue aroused by Forman's movie, the National Commission for the Protection of Human Subjects of Biomedical and Behavioral Research tasked Kenneth Ryan, a Harvard University psychiatrist, with leading an inquiry. The decision to investigate was part of a broad legislative effort to create better oversight of medical research in the wake of the Tuskegee experiment[49] scandal. The conclusions of the report were based on the work of two independent teams. The first, led by psychiatrists Mirsky and Orzack of Boston University, focused on the efficacy and safety of psychosurgical interventions. The second, led by Teuber and Corkin of the Massachusetts Institute of Technology (MIT), was tasked with performing a prospective study, notably of cingulectomy [164]. The studies based on neuropsychological tests and interviews with a limited number of patients concluded that (1) *more than half of the patients improved significantly following psychosurgery, although a few were worse and some unchanged, and* (2) *none of the patients experienced significant neurological or psychological impairment attributable to the surgery* [165]. The historian E.S. Valenstein was then asked to summarize the scientific literature available on the subject. It too was positive [166]. When the commission, which had originally been expected to condemn psychosurgery ahead of a ban, reported its findings to the President in 1977, it had came to a surprising conclusion: *On the basis of data from pilot studies that were conducted under contract to assess the effects of psychosurgery, the Commission has determined unanimously that there are circumstances under which psychosurgical procedures may appropriately be performed* (Fig. 1.19). It also provided a number of recommendations, including a ban on operations on minors, prisoners, and anyone unable to give clear and informed consent. The experts also recommended that interventions only be performed in authorized settings under the guidance of multidisciplinary teams.

---

[49] The Tuskegee experiment, conducted in Alabama between 1932 and 1972, was a clinical study of syphilis: close to 400 poor rural black men were not told of their syphilis diagnosis and were not given treatment for the disease in order to be made unwitting subjects in a study of the natural progression of the disease.

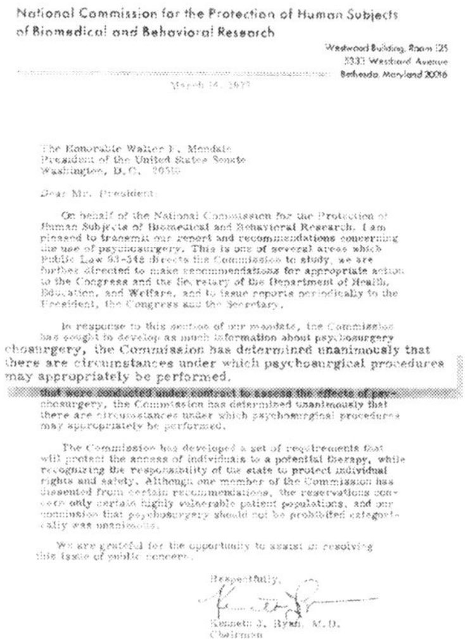

Fig. 1.19 The commission's
report and recommendations
concerning psychosurgery

The Arrival of Neuromodulation

By the end of the 1980s, the public had turned its attention away from psycho-surgery. Only a small number of teams were still performing operations on patients with psychiatric pathologies in a few places around the world: in the United States [167], London [168], Madrid [169], Benelux [170] Sydney [171], Stockholm [172], and Paris [173]. Each center was specialized in a given type of procedure: the cingulectomy[50] at the Massachusetts General Hospital in Boston, the sub-caudate tractotomy[51] at the Brook General Hospital in London, the capsulotomy[52] at the Karolinska Institute or the limbic leucotomy[53] at the Atkinson Morley's Hospital in the south of London. In a short book on the subject of neurosurgery, Philippon summarizes: *experience with very selective lesions has shown that they can be very effective with a minimum of side effects. This selectivity of the lesions can be achieved both by stereotactic methods associating perfect anatomical definition and by control of the volume of the lesion, whether it is obtained through electrocoagulation, refrigeration or through radioactive elements. Lesion sites have also been more precisely defined and mainly concern the inferio-internal part of frontal lobe. Indications must be extremely precise and obsessive neurosis is the best example of this.* In the same 1986 opuscule, the neurosurgeon adds that *the possibility of using techniques for stimulating nerve targets and not destroying them (in a somewhat analogous way to what happened with the surgical treatment*

---

[50] Cf. p. 173.

[51] Cf. p. 180.

[52] Cf. p. 167 and concerning gamma-capsulotomy, p. 188.

[53] Cf. p. 182.

Table 1.2 Summary of important events in the history of psychosurgery

1888	*Burckhardt* performs the first **topectomy** (p. 6)
1906	*Puusepp* performs cuts in the frontal white matter in order to calm agitation in maniacal patients [21, 22]
1935	*Fulton* and *Jacobsen* alongside *Vincent* present various findings on the **function of the frontal lobes** during the Neurological Congress held in London (p. 11) [34, 35]
	Moniz and *Lima* perform the **first frontal leucotomy** (p. 12) [40]
1936	*Freeman* and *Watts* begin developing Moniz's technique in the United States [53] at a time when asylums are overpopulated (p. 15)
1946	The transorbital lobotomy, the so-called **ice pick** technique, which can be performed on an ambulatory basis, is popularized by *Freeman*. Its popularity will lead to abuses (p. 20) [183]
1947	*Wycis* and *Spiegel* perfect **stereotaxy** for use in thalamotomies (p. 143) [111]. Many neurosurgeons like Scoville begin advocating more targeted techniques
1948	*Cairn, Pool* and *Le Beau* develop the **cingulectomy** (p. 26)
1949	*Moniz* receives the **Nobel Prize** for his "discovery of the therapeutic value of leucotomy in certain psychoses" (p. 23). This marks the golden age of psychosurgery
	Talairach and *Leksell* use the new stereotaxy method to target the anterior limb of the internal capsule in a technique called a **capsulotomy** (p. 27) [113]
1952	*Delgado* perfects a **brain stimulation and recording** technique for therapeutic use in psychotic patients (p. 38) [118], Heath undertakes similar research, eventually leading to misconduct [145]
	Laborit, Delay and *Deniker* develop the **first neuroleptic** (p. 32) [133]. The discovery of this and numerous other psychoactive drugs mark the decline of psychosurgery
1959	Film adaptations of Tennessee Williams's play Suddenly, Last Summer [135], and Ken Kesey's novel One Flew Over the Cuckoo's Nest [136] turn **public opinion** against psychosurgery (p. 33)
1964	*Knight* performs the first **subcaudate tractotomy** (p. 157) [184]
1967	*Ballantine* develops **cingulectomy by thermocoagulation** (p. 151)
1973	*Kelly* suggests use of the **limbic leucotomy**, a blend of cingulectomy and subcaudate tractotomy (p. 159) [185]
1976	A report commissioned by the United States Senate concludes in favor of psychosurgery (p. 40) [164]
1978	*Leksell* performs the first **capsulotomy by radiosurgery** (p. 163) [143]
1987	First instance of **deep brain stimulation**, used in the treatment of Parkinson's disease by *Benabid* (p. 169).
1999	*Nuttin* accomplishes the first successful treatment using deep brain stimulation of the anterior limb of the internal capsule in a patient with **OCD** [179]. *Visser-Vandewalle* uses the same technique to target the thalamus of a patient suffering from **Gilles de la Tourette** syndrome [180]
2000	**Stimulation of the vagus nerve** is suggested/used for treating depression (p. 212) [186, 187]
2002	**In France**, the *Comité National Consultatif d'Ethique* **rules in favor** of continued development of psychosurgery [188]
2005	*Mayberg* et *Lozano* publishes his first results of the treatment of **depression** through stimulation of the subgenual cortex (p. 195) [189]
2007	An **alcoholic patient is weaned off alcohol** for the first time through stimulation of the nucleus accumbens (p. 328) [190]
2008	A team led by *Lozano* investigating a treatment for obesity finds that stimulation of the hypothalamus leads to **improved memory** (p. 336) [191]
2010	First study of **cortical stimulation** in the treatment of depression (p. 202) [192]

of pain[54]*) remains purely theoretical for now* [174]. Nonetheless, that same year a French team headed by the neurosurgeon A.-L. Benabid, managed to effectively treat patients with Parkinson's disease by implanting electrodes in the thalamus [175]. This success was followed by treatments for tremor [176, 177] and generalized dystonia [178]. In this new techniques, stimulation electrodes are put in place stereotactically and, thanks to advances in minituarization, are connected to a control box implanted under the skin. The Grenoble school has shown that a high-frequency electrical stimulation can have an effect similar to a lesion.[55] This new technique is superior to classical psychosurgical lesioning techniques in that its effect is reversible and adaptable. The Belgian neurosurgeon Nuttin, seeing the potential for this technology, was the first along with his team in Leuven to undertake the treatment of a patient with obsessive compulsive disorder[56] through deep brain stimulation in 1999 [179]. For this treatment, the team from Leuven targeted the anterior limb of the internal capsule described exactly 50 years earlier by Talairach and Leksell. The same year, an international team led by Visser-Vandewalle obtained encouraging clinical results after stimulating the thalamus of a patient suffering from Gilles de la Tourette syndrome[57] [180]. With these two successful interventions, a new era in psychosurgery was begun, the era of neuromodulation (Table 1.2).

References

1. Alt KW, Jeunesse C, Buitrago-Tellez CH, Wachter R, Boes E, Pichler SL (1997) Evidence for stone age cranial surgery. Nature 387(6631):360. doi:10.1038/387360a0
2. Piek J, Lidke G, Terberger T, von Smekal U, Gaab MR (1999) Stone age skull surgery in Mecklenburg-Vorpommern: a systematic study. Neurosurgery 45(1):147–151; discussion 51
3. Swayze VW 2nd (1995) Frontal leukotomy and related psychosurgical procedures in the era before antipsychotics (1935–1954): a historical overview. Am J Psychiatry 152(4):505–515
4. Valenstein ES (1997) The history of psychosurgery. The history of neurosurgery. Park Ridge, AANS
5. Salcman M (2006) The cure of folly or the operation for the stone by Hieronymus Bosch (C. 1450–1516). Neurosurgery 59(4):935–937. doi:10.1227/01.NEU.0000242109.97950.9F (pii:00006123-200610000-00028)
6. Gross CG (1999) 'Psychosurgery' in renaissance art. Trends Neurosci 22(10):429–431. doi:S0166223699014885 (pii)
7. Sullivan MA (1977) Madness and folly: Peter Bruegel the elder's Dulle Griet. Art Bull 59:55–66

---

[54] Philipon is here referring to stimulation through an implanted electrode of the posterior columns of the spinal cord, which is effective in the treatment of chronic pains primarily in the limbs.

[55] Cf. principle of deep brain stimulation p. 197.

[56] Cf. p. 271.

[57] Cf. p. 296.

8. Brink A (1979) Depression and loss: a theme in Robert Burton's "Anatomy of melancholy" (1621). Can J Psychiatry 24(8):767–772
9. Fara P (2005) The melancholy of anatomy. Endeavour 29(1):20–21. doi:S0160-9327(05)00002-5 (pii:10.1016/j.endeavour.2004.10.009)
10. Paillas JE (1953) Leçon inaugurale de la chaire de neurochirurgie de la faculté de médecine de Marseille
11. Harlow J-M (1848) Recovery from the passage of an iron bar through the head. Boston Med Surg J 389–392
12. Harlow HF (1868) Recovery from the passage of an iron bar through the head. Read before the Massachusetts Medical Society, 3 June 1868
13. Muller C (1958) Gottlieb Burckhardt, the father of topectomy. Rev Med Suisse Romande 78(11):726–730
14. Stone JL (2001) Dr. Gottlieb Burckhardt: the pioneer of psychosurgery. J Hist Neurosci 10(1):79–92
15. Manjila S, Rengachary S, Xavier AR, Parker B, Guthikonda M (2008) Modern psychosurgery before Egas Moniz: a tribute to Gottlieb Burckhardt. Neurosurg Focus 25(1):E9. doi:10.3171/FOC/2008/25/7/E9
16. Mairet A (1883) De la démence mélancolique: contribution à l'étude de la péri-encéphalite localisée et à l'étude des localisation cérébrale d'ordre psychique. Masson
17. Joanette Y, Stemmer B, Assal G, Whitaker H (1993) From theory to practice: the unconventional contribution of Gottlieb Burckhardt to psychosurgery. Brain Lang 45(4):572–587. doi:S0093-934X(83)71061-8 (pii:10.1006/brln.1993.1061)
18. Luigjes J, de Kwaasteniet BP, de Koning PP, Oudijn MS, van den Munckhof P, Schuurman PR et al (2012) Surgery for psychiatric disorders. World Neurosurg. doi:S1878-8750(12)00412-3 [pii]
19. Kotowicz Z (2005) Gottlieb Burckhardt and Egas Moniz-two beginnings of psychosurgery. Gesnerus 62(1–2):77–101
20. Semelaigne R (1895) Sur la chirurgie cérébrale dans les aliénations mentales. Ann Med Psychol (Paris) 394–420
21. Raudam E, Kaasik AE (1981) Ludwig Puusepp 1875–1942. Surg Neurol 16(2):85–87
22. Puusepp L (1937) Alcune considerazioni sugli interventi chirurgici nelle malattie mentali. G Acad Med Torino 100:3–16
23. Doyen E (1907) La crâniectomie chez les enfants arriérés. Archives de neurologie 93
24. Wagner-Jauregg J, Bruetsch WL (1946) The history of the malaria treatment of general paralysis. Am J Psychiatry 102:577–582
25. Sakel M (1937) The origin and nature of the hypoglycemic therapy of the psychoses. Bull NY Acad Med 13(3):97–109
26. Sakel M (1938) Insulin therapy in the future of psychiatry. Can Med Assoc J 39(2):178–179
27. Meduna L (1990) The use of Metrazol in the treatment of patients with mental diseases. Convuls Ther 6(4):287–298
28. Babinski J (1903) Guérison d'un cas de mélancolie à la suite d'un accés provoqué de vertige voltaïque. Revue Neurologique. Société de neurologie de Paris, séance du 7 mai
29. Rasmussen K (2002) The practice of electroconvulsive therapy: recommendations for treatment, training, and privileging (second edition). J ECT 18(1):58–9
30. Puech P, Guilly P, Lairy-Bounes GC (1950) Introduction à la psychochirurgie. Masson
31. Penfield WE (1935) The frontal lobe in man: a clinical study of maximal removals. Brain 58:115–133
32. Wertheimer P (1951) Justification et résultat d'une psychochirurgie. Rev Philos VII à IX(907):337–351
33. Fulton JF, Sheehan D (1935) The uncrossed lateral pyramidal tract in higher primates. J Anat 69(2):181–187
34. Fulton JJ, Jacobsen CF (1935) The functions of the frontal lobes: a comparative study in monkeys, chimpanzees, and man. Abstr Second Int Neurol Congr 70–71
35. Guiot G (1973) Clovis vincent. 1879–1947. Surg Neurol 1(4):189–190

36. Ferro JM (2003) Egas Moniz (1874–1955). J Neurol 250(3):376–377
37. Kyle RA, Shampo MA (1979) Egas Moniz. JAMA 241(6):640
38. Fusar-Poli P, Allen P, McGuire P (2008) Egas Moniz (1875–1955), the father of psychosurgery. Br J Psychiatry 193(1):50. doi:193/1/50 (pii:10.1192/bjp.193.1.50)
39. Brickner R (1932) An interprétation of function based on the study of a case of bilatéral frontal lobectomy. In: Proceedings of the Association for Research in Nervous and Mental Disorders, vol 13, pp 259–351
40. Moniz E (1936) Essai d'un traitement chirurgical de certaines psychoses. Bull Acad Med 385–393
41. Antunes JL (1979) Pedro Almeida Lima. Surg Neurol 11(6):405–406
42. Antunes JL (2010) Egas Moniz: Uma Biografia. Publicacoes, Gradiva
43. Moniz E (1936) Tentatives opératoires dans le traitement de certaines psychoses. Masson
44. Vaysettes A (1976) Contribution à l'étude des résultats à long terme de la psychochirurgie. Université Paul Sabatier, Toulouse
45. Xiao W (2011) Psychosurgery. Chinese neurosurgeons quietly push for easing of brain operation ban. Science 332(6027):294. doi:332/6027/294 (pii:10.1126/science.332.6027.294)
46. Kotowicz Z (2008) Psychosurgery in Italy, 1936–39. Hist Psychiatry 19(76 Pt 4):476–489
47. Juckel G, Uhl I, Padberg F, Brune M, Winter C (2009) Psychosurgery and deep brain stimulation as ultima ratio treatment for refractory depression. Eur Arch Psychiatry Clin Neurosci 259(1):1–7. doi:10.1007/s00406-008-0826-7
48. Decaris F (1978) La Psychochirurgie réflexions sur son évolution et ses indications actuelles, à propos de dix observations. (S.l.n.d.)
49. Mashour GA, Walker EE, Martuza RL (2005) Psychosurgery: past, present, and future. Brain Res Brain Res Rev 48(3):409–419. doi:S0165-0173(04)00129-8 (pii:10.1016/j.brainresrev.2004.09.002)
50. Pressman JD (2002) Last resort: psychosurgery and the limits of medicine. Cambridge University Press, Cambridge
51. Fulton JF (1948) The frontal lobes: research publication for the association for research in nervous and mental disease. Baltimore
52. Diefenbach GJ, Diefenbach D, Baumeister A, West M (1999) Portrayal of lobotomy in the popular press (1935–1960). J Hist Neurosci 8(1):60–69. doi:10.1076/jhin.8.1.60.1766
53. Freeman WW (1942) Psychosurgery. Charles C. Thomas, Baltimore
54. Ferdière G (1940) Résultats immédiats de la leucotomie préfrontale dans un cas de schizophrénie avec stupeur catatonique. Ann Med Psychol (Paris) XV(I):81–89
55. Venet E (2006) Ferdière, psychiatre d'Antonin Artaud. Verdier Lagrasse
56. Puech P (1941) De l'intérêt d'une liaison entre neuro-psychiatrie et neurochirurgie, par Pierre Puech. Masson
57. David M, Guilly P (1970) La Neurochirurgie. Que sais-je?, vol 1369. Presses Universitaires de France, Paris
58. Missa J-N (2001) Psychochirurgie. In: Hautois GM, J-N (ed) Nouvelle encyclopédie de bioéthique médecine, environnement, biotechnologie avec la collab. de Marie-Geneviève Pinsart et Pascal Chabot. Bruxelles [Paris]: De Boeck Université, pp 922
59. Guenot M (2011) La lobotomie, une pratique barbare ou une avancée thérapeutique? Le Nouvel Observateur, Paris. http://leplus.nouvelobs.com/contribution/225452-la-lobotomie-une-pratique-barbare-ou-une-avancee-therapeutique.html. Accessed 23 Dec 2011
60. David M, Sauguet J, Hecaen H, Talairach J (1953) Follow-up of 78 cases of psychosurgery a year after the operation. Rev Neurol (Paris) 89(1):3–21
61. Talairach MJ (1952) Anatomic-physiological reflections on psychosurgery. Rev Neurol (Paris) 87(6):554–557
62. Wertheimer P (1953) Indications for and results of lobotomy. Lyon Med 188(13):272
63. Le Beau J (1951) The surgical uncertainties of prefrontal topectomy and leucotomy (observations on 100 cases). J Ment Sci 97(408):480–504

64. Neimat JS, Hamani C, Giacobbe P, Merskey H, Kennedy SH, Mayberg HS et al (2008) Neural stimulation successfully treats depression in patients with prior ablative cingulectomy. Am J Psychiatry 165(6):687–693. doi:165/6/687 (pii:10.1176/appi.ajp.2008.07081298)
65. Poppen JL, Dynes JB, Weadon PS (1948) Prefrontal lobotomy; general impressions based on results in 470 patients subjected to this procedure. Surg Clin North Am 28:811–816
66. Poppen JL (1948) Technic of prefrontal lobotomy. J Neurosurg 5(6):514–520. doi:10.3171/jns.1948.5.6.0514
67. Grant FC (1950) The value of psychosurgery in mental disease. Pa Med J 53(5):478–482
68. Pool JL (1949) Topectomy; the treatment of mental illness by frontal gyrectomy or bilateral subtotal ablation of frontal cortex. Lancet 2(6583):776–781
69. Lyerly JG (1952) Results of lobotomy in mental disorders. South Med J 45(9):793–798
70. Deutsch A (1948) The shame of the States, 1st edn. Harcourt, New York
71. McKissock W (1959) Discussion on psychosurgery. Proc R Soc Med 52(3):206–209
72. Wilson IW, Warland EH (1947) Pre-frontal leucotomy in 1000 cases. Lancet 2(252):584–594
73. Valenstein ES (1986) Great and desperate cures: the rise and decline of psychosurgery and other radical treatments for mental illness. Basic Books, New York
74. Fiamberti AM (1952) Ce qu'il faut préciser à propos de la méthode originale de la leucotomie transorbitaire. Méd Hyg 10(195):1–4
75. Saltuk E (1951) Psychosurgery in the world and in Turkey. Turk Tip Cemiy Mecm 17(4):171–178
76. Zahmacioglu O, Dinc G, Naderi S (2009) The history of psychosurgery in Turkey. Turk Neurosurg 19(3):308–314
77. Laboucarié J (1971) Le problème actuel de la Leucotomie préfrontale d'après une expérience thérapeutique de vingt ans (1949–1969). Rev Med Toulouse (VII):187–201
78. Lichterman BL (1993) On the history of psychosurgery in Russia. Acta Neurochir (Wien) 125(1–4):1–4
79. Likhterman LB, Likhterman BL (2001) History on ban of psychosurgery in the USSR. Zh Vopr Neirokhir Im NN Burdenko 2:35–38; discussion 8–9
80. Sano K (2002) Development of Japanese neurosurgery: from the Edo era to 1973. Neurosurgery 51(4):861–863
81. Masiero AL (2003) Lobotomy and leucotomy in Brazilian mental hospitals. Hist Cienc Saude Manguinhos 10(2):549–572
82. Heller AC, Amar AP, Liu CY, Apuzzo ML (2006) Surgery of the mind and mood: a mosaic of issues in time and evolution. Neurosurgery 59(4):720–733; discussion 33–9. doi:10.1227/01.NEU.0000240227.72514.27 00006123-200610000-00003 [pii]
83. Winn HR, Youmans JR (2011) Youmans' neurological surgery, 6th edn. Saunders, Philadelphia, London
84. Feldman RP, Goodrich JT (2001) Psychosurgery: a historical overview. Neurosurgery 48(3):647–657; discussion 57–59
85. Fins JJ (2003) From psychosurgery to neuromodulation and palliation: history's lessons for the ethical conduct and regulation of neuropsychiatric research. Neurosurg Clin N Am 14(2):303–319, ix–x
86. Black DW (1982) Psychosurgery. South Med J 75(4):453–457
87. Bucy PB (1973) Percival Bailey 1892–1973. Surg Neurol 1(5):311
88. (1936) Lobotomy: cutting the ability to worry out of the brain. Time, 30 Nov 1936, pp 68–77
89. Kill or cure. Time 1946, 23 Dec 1946, pp 66–77
90. (1949) Mental aid found in brain surgery. New York Times, pp 26
91. Kaempffert W (1941) Turning the mind inside out. Saturday Evening Post (213):213, 18–19, 69, 71–72, 74
92. Laurence WL (1951) Big advances seen in brain surgery. New York Times

93. Robison RA, Taghva A, Liu CY, Apuzzo ML (2012) Surgery of the mind, mood, and conscious state: an idea in evolution. World Neurosurg. doi:S1878-8750(12)00345-2 (pii:10.1016/j.wneu.2012.03.005)
94. Nijensohn DE, Savastano LE, Kaplan AD, Laws ER Jr (2012) New evidence of prefrontal lobotomy in the last months of the illness of Eva Peron. World Neurosurg 77(3–4):583–590. doi:S1878-8750(11)00190-2 (pii:10.1016/j.wneu.2011.02.036)
95. Ligon BL (1998) The mystery of angiography and the "unawarded" Nobel prize: Egas Moniz and Hans Christian Jacobaeus. Neurosurgery 43(3):602–611
96. Gross D, Schafer G (2011) Egas Moniz (1874–1955) and the "invention" of modern psychosurgery: a historical and ethical reanalysis under special consideration of Portuguese original sources. Neurosurg Focus 30(2):E8. doi:10.3171/2010.10.FOCUS10214
97. Le Bau JM, D. (1950) Sur les indications de la neuro-chirurgie du lobe pré-frontal dans les effections mentales, d'après 97 cas personnels. Bull Mémoires Soc méd Hôpitaux Paris 17:763–778
98. Rylander G (1939) Personality changes after operationson the frontal lobes. Acta Psychiatrica et Neurologica 1(Supplément 20):81
99. Scoville WB (1949) Selective cortical undercutting as a means of modifying and studying frontal lobe function in man; preliminary report of 43 operative cases. J Neurosurg 6(1):65–73. doi:10.3171/jns.1949.6.1.0065
100. Scoville WB, Wilk EK, Pepe AJ (1951) Selective cortical undercutting; results in new method of fractional lobotomy. Am J Psychiatry 107(10):730–738
101. Le Beau JP (1949) L'évolution de la psycho-chirugie. La semaine des Hôpitaux de Paris 94:1–7
102. Krayenbuhl H, Stoll W (1950) Prefrontal leucotomy and topectomy for the treatment of irreducible pain. Rev Neurol (Paris) 83(1):40–41
103. Constans JP (1960) Frontal surgery for pain. Acta Neurochir (Wien) 8:251–281
104. Scoville WB (1951) Research project of undercutting of the medial-cingulate gyrus Brodmann's area 24 and 32. Trans Am Neurol Assoc 56:226–227
105. Le Beau J (1952) Selective prefrontal surgery; topectomy of the convexity and cingulectomy. Rev Neurol (Paris) 86(6):699
106. Brotis AG, Kapsalaki EZ, Paterakis K, Smith JR, Fountas KN (2009) Historic evolution of open cingulectomy and stereotactic cingulotomy in the management of medically intractable psychiatric disorders, pain and drug addiction. Stereotact Funct Neurosurg 87(5):271–291. doi:000226669 (pii:10.1159/000226669)
107. Mac LP (1949) Psychosomatic disease and the "visceral brain" recent developments bearing on the Papez theory of emotion. Psychosom Med 11(6):338–353
108. Paillas JE (1951) Aperçu général sur la psychochirurgie. Bio Méd 2(Mars–Avril):59
109. David MP (1961) Neurochirurgie. Collection médico-chirurgicale à révision annuelle. Flammarion édit, Paris
110. Horsley VC, Clarke RH (1908) The structure and functions of the cebellum examined by a new method. Brain 31:45–124
111. Spiegel EA, Wycis HT, Marks M, Lee AJ (1947) Stereotaxic apparatus for operations on the human brain. Science 106(2754):349–350. doi:106/2754/349 (pii:10.1126/science.106.2754.349)
112. Rahman M, Murad GJ, Mocco J (2009) Early history of the stereotactic apparatus in neurosurgery. Neurosurg Focus 27(3):E12. doi:10.3171/2009.7.FOCUS09118
113. Talairach J, Hecaen H, David M (1949) Lobotomies prefrontal limitee par electrocoagulation des fibres thalamo-frontales à leur emergence du bras anterieur de la capsule interne. In: Proceedings IV congress neurologique international, Paris
114. Gildenberg PL (2003) History repeats itself. Stereotact Funct Neurosurg 80(1–4):61–75. doi:10.1159/000075162 75162 [pii]
115. Gildenberg PL (2005) Evolution of neuromodulation. Stereotact Funct Neurosurg 83(2–3):71–79. doi:86865 (pii:10.1159/000086865)

116. Hariz MI (2008) Psychosurgery, deep brain stimulation, and the re-writing of history. Neurosurgery 63(4):E820 (author reply E). doi:10.1227/01.NEU.0000325681.70894.91 00006123-200810000-00039 [pii]

117. Delgado JM (1952) Permanent implantation of multilead electrodes in the brain. Yale J Biol Med 24(5):351–358

118. Delgado JM, Hamlin H, Chapman WP (1952) Technique of intracranial electrode implacement for recording and stimulation and its possible therapeutic value in psychotic patients. Confin Neurol 12(5–6):315–319

119. Delgado JM, Hamlin H, Koskoff YD (1955) Electrical activity after stimulation and electrocoagulation of the human frontal lobe. Yale J Biol Med 28(3–4):233–244

120. Crow HJ, Cooper R, Phillips DG (1961) Controlled multifocal frontal leucotomy for psychiatric illness. J Neurol Neurosurg Psychiatry 24:353–360

121. Cooper R, Winter AL, Crow HJ, Walter WG (1965) Comparison of subcortical, cortical and scalp activity using chronically indwelling electrodes in man. Electroencephalogr Clin Neurophysiol 18:217–228

122. Valenstein ES (1974) Brain control. Wiley, New York

123. Lazorthes GG, Anduze-Acher H (1971) Bilan de quinze années de psychochirurgie (1954–1969). Rev Med Toulouse (VII):177–201

124. Freeman W (1954) Psychosurgery. Am J Psychiatry 110(7):511–2

125. El-Hai J (2005) The lobotomist: a maverick medical genius and his tragic quest to rid the world of mental illness. Wiley, Hoboken

126. Freeman W (1958) Psychosurgery; present indications and future prospects. Calif Med 88(6):429–434

127. Freeman W (1965) Recent advances in psychosurgery. Med Ann Dist Columbia 34:157–160 (PASSIM)

128. Lewis ND (1949) General clinical psychiatry, psychosomatic medicine, psychotherapy, group therapy and psychosurgery. Am J Psychiatry 105(7):512–517

129. Hoffman J (1950) A clinical appraisal of frontal lobotomy in the treatment of the psychoses. Psychiatry 13(3):355–356

130. Rosvold HM, Mishkin M (1950) Evaluation of the effects of prefrontal lobotomy on intelligence. Can J Psychol 4(3):122–126

131. Fernandes B (ed) (1950) Anatomophysiologie cérébrale et fonctions psychiques dans la leucotomie préfrontale. Comtpe-rendu du 1er Congrès International de Psychiatrie, Hermann, Edit, Paris, 19–27 Sept 1950

132. Le Beau JCM, Gaches J, Rosier M (1954) Psycho-chirurgie et fonctions mentales: techniques—résultats applications physiologiques. Masson, Paris

133. Delay J, Deniker P, Harl JM (1952) Therapeutic use in psychiatry of phenothiazine of central elective action (4560 RP). Ann Med Psychol (Paris) 110(21):112–117

134. Divry P, Bobon J, Collard J, Pinchard A, Nols E (1959) Study and clinical trial of R 1625 or haloperidol, a new neuroleptic and so-called neurodysleptic agent. Acta Neurol Psychiatr Belg 59(3):337–366

135. Williams T, Guicharnaud J, Arnaud M (2003) Soudain l'été dernier: suivi de Le train de l'aube ne s'arrête plus ici 10–18

136. Kesey K (2002) Vol au-dessus d'un nid de coucou: roman. Stock

137. Le Bau JW, Wollinetz E, Choppy M, Gaches J (1970) Position actuelle de la psychochirurgie. Cahiers Méd 11(4):289–298

138. Hitchcock ER, Laitinen L, Vaernet K (eds) (1970) Psychosurgery. In: Proceedings of International conference on psychosurgery. Springfield, Ill, Copenhagen, Denmark

139. Lipsman N, Meyerson BA, Lozano AM (2012) A narrative history of the international society for psychiatric surgery: 1970–1983. Stereotact Funct Neurosurg 90(6):347–355. doi:10.1159/000341082

140. Talairach J (2007) Souvenirs des études stéréotaxiques du cerveau humain: Une vie, une équipe, une méthodologie: L'Ecole de Sainte-Anne. John Libbey Eurotext

141. Leksell L (1951) The stereotaxic method and radiosurgery of the brain. Acta Chirurgica Scandinavica 102:316–319
142. Meyerson BA, Linderoth B (2009) History of stereotactic neurosurgery in the Nordic countries. In: Lozano A (ed) Textbook of stereotactic and functional neurosurgery, 2nd edn. Springer, New York
143. Leksell L, Backlund EO (1978) Strålkirurgisk kapsulotomi—en oblodig operationsmetod för psykiatrisk kirurgi Radiosurgical capsulotomy—a closed surgical method for psychiatric surgery). Läkartidningen 75:546–547
144. Hariz MB P, Zrinzo L (2010) Deep brain stimulation between 1947 and 1987: the untold story. Neurosurg Focus 29(2):E1
145. Baumeister AA (2000) The tulane electrical brain stimulation program a historical case study in medical ethics. J Hist Neurosci 9(3):262–278. doi:10.1076/jhin.9.3.262.1787
146. Heath RB (1954) Studies in Schizophrenia (The initial report of findings in 26 patients prepared with depth electrodes was made in 1952 at a meeting in New Orleans, Louisiana). Harvard University Press, Cambridge
147. Butler M (2008) History of the therapeutic use of electricity on the brain and the development of deep brain stimulation. In: Tarsy D (ed) Deep brain stimulation in neurological and psychiatric disorders, Humana Press, Totowa, p xv, p 601, [5] leaves of plates
148. Heath RG, Rouchell AM, Goethe JW (1981) Cerebellar stimulation in treating intractable behavior disorders. Curr Psychiatr Ther 20:329–336
149. Heath RG, Monroe RR, Mickle WA (1955) Stimulation of the amygdaloid nucleus in a schizophrenic patient. Am J Psychiatry 111(11):862–863
150. Heath RG (1972) Pleasure and brain activity in man. Deep and surface electroencephalograms during orgasm. J Nerv Ment Dis 154(1):3–18
151. Heath RG (1963) Electrical self-stimulation of the brain in man. Am J Psychiatry 120:571–577
152. Moan CH R (1972) Septal stimulation for the initiation of heterosexual behavior in a homosexual male. Exp Psychiatry 3(1):23–26
153. Breggin P (1972) Lobotomy—it's coming back. Liberation 17(7):15–6, 3–5
154. Breggin P (1972) Lobotomies are still bad medicine. Med Opin 8:32–36
155. Hariz M (2012) History of "Psychiatric" deep brain stimulation: a critical appraisal. In: Denys D, Feenstra M, Schuurman R (eds) Deep brain stimulation: a new frontier in psychiatry. Verlag, pp 289–294
156. Laitinen LV (1977) Neurosurgical treatment in psychiatry, pain, and epilepsy. Neurosurgical treatment in psychiatry, pain, and epilepsy. University Park Press, Baltimore
157. Delgado JM, Mark V, Sweet W, Ervin F, Weiss G, Bach YRG et al (1968) Intracerebral radio stimulation and recording in completely free patients. J Nerv Ment Dis 147(4):329–340
158. Osmundsen J (1965) Matador with a radio stops bull. New York Times 17(1965):1
159. Delgado JMR (1969) Physical control of the mind; toward a psychocivilized society. 1st edn. World perspectives, vol 41. Harper & Row, New York
160. Mark VHE, Frank R (1970) Violence and the brain, 1st edn. Medical Dept, New York
161. Aarons L (1972) Brain surgery is tested on three California convicts. Washington post, 25 Feb 1972, p 1
162. Shuman SI (1977) Psychosurgery and the medical control of violence: autonomy and deviance. Wayne State University Press, Detroit
163. Hochmann J (2011) Histoire de la psychiatrie, 2e édn. Mise à jour ed. Que sais-je?, vol 1428. Presses universitaires de France, Paris
164. Culliton BJ (1976) Psychosurgery: national commission issues surprisingly favorable report. Science 194(4262):299–301
165. (1977) United States. National commission for the protection of human subjects of biomedical and behavioral research. Psychosurgery: report and recommendations. DHEW publication no (OS) 77-0001. xviii, p 76

166. Valenstein ES (1980) The psychosurgery debate: scientific, legal, and ethical perspectives. A series of books in psychology. W.H. Freeman, San Francisco
167. Ballantine HT Jr, Bouckoms AJ, Thomas EK, Giriunas IE (1987) Treatment of psychiatric illness by stereotactic cingulotomy. Biol Psychiatry 22(7):807–819. doi:0006-3223(87) 90080-1 [pii]
168. Bridges PK (1987) Psychosurgery: historical interest only or contemporary relevance. Br J Hosp Med 37(4):283
169. Burzaco J (1981) Stereotactic surgery in the treatment of obsessive-compulsive neurosis. In: Elsevier (ed) Biological psychiatry. Elsevier, Amsterdam, pp 1103–1109
170. Cosyns P, Caemaert J, Haaijman W, van Veelen C, Gybels J, van Manen J et al (1994) Functional stereotactic neurosurgery for psychiatric disorders: an experience in Belgium and the Netherlands. Adv Tech Stand Neurosurg 21:239–279
171. Hay PJ, Sachdev PS (1992) The present status of psychosurgery in Australia and New Zealand. Med J Aust 157(1):17–19
172. Mindus P, Rasmussen SA, Lindquist C (1994) Neurosurgical treatment for refractory obsessive-compulsive disorder: implications for understanding frontal lobe function. J Neuropsychiatry Clin Neurosci 6(4):467–477
173. Polosan MM, Millet B, Bougerol T, Olié J-P, Devaux B (2003) Traitement psychochirurgical des TOC malins: à propos de trois cas. L'Encéphale. XXIX(Cahier 1):514–552
174. Philippon J (1988) La Neurochirurgie. Que sais-je?, vol 1369. Presses universitaires de France, Paris
175. Benabid AL, Pollak P, Louveau A, Henry S, de Rougemont J (1987) Combined (thalamotomy and stimulation) stereotactic surgery of the VIM thalamic nucleus for bilateral Parkinson disease. Appl Neurophysiol 50(1–6):344–346
176. Benabid AL, Pollak P, Gervason C, Hoffmann D, Gao DM, Hommel M et al (1991) Long-term suppression of tremor by chronic stimulation of the ventral intermediate thalamic nucleus. Lancet 337(8738):403–406. doi:0140-6736(91)91175-T [pii]
177. Benabid AL, Pollak P, Seigneuret E, Hoffmann D, Gay E, Perret J (1993) Chronic VIM thalamic stimulation in Parkinson's disease, essential tremor and extra-pyramidal dyskinesias. Acta Neurochir Suppl (Wien) 58:39–44
178. Coubes P, Roubertie A, Vayssiere N, Hemm S, Echenne B (2000) Treatment of DYT1-generalised dystonia by stimulation of the internal globus pallidus. Lancet 355(9222):2220–2221. doi:S0140-6736(00)02410-7 (pii:10.1016/S0140-6736(00)02410-7)
179. Nuttin B, Cosyns P, Demeulemeester H, Gybels J, Meyerson B (1999) Electrical stimulation in anterior limbs of internal capsules in patients with obsessive-compulsive disorder. Lancet 354(9189):1526. doi:S0140-6736(99)02376-4 (pii:10.1016/S0140-6736(99)02376-4)
180. Vandewalle V, van der Linden C, Groenewegen HJ, Caemaert J (1999) Stereotactic treatment of Gilles de la Tourette syndrome by high frequency stimulation of thalamus. Lancet 353(9154):724. doi:S0140673698059649 [pii]
181. Asenjo A (1963) Neurosurgical techniques. Thomas
182. Smith JS, Kiloh LG (1977) Psychosurgery and society: symposium organised by the Neuropsychiatric Institute, Sydney, Pergamon, Oxford, 26–27 Sep 1974
183. Fiamberti M (1950) Transorbital prefrontal leucotomy in psychosurgery. Minerva Med 41(36):131–135
184. Knight GC (1969) Bi-frontal stereotactic tractotomy: an atraumatic operation of value in the treatment of intractable psychoneurosis. Br J Psychiatry 115(520):257–266
185. Kelly D, Richardson A, Mitchell-Heggs N, Greenup J, Chen C, Hafner RJ (1973) Stereotactic limbic leucotomy: a preliminary report on forty patients. Br J Psychiatry 123(573):141–148
186. Harden CL, Pulver MC, Ravdin LD, Nikolov B, Halper JP, Labar DR (2000) A pilot study of mood in epilepsy patients treated with vagus nerve stimulation. Epilepsy Behav 1(2):93–99. doi:S1525-5050(00)90046-5 (pii:10.1006/ebeh.2000.0046)

187. Rush AJ, George MS, Sackeim HA, Marangell LB, Husain MM, Giller C et al (2000) Vagus nerve stimulation (VNS) for treatment-resistant depressions: a multicenter study. Biol Psychiatry 47(4):276–286. doi:S0006-3223(99)00304-2 [pii]

188. France Comité consultatif national d'éthique pour les sciences de la vie et de la santé (2005) Avis sur la neurochirurgie fonctionnelle d'affections psychiatriques sévères. Ethique et recherche biomédicale Rapport 2002. la Documentation française, Paris

189. Mayberg HS, Lozano AM, Voon V, McNeely HE, Seminowicz D, Hamani C et al (2005) Deep brain stimulation for treatment-resistant depression. Neuron 45(5):651–660. doi:S0896-6273(05)00156-X (pii:10.1016/j.neuron.2005.02.014)

190. Kuhn J, Lenartz D, Huff W, Lee S, Koulousakis A, Klosterkoetter J et al (2007) Remission of alcohol dependency following deep brain stimulation of the nucleus accumbens: valuable therapeutic implications? J Neurol Neurosurg Psychiatry 78(10):1152–1153. doi:78/10/1152 (pii:10.1136/jnnp.2006.113092)

191. Hamani C, McAndrews MP, Cohn M, Oh M, Zumsteg D, Shapiro CM et al (2008) Memory enhancement induced by hypothalamic/fornix deep brain stimulation. Ann Neurol 63(1):119–123. doi:10.1002/ana.21295

192. Nahas Z, Anderson BS, Borckardt J, Arana AB, George MS, Reeves ST et al (2010) Bilateral epidural prefrontal cortical stimulation for treatment-resistant depression. Biol Psychiatry 67(2):101–109. doi:S0006-3223(09)01020-8 (pii:10.1016/j.biopsych.2009.08.021)

Chapter 2
The Neuroanatomy of Emotions

Abstract Common to many mammalians, the limbic system is a set of anatomical structures involved in emotions. Theorized in the last century by Papez and Mc Lean, this system includes the prefrontal cortex—where emotions access consciousness—as well as the hippocampus, amygdala, and hypothalamus. The hypothalamus and its extension, the pituitary gland, causes the visceral manifestations associated with these emotions. These emotional manifestations can be triggered by consciousness, but inversely, physical states can be made conscious thanks in part to the insula. The regulation of these emotional responses is also accomplished by subcortical structures: the basal ganglia. These nuclei—composed of the thalamus, striatum, globus pallidus as well as the subthalamic and accumbens nuclei—are linked to the cortex by loop circuits. These loops act as interfaces between the different components—emotional, cognitive, and motor—of our behavior.

> Man should know that joy, fun, laughter and entertainment, grief, sorrow and tears of discouragement can only come from the brain [...]. This is because the same body as you can go crazy and insane and that the fear and anxiety attack us. All this happens when the brain is sick. I believe that the brain has the greatest power of man.

> *The Sacred Disease, Hippocrates,* 460–377 *av* [1].

In this excerpt, the father of medicine postulates that the ills of the mind are also those of the brain. Sigmund Freud was convinced that some of his psychoanalytical concepts would later be proven by advances in biology and anatomy: "we must remember that all our provisional ideas in psychology will probably 1 day be based on an organic infrastructure" [2]. Eight years later, in 1920, the Austrian neurologist added that: *the shortcomings of our description probably would fade if we could already establish physiological or chemical terms instead of psychological terms* [2]. Yet, rather than working side-by-side, psychoanalysis and neurobiology have often been at odds due to differing logics. Understanding psychiatry, and presumably psychosurgery, requires a detour through neuroanatomy including the neuroanatomy of emotions. But emotions have long been neglected by anatomists, probably in part because they lend themselves less easily to animal research.

M. Lévêque, *Psychosurgery*, DOI: 10.1007/978-3-319-01144-8_2,   49
© Springer International Publishing Switzerland 2014

As Cabanis succinctly expressed, the brain *secretes thought as the liver secretes bile* [3]. The philosopher and physiologist might have added that the brain colors thoughts with emotions just as bilirubin gives bile its yellowish hue. This emotional component opens us to the joys and tragedies of life, but it is also involved— much more than we think—in our cognitive processes and decision-making.[1] Over the past 60 years, thanks notably to the results of psychosurgery, the development of functional neuroimaging[2] and advances in neurobiology, more has become known about the anatomical structures involved in emotional processes. These structures are regrouped in the *limbic system*, a term coined by the neurologist Paul Broca, from the latin *limbus* meaning "border," to designate the area surrounding the cerebral cortex [4]. Broca attributed our animalistic behavior to this entity, *the great limbic lobe*, as opposed to our nobler intellectual abilities, which seemed to arise in the cortex. The notion of a brain structure devoted to emotions, a limbic system, was most actively put forward in the late 1930s by Papez, and Mac Lean [5, 6]. To the cingulate cortex[3] and hippocampus[4] of the limbic lobe, they added the amygdala[5] and hypothalamus.[6] The prefrontal cortex,[7] central gray nuclei[8] and insula[9] later also joined the machinery of emotions, adding to an increasingly improbable list where *everything is connected to everything,* as neuroanatomists are fond of saying [7]. Our emotional manifestations, whether behavioral, autonomic, or cognitive, are thus supported by a diffuse system which itself interfaces with a great number of other brain functions, such as motor skills,

---

[1] Concepts developed in the work of António Damásio, Californian neurologist, in particular in his book "Descartes' Error: Emotion, Reason and the Human Brain" Odile Jacob, Paris.

[2] For about 30 years new noninvasive technologies have given the possibility of an increasingly detailed mapping of the brain's activity. Thanks to these maps, we have "emotional activation" models, which show activity in brain structures related to different emotions. This is accomplished by external induction (exposing the subject to a stimulus triggering an emotion, like giggling or shocking images) or by internal induction (a depressed patient or a subject suffering painful memories). New imaging technologies include:

- TEP-scan, which uses positron emission. After injection of radioactive glucose, which becomes metabolized by certain brain areas, sensors can identify the activated areas in the subject's brain. The resolution of these images remains relatively coarse.
- Functional MRI (fMRI) is a type of imaging by magnetic resonance that allows visualization of the brain's blood flow in precise areas. The BOLD effect (Blood Oxygen Level Dependant), related to the magnetization of the haemoglobin in red blood cells, reveals which brain areas are being activated.
- Magnetoencephalography (MEG)

[3] Cf. p. 95.

[4] Cf. p. 103.

[5] Cf. p. 98.

[6] Cf. p. 112.

[7] Cf. p. 90.

[8] Cf. p. 122.

[9] Cf. p. 107.

cognition, or the senses. These latter functions will not be addressed herein. We will limit ourselves to detailing the pathways and structures relevant to psychosurgery.

The Organs of Emotion

Let us set the scene: the brain includes the cerebrum, the cerebellum, and brain-stem. All three are contained in the skull and entirely enveloped by meninges. The meninges cover all the nerve tissue and are composed from outside to inside by the dura mater, the arachnoid mater, and the pia mater. In between these last two structures, blood vessels and cerebrospinal fluid (CSF) circulate. This fluid also flows into the brain through four cavities called ventricles. The cerebrum is composed of two hemispheres whose surfaces form the cortex and whose interiors, broadly speaking, form the thalami, basal ganglia, and the hypothalamic-pituitary axis.

The Cerebral Cortex

Abstract The cerebral cortex is the substrate in which consciousness as well as memory, language, and our perceptions take root. Of these two square meters of gray matter folded up against the walls of our skull, three lobes are heavily involved in emotions: the frontal, temporal, and insular lobes. The front of the frontal lobe, the dorsolateral cortex, is involved in the planning of behavior while the orbitofrontal cortex, closer to the middle, is involved in motivation. In the interior, the anterior cingulate cortex is involved in emotional processes. These three regions are each connected to basal ganglia, forming cognitive, and limbic loops. This prefrontal cortex, responsible for a large part of our cognitive processes—and abundantly connected to the rest of the limbic system—is part of the interface between cognition and emotion. The interior face of the temporal lobe shelters the hippocampus and the amygdala. The latter is where information from our senses converges. Depending on the situation, the amygdala will lend this sensory input an innate or acquired charge, such as fear, which the hypothalamus will then convert into autonomic manifestations. Researchers now believe the hippocampus plays a less essential role in emotions but that it is critical to memory. The insula, in turn, is used to analyze changes in our visceral states associated with emotional experience allowing us to consciously perceive this physical state.

The cerebral cortex—meaning "bark" in Latin—is a mantle of gray matter. This gray matter, famously synonymous with intelligence is composed of nerve cells

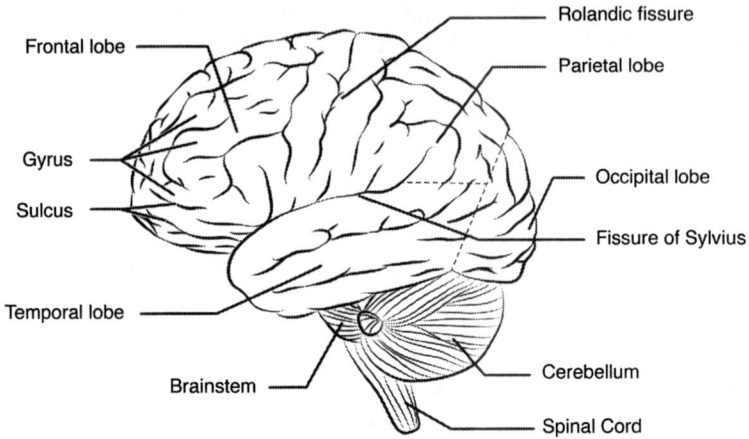

Fig. 2.1 Side view of the brain

called neurons. These cells have a projection, the axon, which allows them to connect to each other and form a network. The folds in the cortex, which greatly increase its surface area, are formed of *gyri*, (Latin *ridges*, sg. *Gyrus)*, surrounded by *sulc*i, (Latin: "furrows", sg. *sulcus*). The deeper furrows which delineate the lobes are called fissures. In general, these fissures vary little from one individual to another. For example, the central, or Rolando's, separates between the frontal lobe, in front and the parietal lobe, in back. The lateral, or Sylvian fissure, divides the temporal lobe (Fig. 2.1).

At the bottom of this fissure is buried the smallest of the lobes, the insula, meaning "island" in Latin (Fig. 2.9, p. 64). The fifth lobe, the occipital lobe, located behind the temporal and parietal lobes, is less clearly demarcated. Within each of these lobes, specific areas called functional areas are devoted to specific functions. Lesioning or destruction of any given area from trauma, tumoral compression, or ischemia causes alteration or loss of that function. In fact, such lesions are what allowed brain functions to be mapped over the centuries. In the early 1950s, researchers, including Montreal neurosurgeon William Penfield, performed experiments on conscious patients in which electrical stimulation of the cerebral cortex triggered certain movements or behaviors and epileptic episodes. These experiments helped further refine the connections between certain functions and areas. They followed on work undertaken half a century earlier by the German neurologist Korbinian Brodmann who had compiled a meticulous survey of these functional areas and assigned each a number. His system is still used today: the numbered Brodmann areas. Now that the stage has been set, we will hereafter emphasize those anatomical structures directly relevant to our subject because of their essential role in emotional processes: the frontal and temporal lobes.

The Frontal Lobe

In 1861, Paul Broca, a neurologist at the Salpêtrière Hospital in Paris, was the first to show through clinical observations combined with subsequent autopsies the important role of the lower, posterior part of the left frontal lobe in articulated language in Genuinely right-handed subjects. This region, areas 44 and 45, according to Brodmann's classification, was named, *Broca's area*. The most posterior part of the lobe, located directly ahead of the central or Sylvian fissure, is the primary motor cortex (area 4). In front of this is the pre-motor area (area 6), which helps plan movements, and ahead of it is area 8, which is responsible for eye movements. The voluminous area in front of the motor region representing almost one-third of the cortical mass is called the *prefrontal cortex*. It is intimately linked with cognitive and emotional processes. Connected to many parts of the brain, the prefrontal cortex receives sensory information already processed in the so-called *associative* regions of the occipital temporal or parietal cortex. Visual information, an image captured by the retina, for example, is transmitted along the primary visual pathway to the occipital cortex, which receives it in "raw" form. The occipital associative cortex is where the various elements composing this "visual stream" transmitted by the primary cortex are recognized and labeled. The same occurs for auditory information in the temporal associative cortex, which among other things, converts sounds into words. The parietal associative cortex, meanwhile, is involved in interpreting tactile information. In addition to being connected to these associative areas, the prefrontal cortex is tightly linked to the rest of the limbic system: the hippocampus, amygdala, hypothalamus, and thalamus especially the dorsal medial nucleus of the thalamus (Fig. 2.2).

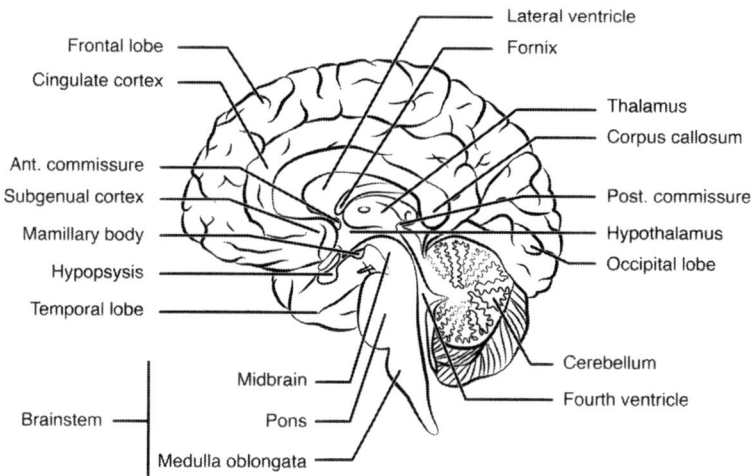

Fig. 2.2 Medial view of the brain

Additionally, there are projections leading toward the basal ganglia and in particular the striatum. These projections are actually part of loops, since once projected onto the striatum and then the pallidum, the information is sent onto the thalamus and from there back to its starting point, the prefrontal cortex. Before discussing,[10] the various cortico-striato-thalamo-cortical (CSCT) loops involved in cognitive functions and the regulation of emotions, the three regions which form the prefrontal cortex must be described: the dorsolateral, orbitofrontal, and cingulate cortices.

The Dorsolateral Cortex

The dorsolateral region of the prefrontal cortex (areas 9, 10 lateral and 46) (Fig. 2.3) is intimately linked to the rest of the prefrontal cortex and to the dorsomedial and ventral anterior nuclei of the thalamus.[11] It extends over the dorsolateral region of the caudate nucleus[12] and is implicated in the *associative*[13] loop (Fig. 2.27, p. 89) [8]. This cortex is involved in tasks requiring spatial memory, concentration, planning, problem solving and the acquisition of rules [9]. In their clinical practice, neuropsychologists call these the *executive functions"* [10]. In a way, they are also what philosophers have referred to as consciousness. As Bergson writes, *consciousness is anticipation of the future… a hyphen between what was and will be"* [11]. Selective lesions of this region cause changes in the executive functions, and inversely, functional imaging reveals activity in this cortex during tasks involving planning. This zone is also active when an individual is attempting to control certain negative emotions. In patients with severe depression, functional imaging studies show little activity in this cortex. Clinically, this translates to psychomotor retardation, including memory and attention disorders and apathy. On the contrary, an increase in activity can be observed in successfully treated patients [12, 13]. In depressive subjects, this dorsolateral cortex seems more active on the right than on the left [14, 15]. Today, repetitive transcranial magnetic stimulation (rTMS)[14] can be used to treat certain depressive patients who do not respond to drug-based treatments. Two protocols exist: either the left dorsolateral cortex can be "woken up" through high frequency rTMS or the right dorsolateral cortex can be inhibited through low-frequency rTMS. Clinical research protocols are currently attempting to determine whether the effect can be sustained over the long term through the implanting of cortical electrodes to maintain stimulation.[15] When a clinical improvement is achieved,

---

[10] Cf. p. 139.

[11] Cf. p. 123.

[12] Cf. p. 128.

[13] Cf. p. 141.

[14] Cf. Indications and principle of the rTMS p. 232.

[15] Cf. Indication and principle of the cortical stimulation p. 236.

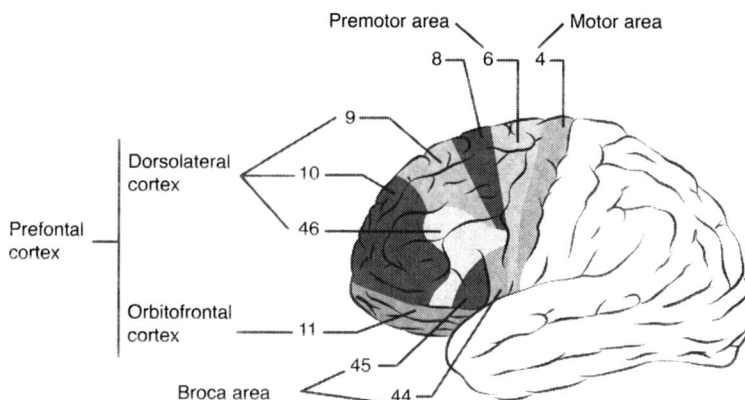

Fig. 2.3 The dorso-lateral prefrontal cortex

functional imaging shows a normalizing of the activity in this region as well as in the related anterior and subgenual cingulate cortex [16, 17].

The Orbitofrontal Cortex

This part of the brain, Brodmann areas 10 medial, 11, 12, and 47, (Fig. 2.4) is located against the skull and above the orbits. Like the dorsolateral cortex, the orbitofrontal cortex is tightly connected to the cingulate cortex, as well as the rest of the associative cortex, the amygdala, and the dorsomedial and ventral anterior nuclei of the thalamus [18]. This cortex projects onto the ventromedial part of the caudate nucleus [8] which is involved in the associative loop[16] and has the particularity of receiving information from all of our five senses [19]. This region and in particular its innermost *medial* part, is implicated in emotional and motivational processes, particularly those involving the notion of reward [20, 21]. Its role, as emphasized by the psychiatrist B. Aouizerate [22], is essential "*in the interpretation of sensory information from the environment by giving it meaning on an emotional and motivational level according the subject's previous experiences,*" which will affect the decision-making process [21]. The lateral part of the cortex is involved in *cognitive*, tasks, mental processes requiring judgment, perseverance or the detection of errors [18]. The orbitofrontal cortex also regulates social behavior as the previously mentioned case of *Phineas Gage*[17] illustrated. Following an accident in which Gage suffered trauma to this part of the brain, he became antisocial, irresponsible, impulsive, and childish [23]. In general, focused lesions in this cortex inhibit the subject's ability to select an appropriate behavioral response based on

---

[16] Cf. p. 142.

[17] Cf. p. 25.

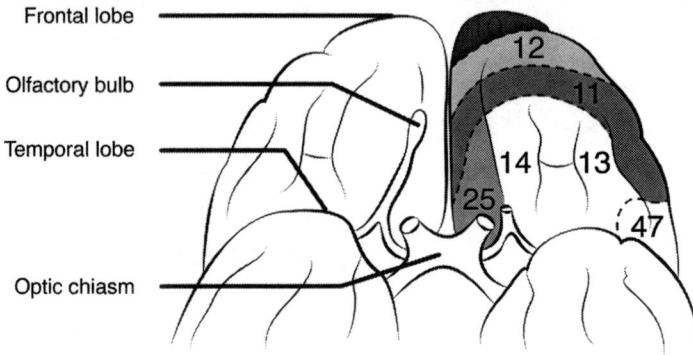

Fig. 2.4 The orbitofrontal (10, 11, and 12) and subgenual (25) cortices

social or emotional cues. Functional imaging reveals increased activity of this region of the cortex [12] in patients suffering from depression or OCD. Here too, normalization has been observed following effective treatment [12, 24–26].

The Anterior Cingulate Cortex

The cingulate gyrus, from *cingulum* meaning "belt" in Latin, wraps around the corpus callosum[18] in the medial part of both hemispheres (Fig. 2.4). As with the orbitofrontal cortex, this cortical area is involved in various motivational, emotional, or cognitive processes, such as attention, working memory, error detection [27], managing conflict situations, and anticipation. The cingulate cortex, particularly its anterior part (areas 24, 32, and 25) (Fig. 2.5), is closely linked to the insula,[19] another structure involved in emotions. According to Damasio, when we experience emotions, "the insula has both a sensorial and motor function though it is focused more on the sensorial aspect of the process, while the anterior cingulate operates as the motor structure" [28]. The anterior cingulate cortex (ACC) is reciprocally linked to the dorsomedial nucleus of the thalamus. The anterior part of the gyrus projects its fibers toward the amygdala, which it holds in check, toward the peri-acqueducale gray matter[20] as well as toward the ventral striatum and nucleus accumbens,[21] thus participating in a *limbic loop*[22] (Fig. 2.28, p. 91) [8].

---

[18] The corpus callosum is a bundle of axons that connect both cerebral hemispheres. It assures the transfer of information between both hemispheres and their coordination (Fig. 2.2, p. 53).

[19] Cf. p. 107.

[20] The periaqueductal gray matter is situated in the midbrain's center around the Sylvius acqueduct connecting the third and the fourth ventricles. This gray substance plays an important role in pain control and defensive behaviors.

[21] Cf. p. 129.

[22] Cf. functional anatomy p. 143.

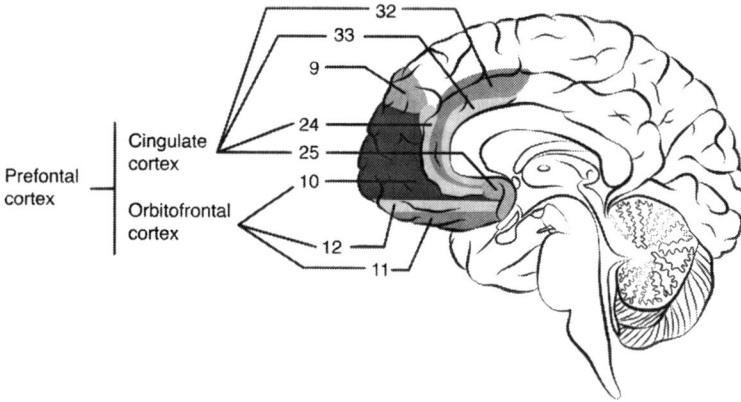

Fig. 2.5 The anterior cingulate and orbitofrontal cortices

These projections are involved in emotional and autonomic responses. Functional imaging reveals increased activity of the cingulate cortex in patients with OCD [12], particularly when these patients undertake tasks in which they must detect errors [22, 27]. A similar hyperactivity has also been noted in its most rostral part, the subgenual area (area 25), in patients with severe depression [29]. As will be discussed in a later section,[23] this finding is what originally led to deep brain stimulation being used during treatment of depressed patients. Significantly, this activity decreases when the depression is successfully treated. Moreover, the presence of such lively activity in the cingulate is a good indicator for the success of a cingulotomy,[24] another psychosurgical procedure used in the treatment of depression and OCD [30].

The Temporal Lobe

Abstract On its inner surface, the temporal lobe is in contact with the hippocampus and the amygdala. All sensory information from the various senses converges on the latter, and depending on the context the amygdala gives it emotional significance—innate or acquired—causing an autonomic response. It is involved in processing the social signals for emotions, especially fear, and the consolidation of emotional memories. By identifying hazards, it plays a fundamental role in preserving the individual. The hippocampus, located further back, places the event back into context and determines the conditions for forming a memory.

---

[23] Cf. p. 334.

[24] Cf. Technique's details p. 285.

The prefrontal cortex then participates in the analysis of these emotional events contrasting the present experience with past ones in order to reach a decision.

This lobe is located underneath the temporal bone, so named because the hairs on the *temples* are the first to suffer the ravages of time (Or in Latin *tempus*) and become gray. The temporal lobe, especially its inner region composed of the amygdala and hippocampus is also involved in many cognitive and emotional processes. In 1937, two American researchers, Klüver and Bucy, observed that primates that underwent bilateral removal of the inner portion of the temporal lobes suffered what they called *psychic blindness*: inability to grasp the emotional significance of sensory information, in particular visual information [31]. The monkeys no longer feared snakes or people and tried to mate with anyone within reach. This lack of discernment was also reflected on an oral level as the animals would try to put everything in their mouths. In addition to these sexual and feeding behaviors, the authors also observed significantly increased docility and placidity, resulting in a marked reduction in the subjects' social interactions [32].

The Amygdala

In 1956, new research on monkeys demonstrated that bilateral ablation centered, more exclusively this time, on the amygdala was enough to cause most of these symptoms [33]. Buried under the cortex, in the medial, anterior part of each temporal lobe, the amygdala takes its name from its almond shape (Fig. 2.6).

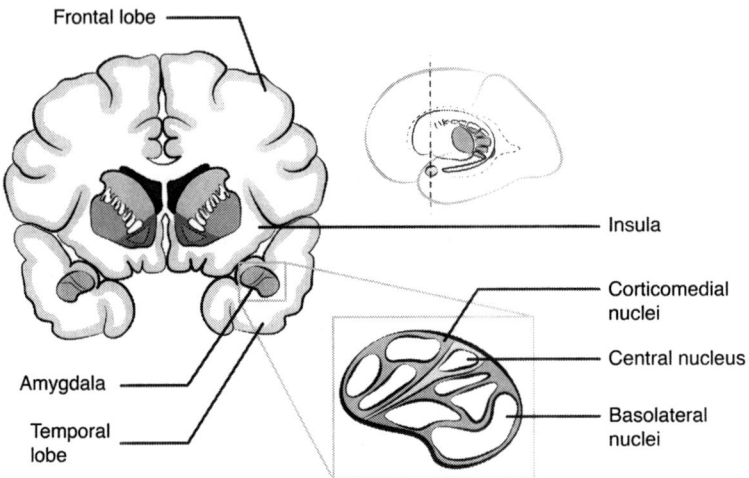

Fig. 2.6 The amygdala

Emotional processes all pass through, some may even arise in, the amygdala, which acts as a relay along numerous pathways. It receives information directly— or via the thalamus—from the associative cortical areas, the medial orbitofrontal cortex, the hippocampus, the basal ganglia, and septal nuclei (Fig. 2.7). After processing this information, the amygdala projects it—via the stria terminalis[25]— toward the hypothalamus[26] and other structures in the brainstem such as the locus coeruleus,[27] which is the source of autonomic and hormonal manifestations of certain emotions. As the neurologist Gil notes, "the amygdala is where the emotional component of the information conveyed by the sensory and sense pathways is integrated, and in conjunction with memory, where meaning is identified and biological and behavioral responses are modulated" [34]. The amygdaloid complex, through its connections, is composed of three nuclei groups. The corticomedial nuclei receive information from the olfactory bulb and project toward the hypothalamus. The basolateral nuclei, receive information from the associative

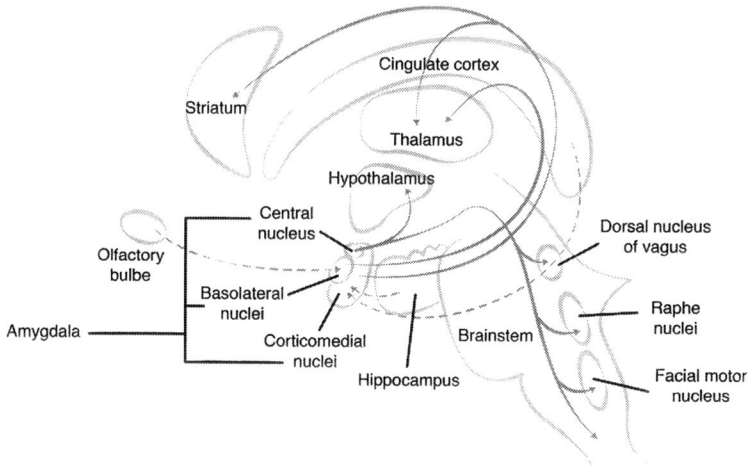

Fig. 2.7 The connections of the amygdala nuclei

---

[25] The stria terminalis runs in a trajectory parallel to fornix's from the amygdala to the hypothalamus, the septal area and passes over the "bed nucleus of the stris terminalis," a group of neurons directly behind the anterior commissure. This bundle of neurons is usually considered an extension of the amygdala, and more precisely of its central nucleus, for histological reasons and because of its multiple connections with the hypothalamus, the brainstem nuclei and in particular the ventral tegmental area (VTA). Its activity also seems modulated by the orbifrontal cortex. This structure has attracted the attention of an increasing number of researchers. It occupies a strategic anatomical position which enables regulation of the stress and reward centers.

This nucleus actually projects to one of the major reward centers (the VTA) and to the hypothalamic paraventricular nucleus (p. 112), which is essential to the activation of the corticotropic axis (p. 146).

[26] Cf. p. 112.

[27] Cf. Norepinephrin and the stress circuit p. 150.

sensory cortex and hippocampus and project toward the ventral striatum ventral, accumbens nucleus, and the dorsal medial nucleus of the thalamus.[28] Finally, the central nucleus, which is connected to the associative sensory areas through its links with the basolateral and cortico medial nuclei, receives information on the visual, auditory, tactile, and olfactory environment of the individual [35]. This nucleus sends information onto the hypothalamus and brainstem where the dorsal nucleus of the vagus nerve[29]—the source of parasympathetic responses—is located. From there information travels to the motor nuclei of the facial muscles—responsible for facial expression of emotions—the raphe nuclei,[30] the locus cœruleus[31] and nucleus basalis of Meynert.[32] These last three anatomical structures are, respectively, the source of serotoninergic,[33] noradrenergic[34] and cholinergic responses, three neurotransmitters at the heart of emotional processes. At the level of the unconscious, the amygdala sorts this information in terms of the danger it may pose the individual. Its role is therefore crucial in the phenomena of fear and anxiety.[35]

The amygdala contributes to emotional experience—positive or negative— according to the situations and the environment. The sensory and associative *cortex* and the *olfactory bulb* inform the *basolateral complex* and the *cortical* and *medial nuclei* about the environment, related to the memory (*hippocampus*). This information is integrated and transmitted to the *central nucleus* which will produce an emotional response: the *facial motor nucleus* will provoke fear or disgust, the *dorsal nucleus of the vagus nerve* and the hypothalamus will provoke respectively a parasympatic or sympatic response. The *raphe nucleus* will activate a serotonergic stimulation of the encephalus. The basolateral nuclei take action in motivational behaviour through the *ventral striatum* and the orbifrontal cortex.

This implicit, subcortical processing of information, "I act and then I think" lowers the response time necessary for protective behavior by eliminating the need for the information to pass through the cortex [36]. If sensory data conveys a threat, real or imagined, then the connections between the central nucleus of the amygdala and the hypothalamus and brainstem are activated and the individual responds with a series of autonomic reactions: quickening of the pulse, dilation of the pupils, draining of color from the face, and various hormonal responses. These phenomena prime the body for a *fight or flight*, response, according to physiologist Cannon [37].

---

[28] Cf. p. 124.

[29] Details of the vagus nerve and its electrical stimulation in depression treatment. Cf. p. 241.

[30] Serotonin producing nucleus cf. p. 149.

[31] Ibid.

[32] In 2008, after a electrode trajectory error, an Italian team recorded the appearance of depression in a dystonia patient following stimulation of this area. This depressive state disappeared after repositioning of the electrode [214].

[33] Cf. p. 149.

[34] Ibid.

[35] Drugs in the benzodiazepine family, like Diazepam(r)®, decrease fear and anxiety responses because the amygdala is rich in receptors for this type of molecule. Efficacy is maintained even after removal of the amygdalae because similar receptors are located in other areas as well.

For example, the sudden appearance of a snake will trigger a biological response putting the organism on high alert and "doping it" in order for it to face the danger or make an escape. The amygdala therefore appears crucial to the preservation of the organism by allowing organisms to identify danger.[36] The detection of danger also occurs more subtly when, for example, an individual reads an expression of fear on someone else's face.[37] Direct electrical stimulation of the amygdala—or seizures, which can be likened to the cortex stimulating itself—produces reactions similar to those displayed when faced with danger. Additionally, these events are often associated with aggressiveness or a feeling of *déjà vu*. In contrast, pathological or surgical destruction of this structure, in addition to inhibiting the expression of fear and the recognition of fear on others' faces, reduces aggressive behavior [38, 39]. Acts of violence or aggression may, therefore, be linked to an imbalance caused by improper prefrontal modulation and amygdala hyperactivity [40]. To test this hypothesis, in the 1960s Narabayashi performed bilateral amygdalotomies in 60 patients with severe aggressive behavior [41, 42]. The Japanese neurosurgeon reported significant improvement in 85 % of the patients. These results are similar to those achieved with hypothalamotomies, another procedure with the same indication, which we will return to later.[38] These two techniques which were practiced until the late 1980s [43–48], have now almost completely disappeared. This decline stemmed from inadequate long-term monitoring, advances in pharmacology and, especially, ethical questions raised by such interventions [49].

More generally, the amygdala contributes to the interpretation of all sensory information with emotional content [50]. Studies in patients with lesions in the amygdala have also shown that this structure [51] intervenes both during the encoding of memories with emotional valence—positive or negative—as well as during recall[39] [52]. The amygdala is also involved (through reciprocal connections between its basolateral nuclei and the nucleus accumbens) when the reward circuit is solicited [53]. As such, it may be implicated in instances of relapse in cases of addiction[40] : the addict may be inclined to take the addictive substance once again when confronted with a situation previously associated with the substance [54].

---

[36] In laboratory tests, the conditioned fear model allowed the role of the amygdala to be understood: a rat is placed in a wire lattice and a signal warns it before each electrical discharge. After multiple sessions, the rat shows signs of anxiety (immobilization, blood pressure increase). These signs disappear after elimination of the amygdalae (LeDoux J. E. 1998. The emotional brain: the mysterious underpinnings of emotional life. Simon & Schuster).

[37] For many years Damásio studied a 28-year-old patient suffering from a bilateral lesion of the amygdalae who was not able to recognize facial expressions like fear, surprise, or disgust.

[38] Cf. p. 364.

[39] An American study of veterans with severe head injuries showed that soldiers with amygdala lesions almost never develop post-traumatic stress disorder (PTSD). In contrast, other victims with this psychiatric disorder showed amygdalar hyperactivity [215]. These observations and animal experimentation data lead certain teams to consider cerebral stimulation of the amygdala as treatment for severe PTSD [216].

[40] Cf. Physiopatholog des addictions p. 359.

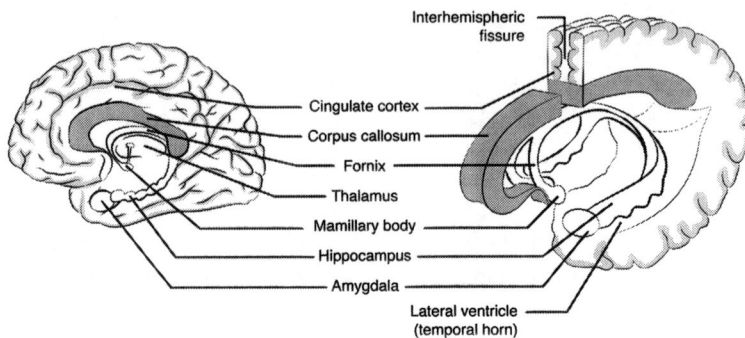

Fig. 2.8 The hippocampus and the hippocampal convolution

The Hippocampus

In behavior based on conditioning, the amygdala interacts closely with the hippocampus[41] a structure located just behind it (Fig. 2.8). Oblong in shape and presenting the appearance of a sea horse, from which it draws its name, this structure maintains close connections with the amygdala as well as with the rest of the associative cortex via the entorhinal cortex.[42] This region, which gathers the cortical information headed to the hippocampus, is also involved in spatial orientation [55]. The hippocampus extends back into the hippocampal gyrus and the fornix. The fibers of the fornix then rejoin the mammillary bodies.[43]

This set of structures plays a crucial role in the declarative memory formation process [56]. *Declarative* memory, refers to consciously accessible information which can be described through language: such as recollecting a history lesson, vocabulary skills (called *semantic* memory, from Greek *semantikos:* "meaning"), as well as remembering events in our life (called *episodic*). The hippocampus, which lies at the heart of the memory circuit (also called the *Papez circuit*[44]) acts as a repeater taking information quickly learned and passing it onto the rest of the cortical mantle, where long-term memory. Neurobiologist Vincent likens it to a mechanism for comparing *the state of the world to its emotional value. Nerve impulses travel around the hippocampal circuits rhythmically at a rate of* 50 *to* 100 *Hz.*

---

[41] To illustrate the complementarity of these structures Damásio gives the example of an individual without amygdalae but with his hippocampus intact who, although he remembered a traumatic event, did not show any fear when confronted with similar circumstances. In contrast, the neuroscientist presents another case of a patient without his hippocampus but with his amygdalae who experienced terror while not being able to remember the cause [217].

[42] This appears to be the first area affected by Alzheimer's disease.

[43] Cf. p. 112.

[44] Cf. Anatomic description of this circuit. p. 133.

This oscillating electrical activity plays an important part in the formation of memories; present during learning it reappears strongly during dreaming, incidentally showing the probable relationship between memory and dream [57]. Long-term memory storage occurs throughout the cortex. Semantic memory resides predominantly in the frontal and temporal cortex of the dominant hemisphere, while episodic memory utilizes more the frontal lobes[45] [58]. In addition to memorization, the hippocampus is also involved in the recall of stored memories. Recall can be initiated by the cortex in response to a cognitive process, but it can also be initiated directly in the olfactory pathway which is located very close to the hippocampus. *And as soon as I had recognized the taste of the piece of madeleine soaked in her decoction of lime-blossom which my aunt used to give me (although I did not yet know and must long postpone the discovery of why this memory made me so happy) immediately the old grey house upon the street,* [...] and with the house the town, from morning to night and in all weathers, the Square where I used to be sent before lunch, the streets along which I used to run errands, the country roads we took when it was fine."[46] The powerful effect that the madeleine has on Proust clearly demonstrates the anatomical vicinity of the olfactory cortex and the hippocampus, but it also shows the close ties binding emotions to memory.[47] It seems that the hippocampus, particularly its posterior part, is also fundamental to spatial orientation. London taxi drivers are often cited to illustrate this as well as the phenomenon of brain plasticity. Imaging studies have shown that in these drivers the hippocampus is more developed than in the population at large because it is constantly being solicited [59]. Deep brain stimulation in the entorhinal cortex, the gateway to the hippocampus, may also increase spatial memory[48] [60]. Using a video game simulating a taxi in a virtual city, a California team recently demonstrated that stimulation of the entorhinal region of seven epileptic patients as they were learning the various routes was associated with improved recall. This is similar to work accomplished by Lozano, and his team on the stimulation of the fornix.[49] This type of research paves the way for neuroprostheses to treat memory decline observed in some neurodegenerative diseases such as Alzheimer's disease, which affects nearly 40 million people worldwide [61, 62].

---

[45] To this conscious declarative memory at the cortex's surface is opposed the unconscious procedural memory of our abilities (like ridding a bicycle or playing piano) arising in structures like the basal ganglia or the cerebellum. Nonetheless, the connection between both systems and hence the passage from one memory form to the other remains permeable.

[46] Cf. Proust [218].

[47] Cf. Emotional memory p. 135.

[48] A team from Marseille, led by F. Bartholomei and P. Chauvel, observed in 2004 that electrical stimulation of the endonasal cortex provoked "déjà vu," i.e., the feeling of having already experienced something being experienced for the first time. In fact, stimulation of this cortex forces a process of recall in the hippocampus or the rhinencephalon (which also participates in memory encoding). Electrical stimulation or even epileptic seizures can provoke a simultaneous processes of encoding and recall giving the subject the impression of reliving a scene that is being experienced for the first time [219].

[49] Cf. p. 200: plasticity and neurogenesis resulting from DBS.

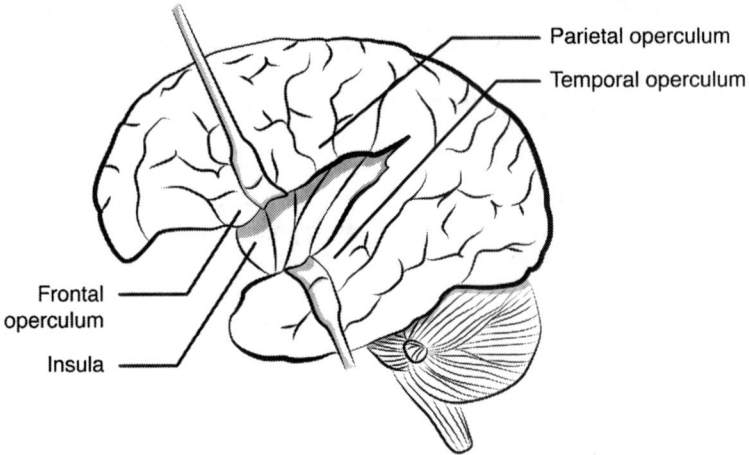

Fig. 2.9 Frontal and temporal lobes are drawn aside showing the insula

The Insula

The edges of the lateral furrow hide a deep depression in the folds of the cortex which contains a triangular lobe (Fig. 2.9). The insular cortex has five small circonvolutions. The cortex is involved in emotions and homeostatic regulation of the body. The anterior part of the insula receives projections directly from the central ventral thalamic nucleus and has reciprocal connections to the amygdala, while the posterior region connects to the associative somatosensory cortex and also receives thalamic afferents.[50]

The anterior portion, which is related to the senses of smell and taste, can trigger certain emotions such as disgust. This protective emotional reaction safeguards the individual against eating spoiled food which has become malodorous. Damasio goes further and considers that disgust—one of the oldest emotions to have evolved—triggered by the insula, may be relatively *developed and applicable to various situations in which the purity of objects or behaviors are compromised and where contamination exists.* [The subjects] *are disgusted by the perception of morally reprehensible actions..* The Californian neurologist adds that, *the insula is an important correlate of all conceivable types of feelings, those emotions associated with those corresponding to all forms pleasure or pain caused by a*

---

[50] The ventral, posterior, inferior, and ventromedial nuclei of the thalamus in particular.

variety of stimuli—hear music you love it or hate it; see images we love, including erotic, be short of drugs and feel lack[51] [63]. The American neurologist devised what is known as the *somatic markers*: hypothesis. According to this hypothesis, the insula maps visceral states associated with emotional experiences and assigns each situation a positive or negative physical response. This mapping allows the brain to very quickly choose between different action scenarios. According to Damasio, these mechanisms reduce the strain on our cognitive processes and allow them to focus on solving the problems for which they are best suited [28]. This assumption is part of a larger theory called *embodied cognition*,[52] which holds that conscious thought cannot be separated from emotions and their physical manifestations. In other words, the amygdala converts some sensory information into somatic responses by sending signals to the autonomic nervous system and endocrine system, which regulate heart rate, perspiration, and hormone secretion. The insula in turn detects these physiological changes and makes the individual conscious[53] of them. As the neuroscientists Ansermet and Magistretti [64] explain, the insula should be seen as a *interoceptive relay in the nervous system that continuously informs the brain on the state of the body. A first loop circuit is thus closed allowing the brain to perceive the somatic state associated with the perception of an external stimulus. The fact that the amygdala and insula are both connected to the prefrontal cortex, which is involved in certain types of memory, allows a second circuit, the memory loop, to be closed: an individual need only recall the source event of the stimulus to again feel the associated physical sensations.* Clinical observations clearly reinforce this theory. For example, the higher up along the spinal cord a lesion is located, the duller the patient's emotional awareness grows due to a lack of autonomic afferents (Fig. 2.10) [65].

---

[51] Functional imaging studies showed lobe activation in drug-addicted subjects (cocaine, alcohol, opiates, and nicotine) exposed to environmental factors associated with their drug habits. Recent work showed that cigarette smokers with lobe damage lose practically all desire to smoke. It also revealed that these individuals were 136 times more likely to lose their tobacco addiction than smokers affected in other areas of the brain [220].

[52] "Embodied cognition."

[53] In some ways, this concept stating that changes in somatic perception modify the conscious perception of an emotion agrees with the "peripheral" theory of James and Langes, two psychologists during the nineteenth century who considered that emotion was a response to physiologic changes (trembling, accelerated cardiac rhythm…). The example of the cobra is often cited to illustrate this theory: the vegetative manifestation unconsciously provoked by the sight of the reptile, not its presence, provokes the fear response. Critics of James and Langes' theory explain that physiologic reaction times are too slow to be the source of sudden emotions and that the range of physiologic manifestations is too limited to portray all emotions. Cannon and Bard formulate the opposite hypothesis. According to their theory, emotional experience is at the origin of physiologic excitation.

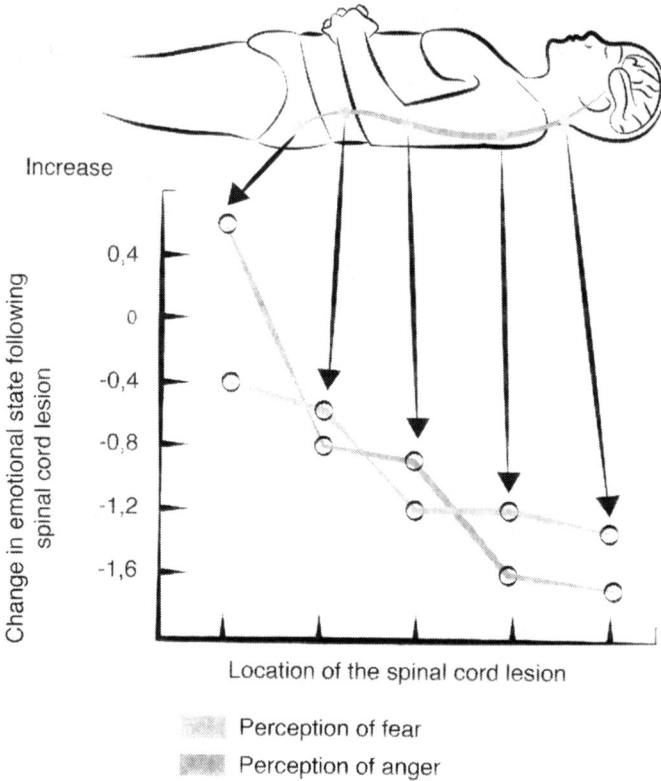

Fig. 2.10 Emotional experience of a person based on the degree of a medullary traumatism. The higher up along the spinal chord the lesion, the weaker the emotional experience, according to [68]

These data are confirmed by functional imaging, which reveals changes in prefrontal activity in these patients [66]. Some authors believe that this mechanism may come into play during the treatment of depression through stimulation of the vagus nerve.[54] By modifying the autonomic *return*, such stimulation may reduce the emotional component of the disease [67]. Indeed, we know that the afferences of this nerve, which terminate in the nucleus of the solitary tract in the brainstem before projecting toward the amygdala and insula, transmit somatic information (Fig. 3.23, p. 163).

The Parietal Lobe

The parietal lobe including areas 3, 1, and 2, which receive somatosensory inputs (touch, position of the muscles and joints, temperature), is located behind the

---

[54] Cf. Vagus nerve stimulation in depression treatment p. 241.

central sulcus. The upper portion of this lobe is also considered a heteromodal associative cortex and plays an important role in the integration of visual, tactile, and auditory (areas 5 and 7) information. This region is involved in spatial perception and motor coordination, also called praxis, but its role in managing emotions remains modest.

The Occipital Lobe

Located in the most posterior part of the brain, the occipital lobe contains the sensory areas for vision. Area 17 is the primary reception center, area 18 is devoted to perception, and area 19, the most peripheral, is devoted to interpretation. This lobe is not directly involved in emotions.

The Hypothalamic-Pituitary Axis and the Septal Area

Abstract The hypothalamus can be seen as an emotional transducer that converts the information received from the amygdala, the insula, the orbitofrontal cortex, and the rest of the limbic system into autonomic (quickening or slowing of heart rate, respiratory changes, digestive changes…) and endocrine responses. The pituitary gland, under the control of the hypothalamus, is involved in the endocrine response including the secretion of corticotropic hormones during stress phenomena.

The hypothalamic-pituitary axis and the neighboring septal area, both belong to the limbic system. The hypothalamic-pituitary axis is an essential region participating in a great number of functions. In particular, it helps maintain the balance—homeostasis of our internal environment by regulating thirst, hunger, body temperature, and sleep, thus ensuring our adaptation to the outside environment. The hypothalamus acts upon the organism through the *autonomic* nervous system, which is *independent* as well as via hormones. It is the pituitary gland, gland under the control of the hypothalamus, which is responsible for this humoral mediation.

The Hypothalamus

The hypothalamus is located at the base of the brain toward the front underneath the thalamus, from which it takes its name. This small 4 cm^3 structure weighing about the same number of grams is involved in many functions. The hypothalamus lines the anterior walls of the third ventricle and contains a dozen nuclei. For the sake of anatomical and functional clarity, we will describe this region from the center to the periphery and from front to back (Fig. 2.11).

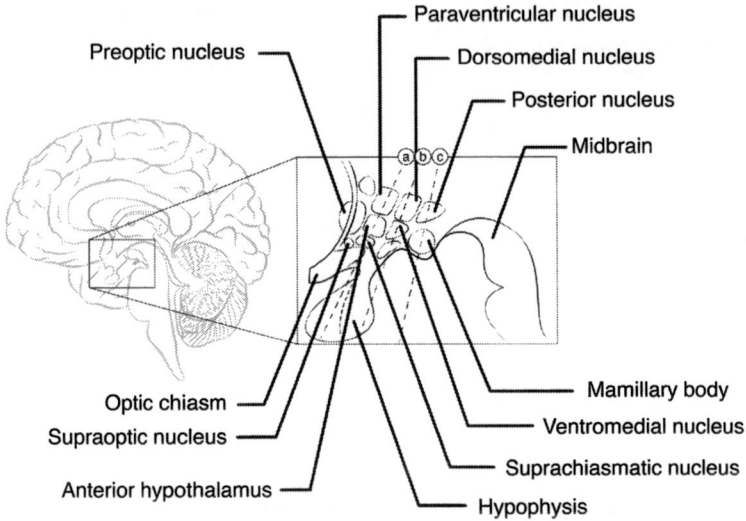

Fig. 2.11 The hypothalamus. General view

From the center outwards, three zones can be distinguished: periventricular, medial, and lateral (Figs. 2.12, 2.13, and 2.14). The periventricular zone, bordering the ventricular walls, regulates hormonal secretion of the anterior pituitary. The medial zone includes the supraoptic and paraventricular nuclei, which both secrete antidiuretic hormones (ADH) and oxytocin, two peptide hormones which are sent to the posterior pituitary to be released (Fig. 2.16, p. 73). The paraventricular nucleus, heavily involved in controlling stress responses, contributes to the secretion of *corticotropin-releasing hormone* (CRH) and regulation of the sympathetic system. This nucleus receives information from the amygdala, hippocampus, prefrontal cortex, and the locus coeruleus.[55] The paraventricular nucleus is therefore an essential relay in the integration of neuroendocrine and autonomic responses to stress. Secretion of CRH, as well as DHA, stimulates synthesis of adrenocorticotropic hormone (ACTH). Stimulation of these neurons during stress causes the release of ACTH, which causes the release of glucocorticoids from the adrenal glands. Glucocorticoids increase the rate at which carbohydrates and proteins are metabolized (Fig. 2.15, p. 73). These various physiological reactions in response to stress are intended to induce the famous "fight or flight" behavior meant to help the organism deal with the stressful stimuli. This can result in aggressive behavior, fear, or even passivity, and may inhibit appetite and reproductive behavior, through disruption of the menstrual cycle and libido. The medial

---

[55] Activation of the locus coeruleus induces the release of norepinephrine in the brain, provoking an increase in attention, memory performances but also anxiety. The "facilitator" effect that norepinephrine has on the hippocampus encourages the remembering of a menacing event's context.

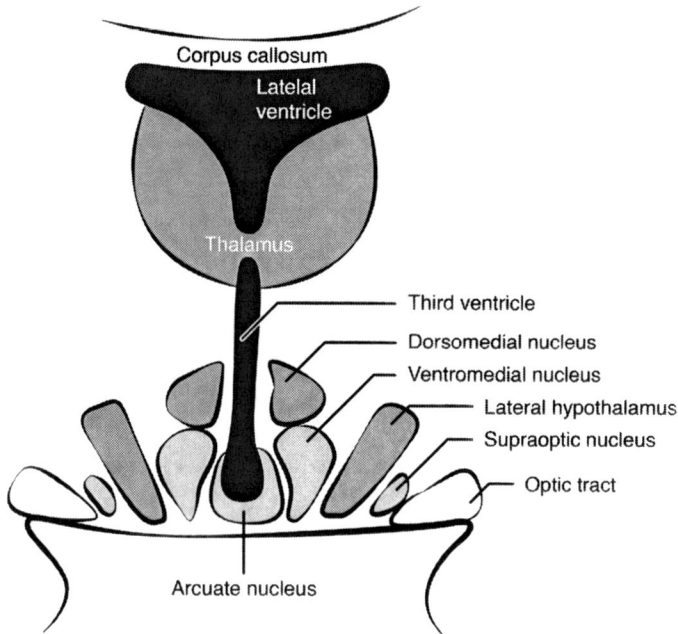

Fig. 2.12 Medial hypothalamus (Section B)

zone is also the location of the dorsomedial and ventromedial nuclei both of which are responsible for behaviors relating to hunger and thirst as the ventromedial nuclei[56] are implicated in sensations of satiety. Surgical lesioning of this structure leads to increased appetite followed by obesity. The opposite occurs following electrical activation of the core: reduction in food intake and body weight and activation of lipolysis [68]. Finally, the lateral zone, under the control of the cortex and amygdala, is also involved in feeding behavior, but its action is opposed to that of the ventromedial nucleus since it promotes consumption. Following lesions in the lateral zone, weight loss [69] and even cachexia have been observed [70–72]. In contrast, electrical stimulation of these areas increases food intake, body weight, and lipogenesis [73]. In 1974, the Dane Quaade, was the first to propose thermal lesioning of the lateral hypothalamus for the treatment of patients with morbid obesity.[57] A *lateral hypothalamotomy* was performed in five patients weighing between 118 and 180 kg. The Copenhagen-based endocrinologist reported a decrease in transit, appetite, and weight in these patients [74]. Some authors believe that the weight gain often observed in patients undergoing stimulation of the subthalamic nucleus may be due to the proximity of this structure to the lateral

---

[56] In the ventromedial nucleus this is controlled by a hormone secreted by the leptin, the white adipose tissue (from the greek λεπτός, leptos, "thin") sometimes called the "hunger hormone."

[57] Cf. p. 374.

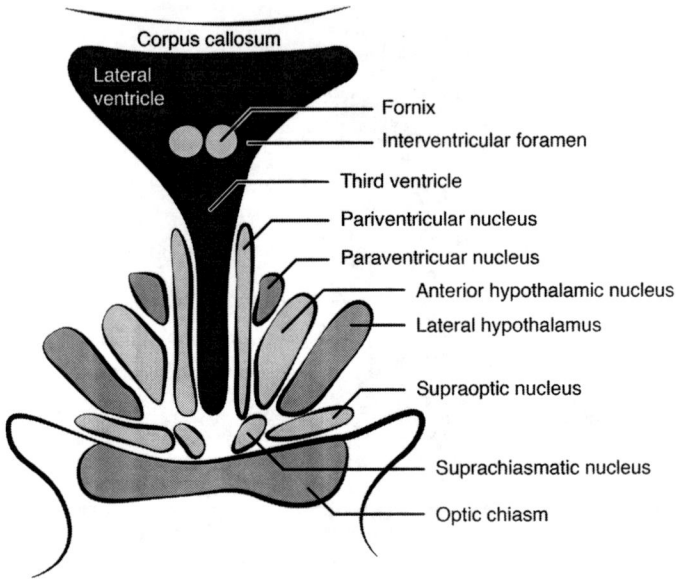

Fig. 2.13 Anterior hypothalamus (Section A)

hypothalamus [75–77]. Current research protocols[58] seek to evaluate the effectiveness of neuromodulation by electrode of the lateral hypothalamus in patients with morbid obesity (IMC > 40 kg/m^2) linked to hyperphagia [78].

To this center-outward segmentation is added a front to back subdivision. The anterior region (Fig. 2.13), located above the optic chiasm, comprises the suprachiasmatic nucleus which along with the pineal gland, helps synchronize the circadian clock to the light–dark cycle. The preoptic nucleus which is involved in thermal regulation and endocrine regulation of sexual behavior. Electrical stimulation of the preoptic nucleus reproduces all the signs of parasympathetic activity.[59]

The posterior region includes the aptly named posterior hypothalamus along with the mammillary bodies which are involved in memorization via the Papez circuit[60] (Fig. 2.14). Given that aggressive behavior results, among other things, in sympathetic manifestations, the neurosurgeon K. Sano proposed in the 1970s to treat patients suffering from hyper-aggressiveness with lesions of the posterior hypothalamus[61] (Fig. 2.15).

---

[58] Cf. p. 375.

[59] Its activation leads to a general slowing of the organism's functions to preserve energy. All that was augmented, dilated, or accelerated by the sympathetic system is now decreased, contracted, and slowed. Only the digestive function and the sexual appetite are favored by the parasympathetic system. The latter is associated with a neurotransmitter, acetylcholine.

[60] Cf. Papez circuit (Fig. 2.24, p. 85).

[61] Cf. section on aggressive behavior disorders p. 352.

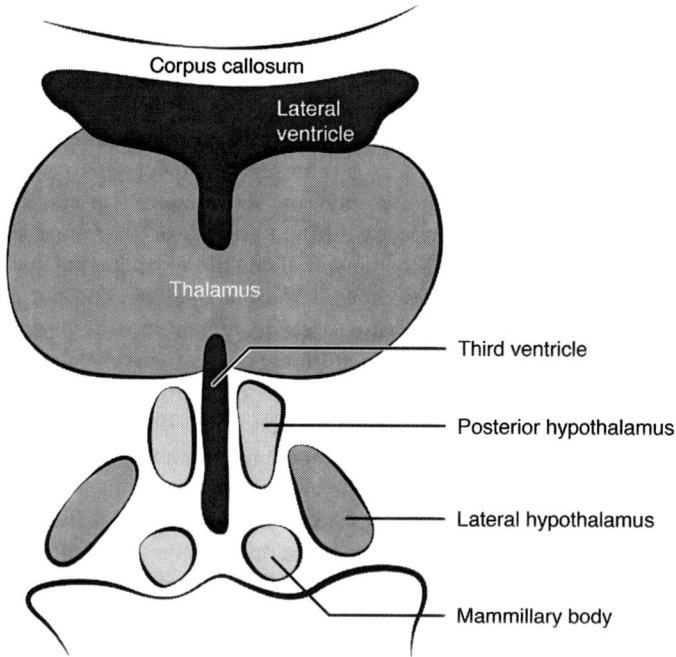

Fig. 2.14 The posterior hypothalamus (Section C)

At first, the Tokyo-based surgeon conducted electrical stimulation of the hypothalamus in patients who, for the most part, had brain damage and mental retardation. After demarcating this *ergotropic*[62] region, a lesion was made bilaterally using thermocoagulation. This *posterior hypothalamotomy*, procedure which he performed on 51 patients led to improvement in 95 % of patients after at least 2 years [79, 80]. Weight gain was probably due to the procedure's impact on the neighboring ventromedial nuclei. More recently, a Paris team led by Agid observed unexpected outbursts of aggression during deep brain stimulation of a patient with Parkinson's [81]. Imaging revealed that the electrodes were not located exactly at the level of the subthalamic nuclei, as the procedure calls for, but in the posterior part of the hypothalamus. In Milan, Franzini and Broggi, have since 2000 been successfully targeting this region for the treatment of patients presenting severe aggressive behavior stemming from brain damage (perinatal toxoplasmosis, head injury, cerebral anoxia...) [51]. This structure has also been targeted for the treatment of *cluster headaches*, excruciatingly severe headaches. Functional imaging studies have revealed that in such patients this region, especially its lower portion, is

---

[62] An "ergotropic" region is a zone controlled by the sympathetic system. Here describing a triangular area of the hypothalamus centered around the "CA-CP" axis connecting the anterior and posterior commissures (Fig. 3.2, p. 109), the top of Sylvius aqueduct and the anterior area of the mammillary bodies (Fig. 2.11, p. 68), this region is also known as "the triangle of Sano."

hyperactive [82]. Curiously though, this hyperactivity is not associated with increased aggressive behavior. Brain stimulation of the posterior hypothalamus is currently being evaluated for use in the treatment of untreatable cluster headaches, which can be so intense as to drive affected people to suicide [51, 83]. The posterior region of the hypothalamus, as we have seen, also contains an extension of the mammillary bodies, the fornix. Research protocols are underway to assess whether stimulation of these bundles improve memory performance. Research began following an unexpected clinical response during a session of deep brain stimulation. In 2008, Lozano and his team in Toronto stimulated the ventromedial nucleus of the hypothalamus of a conscious patient with morbid obesity. The purpose of the procedure was to determine if the patient felt decreased appetite during high-frequency stimulation of one or more of the different parts of the ventromedial nucleus. Instead of the sought-after response, during the procedure the patient keenly recalled a scene in a park with his friends which had occurred 30 years prior. Neuropsychological tests showed significant improvement in biographical memory after each stimulation [61]. Imaging showed that the electrodes were in fact located closer to the fornix than to the ventromedial nuclei. This serendipitous discovery led the Canadian team to explore the approach in the treatment of Alzheimer's patients. Clinical studies[63] have been initiated in the hope that stimulation of the fornix can halt memory loss associated with this disease [62].

The Pituitary Gland

Protruding off the bottom of the hypothalamus, the pituitary gland rests in a small bone cavity and consists of an anterior and posterior portion: the anterior pituitary (also called adenohypophysis) and posterior pituitary. The adenohypophysis is regulated by neurons in the hypothalamus and secretes releasing factors which act on the glands of the body. Thus, luteinizing hormone(LH) and follicle-stimulating hormone (FSH) stimulate release of sex hormones (progesterone, testosterone). Thyrotropin-releasing hormone stimulates the thyroid gland while prolactin contributes alongside oxytocin to lactation. The adrenocorticotropic hormone[64] is a releasing factor for hormones secreted by the adrenal gland. Produced especially during stressful situations, is a releasing factor for hormones secreted by the adrenal gland. Produced especially during stressful situations, prepares the individual to respond to environmental stresses (Fig. 2.15). However, sustained release can have deleterious effects on the hippocampus by causing atrophy and impairing declarative memory[65] as, for example, in cases of sustained stress [77] or Cushing's syndrome, characterized by abnormally high levels of cortisol in the blood [85, 86].

Two hormones synthesized in the hypothalamus are discharged in the posterior pituitary (Fig. 2.16): the antidiuretic hormone, which prevents leakage of water

---

[63] See, p. 200, phenomena of plasticity and neurogenesis related to stimulation.

[64] Cf. p. 113.

[65] Cf. definition p. 135.

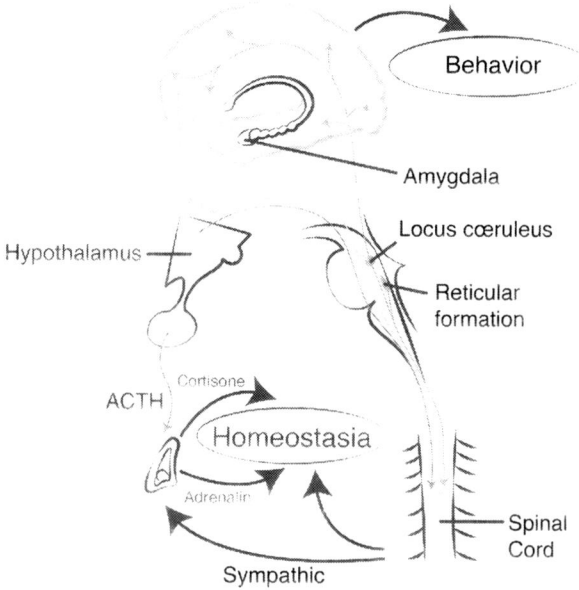

Fig. 2.15 Hypothalamus and stress. Adaptation to stress results in an increase in cardio-respiratory rate, increased blood pressure, analgesia, mobilization of energy—via glucocorti-coids—through increased glucose uptake in muscles. Inhibition of anabolic pathways with slower digestion and growth and decreased immunity and reproduction is also observed

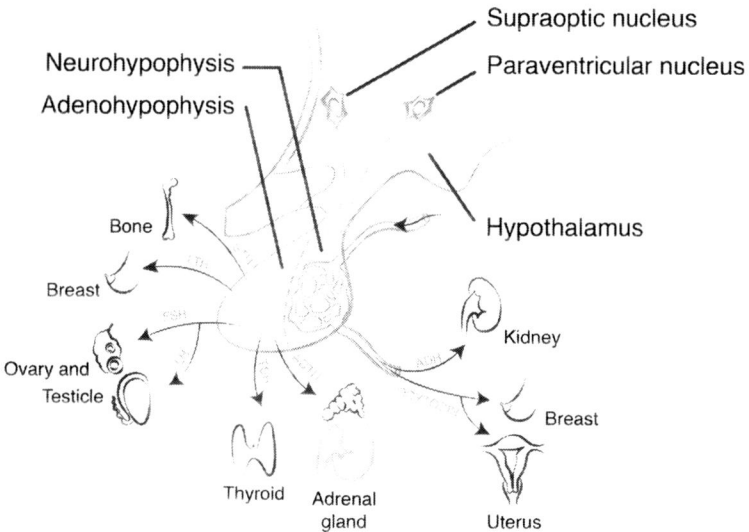

Fig. 2.16 Pituitary gland and hormonal secretions

from the kidney, and oxytocin. This hormone which participates in lactation may also be involved in shaping the mother–child bond, social phenomena, some instances of solidarity, altruism, and trust in others [87]. Intranasal administration of oxytocin could also improve the social behavior of patients with autism or Asperger syndrome [88]. Oxytocin nasal sprays may also be effective against the symptoms of schizophrenia when associated with an antipsychotic treatment [89].

The Septal Area

The septal area is located above the anterior commissure, in front of the thalamus, behind the beak of the corpus callosum, and below the *septum pellucidum*,[66] from which it derives its name. Its exact contour remains open to discussion. Some authors include neighboring lateral structures, such as the nucleus accumbens, or medial structures such as the subgenual cortex (area 25), or even the bed nucleus of the stria terminalis (BNST). The septal nuclei themselves can be divided into two groups: a medial group and a lateral group. Medial nuclei have reciprocal connections to the hippocampus—via the fornix—and receive information from the lateral nuclei. The septal nuclei are reciprocally connected to the lateral hypothalamus and receive information from the cingulate cortex. They have projections to the lateral habenula headed for the ventral tegmental area (VTA)—via the median forebrain bundle (MFB) (Fig. 2.30, p. 93) and the periaqueductal gray matter. This last region is responsible for feelings of well-being or analgesia[67] through the release of endorphins, natural opioids, while the lateral habenula influences the release of dopamine, serotonin and norepinephrine.[68] If we include within the septal area the BNST, the many connections mentioned above, and connections rooted in the amygdala, we see that this region is a strategic node in the modulation of emotions, particularly those associated with positive reinforcement. This region therefore quickly became the focus of research into deep brain stimulation. In 1954, Olds and Milner of McGill University in Montreal, conducted electrical stimulation of this area in rats [90]. The neurophysiologists observed that it caused the animal subject intense pleasure. Such pleasure, in fact, that given the opportunity to stimulate itself, the animal would neglect all other activities to the point of jeopardizing its survival. At the same time, the American Heath announced that a schizophrenic patient with intractable pain caused by a metastatic cancer was soothed by temporary electrical stimulation of this same region [91, 92]. Similar success was subsequently achieved in nonpsychotic patients with chronic pain [93] and since then, stimulation of the septal area has

---

[66] The septum pellucidum is a membrane separating the anterior horns from the lateral ventricles.

[67] The septal nuclei were also targeted for intractable pain treatment.

[68] The lateral habenula, which projects to all three neuromediator circuits, slowing them down, is one of the anatomical targets explored. It will be discussed (p. 226) in the section about chronic depression treatments using deep brain stimulation.

Table 2.1 Studies have described the effects of stimulation of the septal area in humans

Country, year	Number of patients	Clinical effect, (stimulation parameters)
United States, 1960 [98]	52	Feeling of well-being and wanting to continue the stimulation, (50 Hz, 1 ms)
The Netherlands [99]	6	More gay and more alert (1), (2–5 kHz, 0.02–0.06 ms, <12 V)
United States, 1972 [100]	1	Important sexual pleasure
Switzerland, 1985 [95]	10	Feeling of well-being (1 ms)

been offered to a very limited number of patients with intractable neuropathic pain [94] with encouraging results. Stimulation of the PAG could explain this efficacy [94, 95]. Heath and his team in New Orleans continued their "exploration" of this region, primarily in schizophrenic patients, and observed that sensations very similar to an orgasm could be elicited through stimulation [96]. The principal studies on stimulation of this area are summarized in Table 2.1 [97].

The Thalamus and the Basal Ganglia

Abstract The thalamus is a key center in the integration of sensory, motor, cognitive, and emotional information. Three of its nuclei—the anterior, medial dorsal, and ventral anterior nuclei—as well as a structure located at it base, the subthalamic nucleus, are implicated in emotions. The basal ganglia include an internal and external segment of the globus pallidus and the striatum, whose ventral region is involved in cognitive functions. Located at the base of the striatum, the nucleus accumbens is involved in the reward circuit. These different structures are integrated alongside the frontal cortex within circuits: the cortico-striato-thalamo-cortical loops that regulate our motor skill, cognition, and emotions.

The Thalamus

The thalamus (Greek: θάλαμος *thalamos,* inner chamber[69]) is a symmetrical structure located on each side of the brain forming the walls of the third ventricle (Fig. 2.17). Situated between the cortex and the brainstem, this set of nuclei relays and integrates motor, sensory, and sense information—with the exception of smell—and thus has many reciprocal connections to the cortex. We will limit our discussion to the structures involved in emotional: the anterior, ventral anterior, and medial dorsal nuclei.

---

[69] According to the first anatomists, the visual pathways seemed spread over this "bed," the "thalamus nervorum opticorum."

Corpus callosum

Lateral ventricle

Head of the caudate nucleus

Anterior limb
of the internal capsule

Putamen

Globus pallidus

Third ventricle

Tail of the caudate nucleus

Habenula

Insula

Anterior nucleus

Thalamus — Ventral anterior nucleus

Mediodorsal nucleus

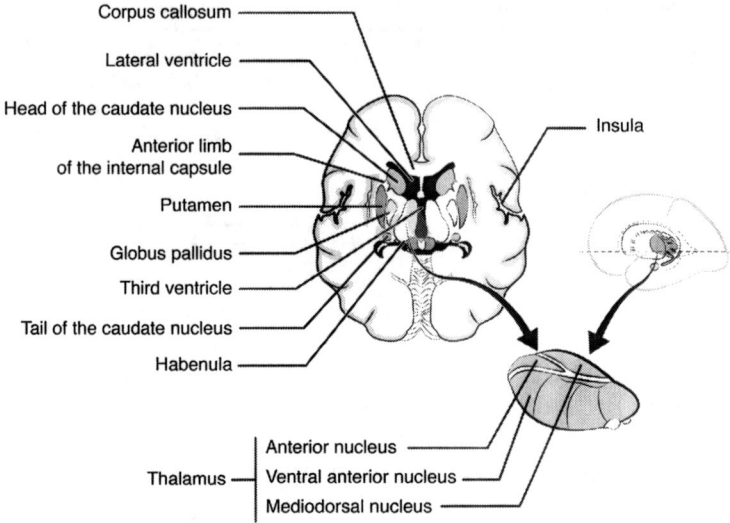

Fig. 2.17 The thalamus

The Anterior Nucleus

The anterior nucleus receives information from the hippocampus via the mammillary bodies[70] which, once integrated, is sent to the cingulate cortex. It is part of
the Papez circuit involved in memory[71] (Fig. 2.24, p. 85). This nucleus is currently
being targeted in DBS research into the treatment of intractable forms of epilepsy
[101–103].

The Ventral Anterior Nucleus

Afferents of the ventral anterior nucleus emanate mainly from the internal globus
pallidus (GPi), while its efferent fibers project toward the dorsolateral and
orbitofrontal cortex. This nucleus is involved in an associative cortico-striato-
thalamo-cortical (CSCT) loop devoted to cognitive processes (Fig. 2.27, p. 89)
[109].

---

[70] Two nuclei of the hypothalamus cf. p. 118.
[71] Cf. the anatomical description of this circuit p. 133.

The Dorsomedial Nucleus

The dorsal medial nucleus receives inputs from the hypothalamus, amygdala, olfactory cortex internal globus pallidus, and the neighboring thalamic nuclei. Once integrated, the information is projected onto the entire prefrontal cortex, and, in particular, the anterior cingulate cortex. This nucleus participates in the CSTC loop (also called "limbic" loop) involved in emotions (Fig. 2.28, p. 91) [104].

The Associative Thalamocortical Connections

These three thalamic nuclei are reciprocally connected to the prefrontal cortex by several thalamocortical tracts that run between the caudate nucleus and the putamen. This band of white matter forms the anterior part of the internal capsule and constitutes its anterior limb. The posterior limb of the internal capsule is composed of a bundle of axons—the pyramidal tract—which originates in the motor center and controls movement on the opposite half of the body (Fig. 2.18).

Within the anterior limb of the internal capsule (ALIC), two thalamocortical tracts are of interest to us: the so-called *associative* tract connecting the orbito-frontal and dorsolateral cortices to the ventral anterior and medial dorsal nuclei of the thalamus, and the *limbic* tract connecting the orbitofrontal and cingulate cortices to the dorsal medial nucleus [105]. These two bundles interest us because they are the targets of two psychosurgical procedures of the ALIC: the anterior capsulotomy[72] which creates lesions in these bundles (Fig. 3.6, p. 114). DBS, which blocks their operation through the application of an electrical current (Fig. 2.19).

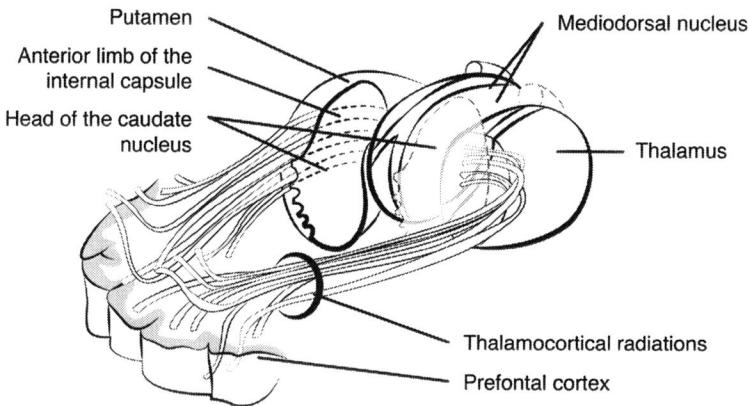

Fig. 2.18 Thalamocortical radiations projecting through the anterior limb of the internal capsule to the prefrontal cortex. According to [112]

---

[72] Cf. the historical p. 51, the thermocoagulation p. 167 or radiosurgery surgical technique p. 188, its results in obsessive–compulsive disorder p. 284 or in depression p. 326.

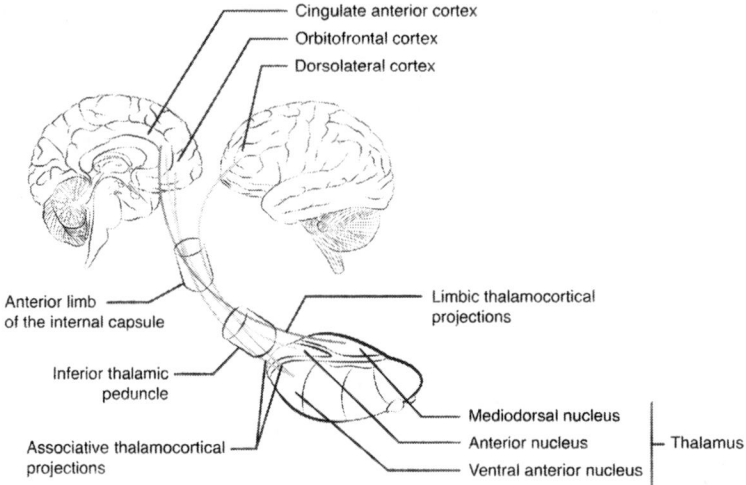

Fig. 2.19 Thalamocortical associative and limbic connections

The Subthalamic Nucleus

This paired nucleus (found on each side of the brain) in the shape of elongated lens of about 150 mm^3 is situated, as its name suggests, on the ventral side of the thalamus. It was discovered by the French neurologist JB. Luys and used to be known as the *corpus Luys* (Fig. 2.20).

The subthalamic nucleus (STN) contains glutamatergic excitatory neurons receiving afferences from the prefrontal cortex, substantia nigra and external globus pallidus. It projects, in turn, primarily onto the internal globus pallidus and thalamus. Involved in various CSTC loops,[73] the STN modulates motor, cognitive, and emotional responses. These three functions correspond to three anatomical areas. The area tasked with emotions, called the limbic area, is situated toward the rear. The cognitive areas occupies the lateral portion of the nucleus [106]. The motor area is the main target for deep brain stimulation used in the treatment of Parkinson's disease and is being evaluated for the treatment of OCD, as discussed in later section.[74] Uncertainty remains as to the exact emotional and cognitive functions of this structure. Nonetheless, some of the undesirable side effects of high frequency electrical stimulation, which is considered to inhibit this structure, may shed some light on the possible role of this nucleus. At the cognitive level,

---

[73] Cf. p. 139.

[74] Cf. p. 292.

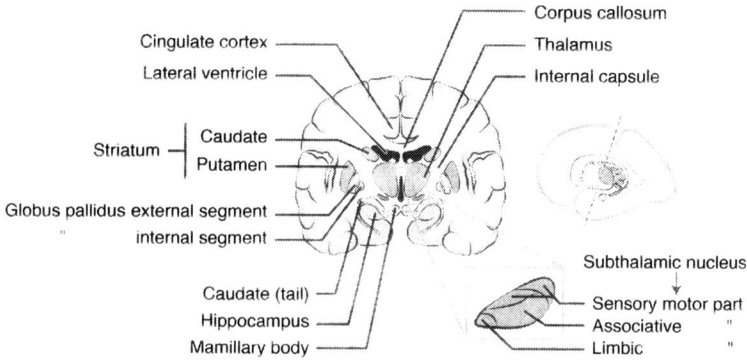

Fig. 2.20 The subthalamic nucleus

DBS of the nucleus can result in decreased verbal memory and fluency [107–116], executive functions [111, 112, 117–120], and attention [121, 122]. In terms of its effects on mood, symptoms can range from mania [115, 123–125], depression [111, 114, 125–139] or even suicide [119, 132, 140] as well as personality disorders [107, 133], increased anxiety [111, 113] and hypersexuality [119, 125, 141–145]. These diverse and sometimes contradictory effects are evidence, on the one hand, of the complexity of the STN, and on the other, of the still poorly understood mechanisms of high frequency stimulation. One may also wonder whether the clinical effects obtained are brought on by the combination of the activation of the fibers surrounding the nucleus and the inactivation of the neurons it contains. The exact position of the electrode within the structure and the electrical parameters also plays a key role.[75]

The Striatum and the Pallidum

The striatum is a striated (hence, its name) paired nerve structure composed of two interconnected dopaminergic entities of identical embryological origin: the caudate nucleus and the putamen. The caudate nucleus, shaped like a horseshoe, wraps around the thalamus (Figs. 2.21, 2.22).

It has a bulbous frontend and elongated body tapering off just behind the amygdala. The head of the nucleus is connected to the putamen by "putamino-caudate," bridges crossing the internal capsule, including the ALIC. The putamen resembles a pyramid and its interior portion faces the pallidum. The pallidum, also

---

[75] Cf. Mysteries of DBS p. 198.

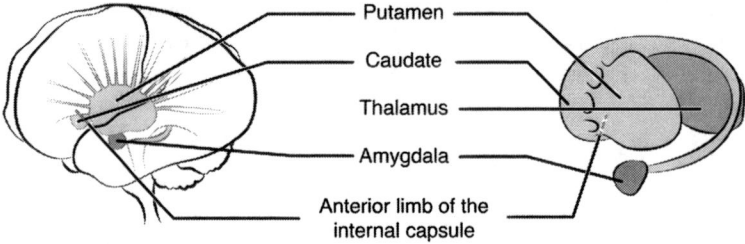

Fig. 2.21 The basal ganglia

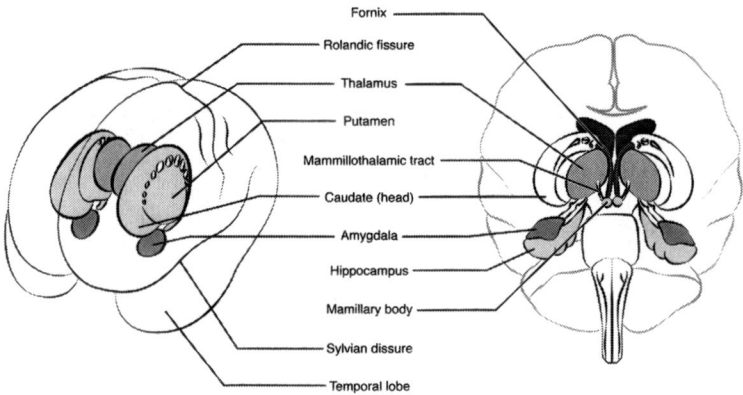

Fig. 2.22 Side and anterior view of the basal ganglia

called globus pallidus, consists of two segments, the external globus pallidus (GPe) and the internal globus pallidus. The motor sector of the GPi includes the lateral, ventral, and posterior portions. The limbic sector follows the anterior ventral–medial axis, and the remaining area is the associative sector. The putamen and pallidum form an anatomic entity: the lenticular nucleus.

The striatum is divided into an upper, dorsal part, and a lower, ventral part. The dorsal striatum is involved in motor control and cognition. Its role appears crucial to routine habits [146, 147]. The ventral striatum, however, takes part in the regulation of emotions and behaviors, especially the initiation and execution of behaviors involving the notion of reward [21]. In front and at the base of the ventral striatum where the putamen and the head of the caudate nucleus meet is located a critical structure, the nucleus accumbens (Fig. 3.3, p. 110).

The striatum is divided into an upper, dorsal part, and a lower, ventral part. The dorsal striatum is involved in motor control and cognition. Its role appears crucial to routine habits [154, 155]. The ventral striatum, however, takes part in the regulation of emotions and behaviors, especially the initiation and execution of behaviors involving the notion of reward [21]. At the bottom and in front of this ventral striatum there is a key structure: the nucleus accumbens, which corresponds to the fusion between the putamen and the caudate nucleus.

The Nucleus Accumbens

Abstract Situated at the base of the ventral striatum, the nucleus accumbens consists of a "core," involved in motor control, and a "shell" connected to the amygdala and the rest of the limbic system. Functioning as a relay within the CSTC loop, this nucleus helps regulate emotions and motivation, and as such, it is considered the interface between desire and action.

Because of its importance in psychosurgery, the nucleus accumbens, situated at the base of the ventral striatum merits particular attention. It is the interface between two fundamental circuits in the regulation of emotions and behavior: the CSTC loops and the reward circuit.[76] For histological reasons, the nucleus accumbens is composed of a "core," and a "shell" [112].

The shell is where the ends of the mesolimbic dopamine[77] releasing neurons come together. Dopamine, the crucial fuel of the reward circuit, is inseparable from the motivational processes of the limbic system. The core of the nucleus is connected to the extrapyramidal motor system responsible for regulating movement via the CSTC motor loop. This core can be likened to a strategic gate between the limbic and extrapyramidal systems, an "interface between motivation and action" [148]. It is possible that overactivity in one of these CSTC loops causes OCD. French and German teams have therefore suggested modulating this system through implantation of stimulation electrodes in the nucleus accumbens[78] [149–151]. The nucleus accumbens also receives excitatory afferents[79] (Fig. 2.23) from the amygdala [152], hippocampus [152–155], thalamus [156, 157] and orbitofrontal cortex [158]. It is believed that the nucleus accumbens integrates environmental information via the hippocampus, information on the emotional context via the amygdala and cognitive data through its connections to the prefrontal cortex. It draws on this information to contribute to the selection of an appropriate behavioral response to a given situation. Its function would appear crucial in motivational behavior—sex, addiction, or stress related. As such, it seems to play an important role in adapting behavior and the learning process [159]. The accumbens nucleus in turn, projects to the ventral pallidum through

---

[76] Cf. p. 146.

[77] Ibid.

[78] Cf. p.291.

[79] These excitative afferents are mediated by glutamate, a neurotransmitter that stimulates the central nervous system (CNS).

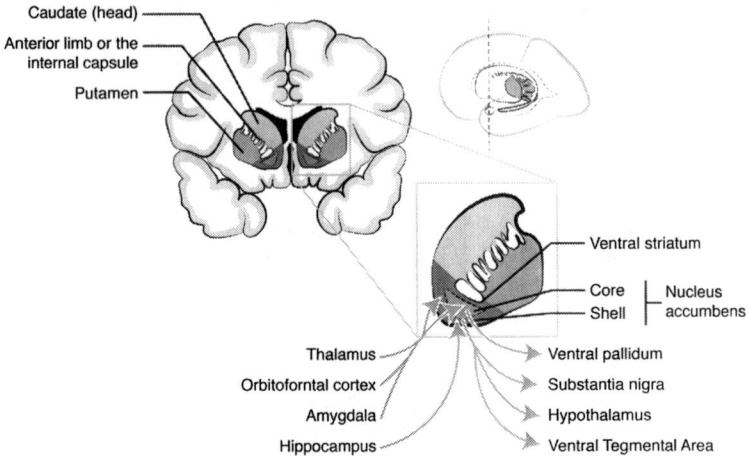

Fig. 2.23 The nucleus accumbens and its connections

inhibitory efferents[80] [160–162] and to the ventral segmental area (VTA) and substantia nigra. The latter two structures are the primary dopamine producing areas [163, 164]. The shell also has efferents to the lateral portion of the hypothalamus [165]. In 1954, a study showed that rats with a stimulating electrode, which they were able to activate themselves, implanted in the VTA resorted to endless sessions of autostimulation, even to the point of compromising their food-intake and starving themselves to death [90]. Similar effects were subsequently obtained when the electrodes were implanted in the nucleus accumbens [166]. The animal subject would stimulate itself up to 20 times a minute [167–169]. The administration of morphine [170, 171], however, reduced the amount of autostimulation. It was later shown that all drugs increase the concentration of neurotransmitter in the shell of the nucleus accumbens [172, 173] which explains why an influx of dopamine decreased the frequency of autostimulation. Similarly, when weaning off an addictive substance, there is a steep reduction in the release of dopamine in the shell [174]. When a male rat is placed in the presence of a female rat in heat the level of dopamine in the shell increases, and if he is able to engage in the reproductive act, it skyrockets. In humans, functional imaging shows activity of the nucleus accumbens when pleasant or erotic scenes are being viewed [175, 176]. This has led some authors to call this nucleus the "pleasure center." This hedonistic[81] attribute has encouraged teams to successfully target this nucleus

---

[80] These inhibitory afferents are mediated by GABA (gamma-aminobutyric acid) a neurotransmitter that inhibits the CNS.

[81] Hedonism comes from the Greek word ηδονή, which means pleasure. It is a doctrine that has as moral principle the search for pleasure and the avoidance of pain.

with deep brain stimulation in order to treat intractable depression[82] [177, 178]. Given that one of the major symptoms of depression is anhedonia,

German researchers have suggested that neuromodulation by stimulation of the nucleus could likely reduce the symptoms resulting from loss of pleasure [179]. From 1970 to 1976, another German team performing subcaudate tractotomies[83] on patients with severe OCD noticed during follow-up that 8 of the 16 patients had developed a severe addiction. In 1998, MRI scans showed that the lesions were in fact located in the ventral striatum and that in six of the patients they were located in the nucleus accumbens [180]. Based on these findings, animal testing and functional imaging data, this nucleus is currently being studied as a target for treatment of certain addictions using deep brain stimulation[84] (Table 4.13, p. 246) [181–185]. It should be noted procedures involving ablation of the nucleus accumbens, though ethically questionable, are also offered to patients addicted to opiates [186].

Emotion and Its Circuits

Abstract Several tightly interconnected neural circuits are involved in emotions. The Papez circuit, which includes the hippocampus, thalamus, and mammillary bodies, is involved in memory. Two other loops connecting the prefrontal cortex to the striatum and thalamus and returning to the cortex also carry cognitive and emotional information. This last loop, the emotional loop, is connected through the nucleus accumbens with the dopamine pathway involved in reward-based motivational processes. Other more diffuse circuits of neurotransmitters—serotonin and norepinephrine—are also involved in the regulation of mood.

A Brief History: The Papez Circuit

In 1937, James Papez theorized a possible circuit to account for emotion [5]. Based on research by Bard, who highlighted the role of the posterior hypothalamus in behavior characteristic of fury through experiments on decerebrated cats [187], Papez suggested that the hippocampus is also involved in emotion. It was known at the time that the hippocampus underwent histological changes in patients with rabies, known for their excessive emotional manifestations characterized notably by bouts of terror. In his original article, the neuroanatomist wrote that all

---

[82] Cf. p. 291.
[83] Subcaudate Tractotomy cf. p. 180.
[84] Cf. p. 193.

information from our senses is directed to the thalamus. There, the information is split into two streams: one for "thought" and the other for "feeling." The first stream heads for the sensory and cingulate cortices to transform sensation into conscious perception (sensory cortex) and thought (cingulate cortex). According to Papez, the cingulate cortex, depending on the emotional charge of the thought, then sends it toward the hippocampus and from there via the fornix, to the mammillary bodies of the hypothalamus. At this stage, the *emotional experience* is converted into a *physical expression*. The second stream heads directly to the mammillary body to convert some of the sensations into physical manifestations. This stream also influences the cingulate cortex which it reaches via the anterior nucleus of the thalamus. Drawing on the theory of Cannon-Bard[85] the American neuroanatomist hypothesized that emotional *experience* born in the cingulate cortex precedes emotional *expression* from the hypothalamus. Papez's theory, however, does not completely preclude James-Langes theory since information from the hypothalamus, i.e., emotional experience, also reaches the cingulate cortex. Ultimately, by describing this hippocampo-mammilla-thalamo-cortical circuit Papez primarily gave his name to a circuit involved in memory (Fig. 2.24). Clinical observation later confirmed the importance of the hippocampus in memory tasks. In 1954, the neurosurgeon W. Scoville performed a bilateral removal of the hippocampi in order to treat an epileptic patient who thereafter became unable to retain any information [188]. This case along with observations of animals showed that a bilateral lesion of one or more parts of the hippocampo-mammilla-thalamo-cortical circuit causes anterograde amnesia. All information from the cortex is funneled through the entorhinal cortex, the "gateway" to the hippocampus. From there, information reaches the mammillary bodies via the fornix and is then redirected to the anterior nucleus of the thalamus through the mamilla–thalamic tract.[86] The thalamus then projects to the cingulate cortex. In turn, the cingulate gyrus returns part of the data to the entorhinal cortex completing the circuit. The cortex is thus the primary input for information, and the Papez circuit projects back to the same cortex through successive iterations, which allow declarative memory[87] to be encoded. The connections between this circuit and the hypothalamus and amygdala explain the strong ties binding memory to emotion. Voltaire wrote, *that which touches the heart is engraved in the memory*. The reader

---

[85] Affective reaction—joy, disgust, enthusiasm, fear, anxiety and others—is a feeling qualified as "emotional experience," and according to Cannon and Bard it also provokes an "emotional expression" that manifests through neurovegetative signs, which become quantifiable. This causality is not unambiguous. As we know from experiments with certain relaxation techniques or meditation, it is possible to reduce the "emotional experience" by attenuating this "emotional expression." See the theory of James and Langes p. 84.

[86] Also known as the Vicq d'Azyr bundle, after the French physician that described it, Félix Vicq d'Azyr, Queen Marie-Antoinette's personal physician.

[87] Cf. its description p. 103.

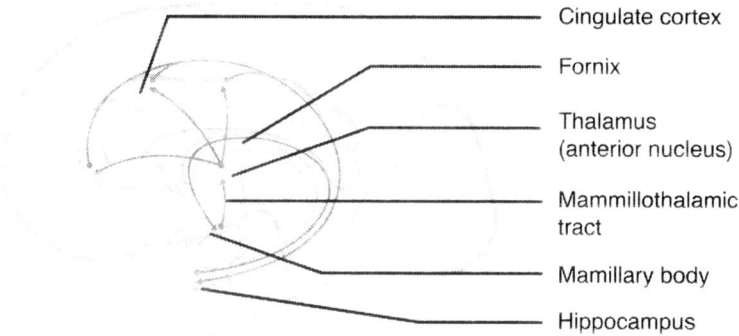

Cingulate cortex

Fornix

Thalamus
(anterior nucleus)

Mammillothalamic
tract

Mamillary body

Hippocampus

Fig. 2.24 Hippocampo-mammillary connections of the memory circuit

will recall precisely where she was on 11 September 2001 when the World Trade Center towers collapsed. The emotional nature of the event led to a "snapshot", which under normal circumstances would quickly be forgotten, being etched into memory [189, 190]. Thus stress resulting from certain events increases the release of norepinephrine and dopamine by the amygdala, which regulates the areas where these neurotransmitters are synthesized. Norepinephrine in turn activates the amygdala [51] with has specific receptors for this neurotransmitter. The amygdala then acts on the hippocampus, making it ready to place the event within the situational context and to assess whether the conditions for long-term memory creation are met or if the emotion-generating event can be forgotten [191]. Dopamine, meanwhile, appears to be more involved in long-term memory. VTA is the source of dopamine [192]. The signal causes increased release of dopamine. This influx of dopamine to the hippocampus improves the transmission of nerve impulses within the structure. Hence, efficacy and therefore memory is enhanced. Conversely, prolonged anxiety or stress negatively impacts declarative memory performance [193]. This memory impairment is related to the effect of gluco-corticoids, hormones secreted during stress, on the hippocampus. Atrophy of the hippocampus can be observed after situations of long-term stress [84, 194] or because of excessive cortisol levels [85, 86]. In cases of extreme stress this can lead to complete loss of memory of the anxiety-causing event. In contrast, the amygdala, which is not affected by the action of these hormones, continues to set these events down in unconscious form as conditioned fear [195]. According to neuroscientist Marc Jeannerod, this phenomenon accounts for, "reactions such as phobias, war neurosis,[88] *panic attacks* [which] *may well find an explanation in this dissociation between amnesia of the circumstances surrounding the trauma and the persistent presence of conditioned fear* [196].

---

[88] Cf. Post-traumatic stress disorder p. 384.

Fig. 2.25 MacLean triune
brain, according to [206]

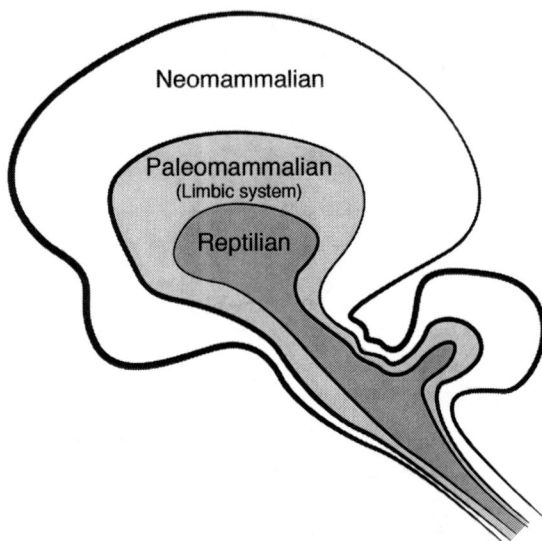

The MacLean Limbic System

In 1949, Paul MacLean offered a different mechanism for the neuroanatomy of
emotions based not only on the Papez circuit but also on Darwinian evolution
[197]. He saw the human brain as a stack of three brains (Fig. 2.25) [6].

According to MacLeans, this triune structure is the result of three concentric
anatomical systems having been sequentially brought together in the course of
evolution. A *reptilian brain*, composed of the basal ganglia and brainstem, controls
functions such as arousal, eating, and reproduction. This primitive structure is
overlaid by a *visceral* or *paleomammalian brain* later named the *limbic brain* [198].
Indeed, he considered that the great limbic lobe, described by Broca in 1878 [4],
winds around the reptilian brain forming a limbic brain. In addition to the great
limbic lobe of Broca[89] he also included the structures added by Papez, the thalamus
and hypothalamus, as well as the prefrontal cortex and amygdala. The American
scientist emphasized the close connections between the amygdala and the Papez
circuit. The amygdala filters the information passing through the Papez circuit and
is, as the psychiatrist Jouvent describes *the true watchman of the internal and
external environment* [...] *giving negative emotional valence, dangerous, or
positive, favorable.* [The Amygdala] *receives information from converging sensory
inputs (lateral nuclei). The sensory thalamus is its privileged partner* [199]. The
connections between the amygdala (central nuclei) and the hypothalamus are

---

[89] The French neurologist associated this great limbic lobe with bestial behavior, opposing it to
the intellectual faculties generated in the rest of the cortex.

responsible both for hormonal reactions, such as the release of glucocorticoid hormones, as well as autonomic responses which can involve the sympathetic or parasympathetic systems. Ultimately, MacLean attributed three functions to the limbic brain: self-preservation, inherent to the amygdalar region, the preservation of the species, i.e., sexuality, based in the septal region,, and finally inter-personal relationships, located within the thalamocingulate complex. According to the Yale researcher, this better evolved structure allows mammals to overcome stereotypical behaviors dictated by their reptilian brain by adding social skills, affective skills like emotions, and motivation. These two ancestral brains supposedly form *the horse*. The rest of the cortex, called neocortex, is the rider atop the horse. In other words, the neocortex represents rational intelligence which seeks to be free from emotions.[90] MacLean's anatomical model of emotion is often cited even though it has been much criticized. For example, it exaggerates the importance of the hippocampus, the mammillary bodies and the anterior thalamus, and underestimates the role of the basal ganglia in emotional processes [189].

The Cortico-Striato-Thalamo-Cortical Loops

MacLean's model leaves little room for the basal ganglia in the regulation of emotions. However, research by Alexander [104] has led to greater awareness of the fundamental role these nuclei have on how we function, especially emotionally. The model suggested by the Baltimore neurologist enables a clearer understanding of the involvement of the basal ganglia in our motor, cognitive, and emotional processes and their intricacies. Alexander has described a system composed of five parallel circuits involving the basal ganglia, the thalamus, and the frontal cortex. These five cortico-striato-thalamo-cortical loops (CSCT) connect the cortical areas to areas in the striatum and pallidum which in turn project back to the cortical areas via the thalamic nuclei. Of these loops, the best known is the one involved in sensorimotor functions. For this reason, it is interesting and informative to examine this loop in more detail. The limbic and cognitive loops of more direct relevance to the subject at hand, function very similarly.

The Motor Loop Circuit as an Example

This motor circuit (Fig. 2.26) involves the frontal motor cortex[91] (areas 4 and 6) and the parietal somatosensory cortex.[92] Both project to the dorsal striatum, or

---

[90] Read the excellent work by R. Jouvent (2009), Le cerveau magicien (The brain as magician) Odile Jacob, Paris.

[91] Cf. p. 90.

[92] Cf. p. 110.

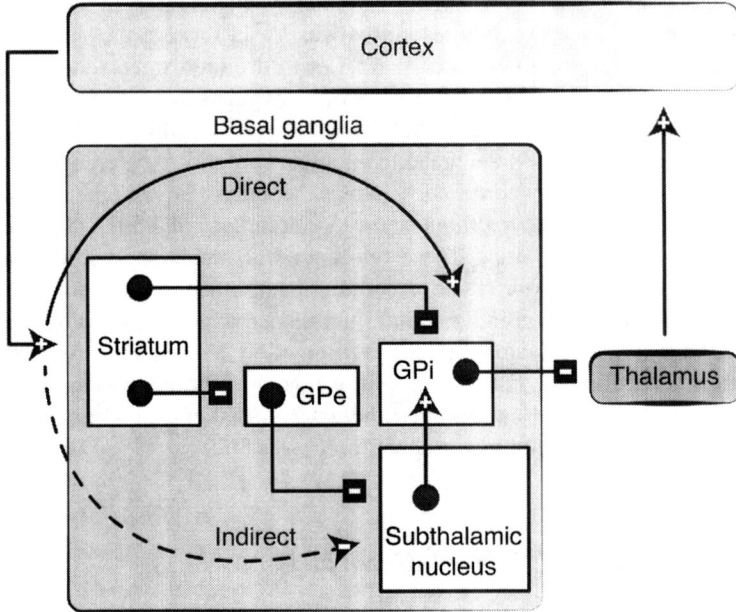

Fig. 2.26 The motor cortico-striato-thalamo-cortical loop (CSTC)

more precisely the putamen and have an excitatory effect through the action of glutamate, an excitatory neurotransmitter. The striatum then projects to the ventral part of the internal globus pallidus (GPi) and the substantia nigra (SN) slowing them both through the inhibitory action of GABA.

The GPi and SN then project to the motor nuclei of the thalamus, which they inhibit through the action of GABA. The thalamus in turn stimulates the cortex through the release of glutamate thus completing the loop. Within this circuit there are two separate pathways along which signals may travel. These two routes rely on different neurotransmitters in the striatum, solicit different structures, and have opposite effects. The first is the *direct route*, in which striatal neurons which synthesize GABA and substance P project an inhibitory input to the GPi and SN. The second is the *indirect route*, in which striatal neurons which synthesize GABA and enkephalin instead of substance P project an inhibitory input to the external globus pallidus (GPe). The GPe in turn projects an inhibitory input to the dorso-lateral part of the subthalamic nucleus[93] (STN), which then projects onto the GPi and SN using glutamate. In the second scenario the GPi and SN receive an excitatory input. Activation of the direct route causes a decrease in the activity of the output nuclei (GPi and substantia nigra) leading to a disinhibition of the activity of the thalamus and thus release of glutamatergic excitatory impulses to

---

[93] Cf. anatomy p.126.

the cortex, which encourages movement. The direct pathway can be likened to the *accelerator pedal* in a car. In contrast, activation of the indirect pathway *brake pedal*. Which pathway is activated depends on the presence of dopamine, in the striatum: dopamine released by the substantia nigra activates the direct route and inhibits the indirect route. The associative and limbic circuits discussed below function according to the same model.

The Associative CSTC Loop

The associative circuit begins in the lateral and dorsolateral[94] orbitofrontal cortices and connects to the striatum near the head of the caudate nucleus and anteromedial portion of the putamen (Fig. 2.27) [8].

It then passes through the GPi and SN, before entering the thalamus through the inferior thalamic peduncle and reaching the ventral anterior[95] and nuclei, which link back to the prefrontal cortex [200]. This pathway corresponds to the *direct route* mentioned above. In the *indirect pathway*, the GPe and ventromedial portion of the STN are interposed between the striatum and the GPi. In terms of cognition, the associative loop seems to be implicated in working memory, spatial orientation, as well as executive functions relating to attention and preparation or initiation of actions. This circuit also intervenes at the emotional level by enabling empathy and appropriate responses during social interactions [200]. Decreased levels of dopamine within this circuit may cause the cognitive slowing and apathy observed in patients with Parkinson's disease [201]. In contrast, increased dopamine levels causes cognitive impulsiveness, tachypsychia, and novelty seeking.

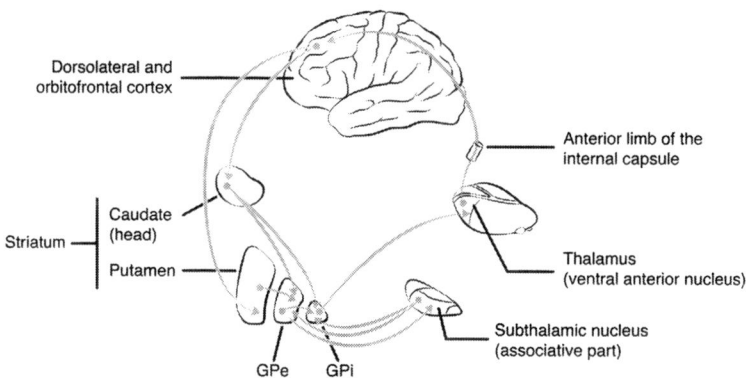

Fig. 2.27 The associative cortico-striato-thalamo-cortical (CSTC) loop. According to [209]

---

[94] Cf. p. 93.

[95] Cf. p. 124.

Psychomotor retardation (Fig. 4.4, p. 216) observed in cases of severe depression is probably related to dysfunction of this circuit [202, 203]. The struggle to push away negative thoughts or to ignore pain could also be related [202–206]. A targeted lesion within these structures, particularly in the orbitofrontal cortex, is likely to lead to personality changes such as impulsiveness, emotional lability, or a lack of "tact" when dealing with others [207, 208]. When instead the lesion is located in the dorsolateral cortex, the patient may exhibit perseveration, impaired planning for and adaption to new tasks, or difficulty blocking out external stimuli [207, 208].

The Limbic CSTC Loop

The limbic circuit begins in the anterior portion of the cingulum[96] (areas 24) and orbitofrontal cortex [8] and projects to the limbic (i.e., ventral) area of the striatum. This area comprises the ventral regions of the caudate nucleus and putamen and the nucleus accumbens (Fig. 2.28).[97]

The ventral striatum also has afferent connections from the amygdala[98], the hippocampus[99], and the entorhinal cortex.[100] Its efferent connections project onto the ventral globus pallidus which acts as a relay within the dorsomedial nucleus of the thalamus.[101] The limbic circuit also contains an *indirect pathway* in which the GPe and the rostral part of the STN intervene between the ventral striatum and the GPi. This loop circuit is involved in motivational aspects of behavior. In Parkinson's patients, low levels of dopamine in the limbic loop—as in the associative loop—causes cognitive slowing and apathy [201]. Extensive bilateral lesioning of the cingulate cortex[102] can lead to varying degrees of diminished motivation including apathy, aboulia, and mutism. In certain instances, verbal expression is limited to monosyllabic responses and the face no longer conveys any emotion, even in response to pain [207–209]. In fact, pain is no longer perceived as suffering. The different loops presented here almost always act in concert and share the same structures and neurotransmitters [200]. Their interrelatedness can be illustrated as follows: if you fancy a lemonade, this implies motivation (limbic loop); planning to reach the bottle (cognitive loop); and motor behavior to pour the lemonade into a glass and drink (motor loop). The STN, which is involved in all three loops, seems to play a key role in interfacing cognitive manifestations,

---

[96] Cf. p. 95.

[97] Cf. p. 129.

[98] Cf. p. 98.

[99] Cf. p. 103.

[100] The entorhinal cortex (areas 28 and 34) is located in the internal part of the temporal lobe, it is an area of convergence for information proceeding from the associative cortex to the hippocampus.

[101] Cf. p. 123.

[102] Cf. p. 95.

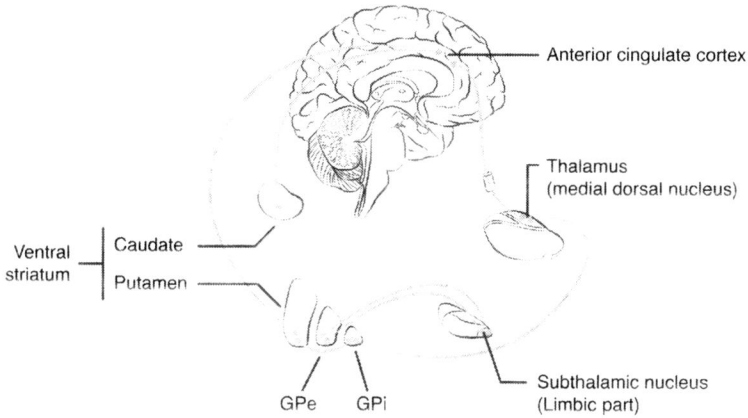

Fig. 2.28 The cortico-striato-thalamo-cortical (CSTC) limbic loop. According to [200]

limbic manifestations, and motor behavior. The same is true of the nucleus accumbens,[103] which is also an important interface between desire and action. The subthalamic nucleus (STN) may also, according to a French team led by B. Bioulac, serve a more complex function as the *central clock of the central basal ganglia* synchronizing the oscillatory activity of these nuclei with the activity in the cortex [210, 211]. These oscillations are essential to brain connectivity and plasticity [212].

The Neurotransmitter Circuits

Abstract Three main neurotransmitters, dopamine, serotonin, and norepineph-rine, all monoamines, are involved in the neurochemical circuitry of the limbic system. Dopamine synthesized in the substantia nigra intervenes in CSTC loops while dopamine secreted by neurons in the ventral tegmental area is involved in the reward circuit. Serotonin synthesized in the raphe nuclei modulates behavior, primarily through inhibition, while noradrenaline synthesized in the locus coeruleus increases attention to external stimuli.

As we saw in the previous section, *dopamine* is at the heart of loop circuits. However, two other neurotransmitters must also be mentioned for their role in the limbic system: *serotonin*, which has an inhibitory effect on behavior, and *nor-epinephrine*, which has an excitatory effect on behavior. These neurotransmitters are primarily synthesized by neurons in the brainstem and released over wide areas of the brain creating a *diffuse regulatory system*.

---

[103] Cf. p. 129.

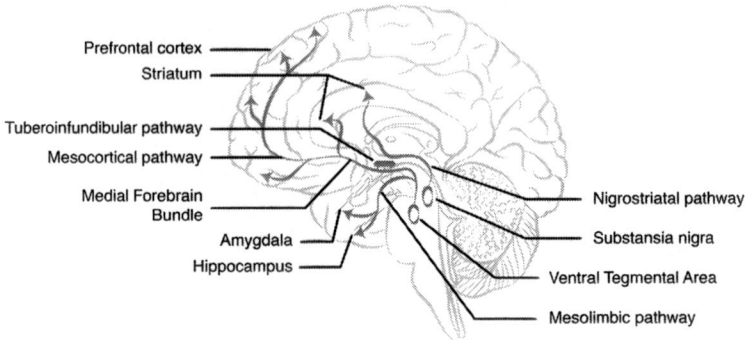

Fig. 2.29 The dopaminergic pathway

Dopamine and the Reward Circuit

Within the brain dopamine plays a critical role in motivity, cognition, motivation, sleep, and memory. Four major dopaminergic pathways can be identified according to where the molecule is being produced and released (Fig. 2.29).

Dopamine is synthesized mainly by neurons in the substantia nigra and the ventral tegmental area (VTA) whose axonal projections target the striatum or the septal nuclei. The dorsal part of the striatum receives dopaminergic projections from the SN along *the nigrostriatal pathway* and is involved in motor control.[104] The ventral striatum, however, receives dopaminergic afferents from the VTA along the medial forebrain bundle[105] (Fig. 2.30).

This second dopaminergic pathway, called *the mesolimbic pathway*, is of more particular interest to us because of its relation to the *limbic system*. The mesolimbic pathway is also called *the reward circuit* because of its involvement in the control of motivational and reward processes: it gives positive reinforcement to pleasurable behavior. In animals, lesions of the VTA result in neglect of the environment and reduced exploratory behavior. However, if electrodes are implanted in the VTA or along the MFB and the animal is allowed to freely auto-stimulate itself, it will engage in this highly gratifying behavior to the point of neglecting its basic

---

[104] Parkinson's disease is an example of a substantia nigra degenerative disease that provokes a rarefaction of dopamine. This deficiency in the cortico-striato-thalamo-cortical loop will generate a rarefaction of movement. In the other loops, associative and limbic (which are also dependent on this neuromediator), this dopamine insufficiency will manifest through cognitive problems (dementia) or psychiatric problems (depression, anxiety) also found in this neurologic disease.

[105] The medial forebrain bundle arises in the deep nuclei of the cerebellum and then becomes the periaqueducal gray matter. It then divides into two branches: an inferior and internal branch going to the lateral hypothalamus and a superior external branch projecting to the nucleus accumbens after transiting through the inferior part of the anterior limb of the internal capsule. This superior external branch projects to the orbitofrontal, dorsolateral and probably the subgenual cortices [221].

Fig. 2.30 Medial forebrain bundles *MFB*—top view of the brain. *VTA* Ventral Tegmental Area; *ALIC* Anterior Limb of the Internal Capsule, *MTC* Mammillothalamic Connections, *SGC* SubGenual Cortex, *NAcc* Nucleus Accumbens, *LH* Lateral Hypothalamus, *STN* SubThalamic Nucleus, *SNR* Substantia Nigra Reticulata, *PAG* Periaqueductal gray matter, 3 V: Third Ventricle. According to [222]

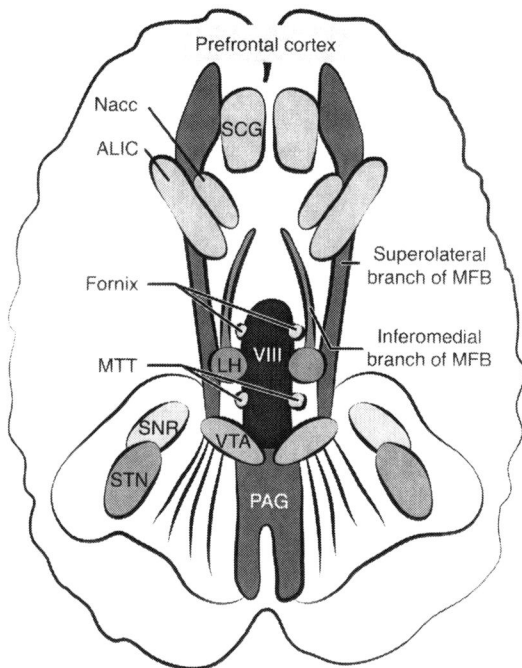

survival activities [90]. Reward and reinforcement phenomena are intended to help the subject delight in behaviors essential to survival such as eating and reproduction. In addition to these motivation and aversion processes, the mesolimbic system is also involved in certain cognitive functions. This circuit is co-opted when an individual takes drugs since all addictions, as discussed earlier have in common that they increase the concentration of dopamine in the nucleus accumbens. This dopamine production, which causes feelings of pleasure, leads to compulsive behavior in which drug-use replaces survival behaviors. The third dopamine pathway, *the mesocortical pathway*, is composed of dopaminergic neurons in the VTA whose axons project to the prefrontal cortex and in particular the anterior cingulate cortex. It is implicated in concentration and executive functions such as memory. The final bundle of dopaminergic neurons, the *tuberoinfundibular pathway*, arises in the hypothalamus and inhibits prolactin secretion in the anterior pituitary. Dopamine binds to two classes of receptors: D1 and D2 [213]. The D1-class is composed of post-synaptic receptors with excitatory effects. It includes the D1 receptors in the striatum, nucleus accumbens and cortex, and D5 receptors in the hippocampus and hypothalamus. The D2-class, pre- and post-synaptic, is inhibitory and includes the D2 receptors in the striatum, nucleus accumbens, d cortex and anterior pituitary, D3 in the ventromedial striatum and nucleus accumbens, and D4 in the cortex and the hippocampus. These last two receptors are less abundant in the brain. In schizophrenia, hyperactivity of the mesolimbic pathway may, among other things,[106] be responsible for symptoms such as delusions and hallucinations. Conventional neuroleptics have the effect of blocking D2 receptors, thus reducing hallucinatory and delusional symptoms. However, these molecules have the disadvantage of binding to other pathways like the nigrostriatal pathway causing movement disorders (dyskinesia), or the meso-cortical pathway, causing cognitive slowing, and the tuberoinfundibular pathway causing increased levels of prolactin.

Serotonin

All the neurons producing serotonin [5-hydroxytryptamine (5-HT)] within the brain are located in the medial part of the brainstem. They are the raphe nuclei (Fig. 2.31).

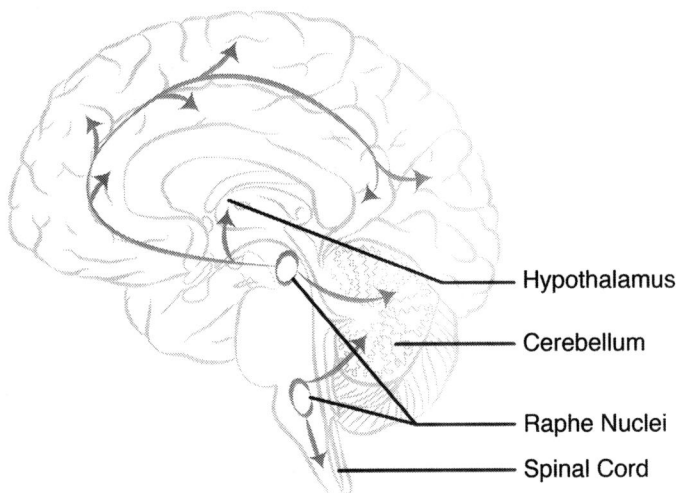

Fig. 2.31 The serotonergic pathway

[106] Multiple neurobiological hypothesis try to explain the symptoms of schizophrenia. Dopaminergic hypothesis, formulated in 1973, comes from the efficiency of chlorpromazine, which changed, as we saw, the way of dealing with this psychosis in the 1950s. The serotoninergic hypothesis is nowadays confronted by the fact that another drug—clozapine— efficient in treating delusional symptoms, possesses more affinity for certain serotonin receptors than for dopamine's. This is why it has the advantage of not provoking undesirable motor effects of first-generation neuroleptics. The glutamate, which plays a role in memorization, learning and brain development, like GABA, inhibitor neurotransmitter, were also involved. To this we can add neurodevelopmental hypothesis. Brain imaging developed the idea that schizophrenia could be a problem of cortical function. Events during pregnancy could disturb multiplication and neuronal migration as well. Genetic, as well as environmental factors, are also explored, given that 15 % of schizophrenias are congenital.

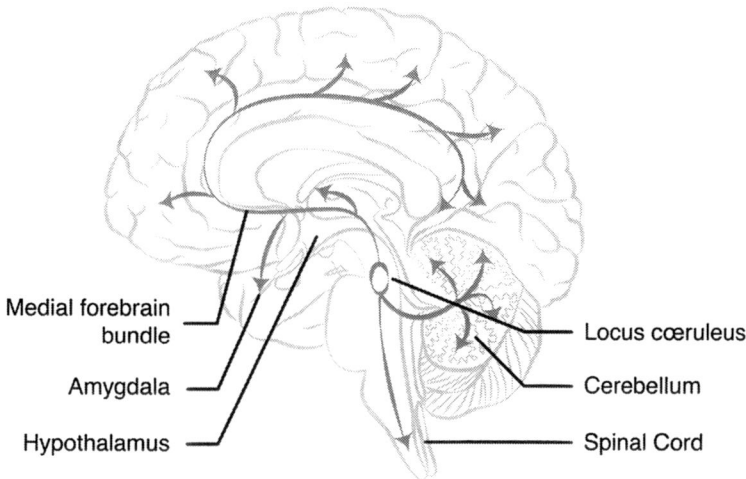

Fig. 2.32 The noradrenergic pathway

   Their projections irrigate the entire central nervous system. In the lower part of the brainstem, these projections reach the spinal cord and modulate pain messages. Neurons in the upper part project throughout the brain and are involved in thermoregulation, regulation of mood, and the sleep–wake cycle.

Norepinephrine and the Stress Circuit

The nuclei secreting neurons are primarily located in a nucleus in the brainstem: thee locus cœruleus (Fig. 2.32).

   This nucleus, which has close ties with the amygdala projects axons to almost all of the brain through a network of channels in common with dopaminergic neurons, within the MFB and serotonergic neurons. As with the amygdala, stimulation of the locus coeruleus causes anxiety behavior in animals, and conversely, the tranquilizing substances such as benzodiazepines, alcohol, or opiates decrease its activity. Norepinephrine is involved in operation of the body's alarm system via the sympathetic nervous system and the hypothalamic–pituitary–adrenal axis (Fig. 2.15, p. 73). Norepinephrine is also involved alongside serotonin, in the regulation of attention and vigilance. Noradrenergic hyperactivity can lead to anxiety and hypoactivity to depression.

References

1. Hippocrate, Jouanna J (2003) La maladie sacrée texte établi et trad. par Jacques Jouanna. Hippocrate Tome II, vol 3. les Belles lettres, Paris
2. Freud S, Frossard J, classiques La (2010) Au-delà du principe de plaisir texte intégral [Enregistrement sonore]. [Caen]: Alexis Brun productions
3. Cabanis P-J-G (1823) Oeuvres complètes de Cabanis. Bossange frères, Paris
4. Broca P (1878) Anatomie comparée des circonvolutions cérébrales: le grand lobe limbique. Rev Anthropol 1:385–498
5. Papez JW (1937) A proposed mechanism of emotion. Arch Neurol Psychiatry 38(1):725–743
6. MacLean P (1949) Psychosomatic disease and the "visceral brain" recent developments bearing on the Papez theory of emotion. Psychosom Med 11(6):338–353
7. Kotter R, Stephan KE (1997) Useless or helpful? The "limbic system" concept. Rev Neurosci 8(2):139–145
8. Burruss JW, Hurley RA, Taber KH, Rauch RA, Norton RE, Hayman LA (2000) Functional neuroanatomy of the frontal lobe circuits. Radiology 214(1):227–230
9. Pirot S (2003) L'anatomie fonctionnelle du cortex préfrontal: du singeà l'homme. Encephale 20:27–31
10. Fuster JM (2001) The prefrontal cortex–an update: time is of the essence. Neuron 30(2):319–333. doi:S0896-6273(01)00285-9 [pii]
11. Bergson H (1911) L'énergie spirituelle. Ed. Alcan, Paris
12. Rauch SL, Dougherty DD, Malone D, Rezai A, Friehs G, Fischman AJ et al (2006) A functional neuroimaging investigation of deep brain stimulation in patients with obsessive-compulsive disorder. J Neurosurg 104(4):558–565. doi:10.3171/jns.2006.104.4.558
13. Drevets WC (1998) Functional neuroimaging studies of depression: the anatomy of melancholia. Annu Rev Med 49:341–361. doi:10.1146/annurev.med.49.1.341
14. Baxter LR Jr, Schwartz JM, Phelps ME, Mazziotta JC, Guze BH, Selin CE et al (1989) Reduction of prefrontal cortex glucose metabolism common to three types of depression. Arch Gen Psychiatry 46(3):243–250
15. Mottaghy FM, Keller CE, Gangitano M, Ly J, Thall M, Parker JA et al (2002) Correlation of cerebral blood flow and treatment effects of repetitive transcranial magnetic stimulation in depressed patients. Psychiatry Res 115(1–2):1–14. doi:S092549270200032X [pii]
16. Kito S, Fujita K, Koga Y (2008) Changes in regional cerebral blood flow after repetitive transcranial magnetic stimulation of the left dorsolateral prefrontal cortex in treatment-resistant depression. J Neuropsychiatry Clin Neurosci 20(1):74–80. doi:10.1176/appi.neuropsych.20.1.74
17. Richieri R, Adida M, Dumas R, Fakra E, Azorin JM, Pringuey D et al (2010) Affective disorders and repetitive transcranial magnetic stimulation: therapeutic innovations. Encephale 36(Suppl 6):S197–S201. doi:10.1016/S0013-7006(10)70057-9
18. Bechara A, Damasio H, Damasio AR (2000) Emotion, decision making and the orbitofrontal cortex. Cereb Cortex 10(3):295–307
19. Ollat HP S (2004) Cortex orbitofrontal, comportement et émotions. Encéphale. 25:25–33
20. Rolls ET (2004) The functions of the orbitofrontal cortex. Brain Cogn 55(1):11–29. doi:10.1016/S0278-2626(03)00277-X
21. Tremblay L, Schultz W (1999) Relative reward preference in primate orbitofrontal cortex. Nature 398(6729):704–708. doi:10.1038/19525
22. Aouizerate BM-G C, Cuny E, Guehl D, Amieva H, Benazzouz A, Fabrigoule C, Allard M, Rougier A, Burbaud P, Tignol J, Bioulac B (2005) Stimulation cérébrale profonde du striatum ventral dans le traitement du trouble obsessionnel-compulsif avec dépression majeure. Médecine et Sciences 21(10):811–813
23. Damasio H, Damasio AR (1989) Lesion analysis in neuropsychology. Oxford University Press, New York

24. Baxter LR Jr (1994) Positron emission tomography studies of cerebral glucose metabolism in obsessive compulsive disorder. J Clin Psychiatry 55(Suppl):54–59
25. Swedo SE, Pietrini P, Leonard HL, Schapiro MB, Rettew DC, Goldberger EL et al (1992) Cerebral glucose metabolism in childhood-onset obsessive-compulsive disorder Revisualization during pharmacotherapy. Arch Gen Psychiatry 49(9):690–694
26. Trivedi MH (1996) Functional neuroanatomy of obsessive-compulsive disorder. J Clin Psychiatry 57(8):26–35 (discussion 6)
27. Brown JW, Braver TS (2005) Learned predictions of error likelihood in the anterior cingulate cortex. Science 307(5712):1118–1121. doi:10.1126/science.1105783
28. Damasio AR, Blanc M (1995) L' erreur de Descartes la raison des émotions trad. de l'anglais... par Marcel Blanc. O. Jacob, Paris
29. Mayberg HS, Liotti M, Brannan SK, McGinnis S, Mahurin RK, Jerabek PA et al (1999) Reciprocal limbic-cortical function and negative mood: converging PET findings in depression and normal sadness. Am J Psychiatry 156(5):675–682
30. Dougherty DD, Weiss AP, Cosgrove GR, Alpert NM, Cassem EH, Nierenberg AA et al (2003) Cerebral metabolic correlates as potential predictors of response to anterior cingulotomy for treatment of major depression. J Neurosurg 99(6):1010–1017. doi:10.3171/jns.2003.99.6. 1010
31. Kluver HB (1937) P. C. Psychic 'blindness' and other symptoms following bilateral temporal lobectomy. Am J Physiol 119:254–284
32. Clarac F, Ternaux J-P, Buser P (2008) Encyclopédie historique des neurosciences du neurone à l'émergence de la pensée avant-propos de Dominique Wolton préface de Pierre Buser. Neurosciences et cognition. De Boeck, Bruxelles (Paris)
33. Weiskrantz L (1956) Behavioral changes associated with ablation of the amygdaloid complex in monkeys. J Comp Physiol Psychol 49(4):381–391
34. Gil R Lamoglia E (2010) Neuropsychologie. Elsevier Health Sciences France
35. Martin JH (2003) Neuroanatomy: text and atlas. McGraw-Hill
36. Kunst-Wilson WR, Zajonc RB (1980) Affective discrimination of stimuli that cannot be recognized. Science 207(4430):557–558
37. Cannon WB (1931) Again the James-Lange and the thalamic theories of emotion. Psychol Rev 38(4):281–295
38. Adolphs R, Tranel D, Damasio H, Damasio A (1994) Impaired recognition of emotion in facial expressions following bilateral damage to the human amygdala. Nature 372(6507): 669–672. doi:10.1038/372669a0
39. LeDoux JE (1999) The emotional brain : the mysterious underpinnings of emotional life. Phoenix, London
40. Siever LJ (2008) Neurobiology of aggression and violence. Am J Psychiatry 165(4):429–442. doi:10.1176/appi.ajp.2008.07111774
41. Narabayashi H, Uno M (1966) Long range results of stereotaxic amygdalotomy for behavior disorders. Confin Neurol 27(1):168–171
42. Narabayashi H, Nagao T, Saito Y, Yoshida M, Nagahata M (1963) Stereotaxic amygdalotomy for behavior disorders. Arch Neurol 9:1–16
43. Balasubramaniam V, Ramamurthi B (1970) Stereotaxic amygdalotomy in behavior disorders. Confin Neurol 32(2):367–373
44. Hitchcock E, Cairns V (1973) Amygdalotomy. Postgrad Med J 49(578):894–904
45. Small IF, Heimburger RF, Small JG, Milstein V, Moore DF (1977) Follow-up of stereotaxic amygdalotomy for seizure and behavior disorders. Biol Psychiatry 12(3):401–411
46. Mempel E, Witkiewicz B, Stadnicki R, Luczywek E, Kucinski L, Pawlowski G et al (1980) The effect of medial amygdalotomy and anterior hippocampotomy on behavior and seizures in epileptic patients. Acta Neurochir Suppl (Wien) 30:161–167
47. Jacobson R (1986) Disorders of facial recognition, social behaviour and affect after combined bilateral amygdalotomy and subcaudate tractotomy–a clinical and experimental study. Psychol Med 16(2):439–450

48. Ramamurthi B (1988) Stereotactic operation in behaviour disorders. Amygdalotomy and hypothalamotomy. Acta Neurochir Suppl (Wien) 44:152–157
49. Fountas KN, Smith JR (2007) Historical evolution of stereotactic amygdalotomy for the management of severe aggression. J Neurosurg 106(4):710–713. doi:10.3171/jns.2007.106.4.710
50. Anderson AK, Phelps EA (2001) Lesions of the human amygdala impair enhanced perception of emotionally salient events. Nature 411(6835):305–309. doi:10.1038/35077083
51. Franzini A, Ferroli P, Leone M, Broggi G (2003) Stimulation of the posterior hypothalamus for treatment of chronic intractable cluster headaches: first reported series. Neurosurgery 52(5):1095–1099 (discussion 9–101)
52. Cahill L, Babinsky R, Markowitsch HJ, McGaugh JL (1995) The amygdala and emotional memory. Nature 377(6547):295–296. doi:10.1038/377295a0
53. Ambroggi F, Ishikawa A, Fields HL, Nicola SM (2008) Basolateral amygdala neurons facilitate reward-seeking behavior by exciting nucleus accumbens neurons. Neuron 59(4):648–661. doi:10.1016/j.neuron.2008.07.004
54. Frenois F, Stinus L, Di Blasi F, Cador M, Le Moine C (2005) A specific limbic circuit underlies opiate withdrawal memories. J Neurosci 25(6):1366–1374. doi:10.1523/JNEUROSCI.3090-04.2005
55. Hafting T, Fyhn M, Molden S, Moser MB, Moser EI (2005) Microstructure of a spatial map in the entorhinal cortex. Nature 436(7052):801–806. doi:10.1038/nature03721
56. Bear MF, Connors BW, Paradiso MA, Nieoullon A (2007) Neurosciences à la découverte du cerveau traduction et adaptation françaises, André Nieoullon. 3e éd. Rueil-Malmaison: Pradel
57. Vincent J-DL P-M (2012) Le cerveau sur mesure. Odile Jacob, Paris
58. Bontempi B, Laurent-Demir C, Destrade C, Jaffard R (1999) Time-dependent reorganization of brain circuitry underlying long-term memory storage. Nature 400(6745):671–675. doi:10.1038/23270
59. Maguire EA, Frackowiak RS, Frith CD (1997) Recalling routes around london: activation of the right hippocampus in taxi drivers. J Neurosci 17(18):7103–7110
60. Suthana N, Haneef Z, Stern J, Mukamel R, Behnke E, Knowlton B et al (2012) Memory enhancement and deep-brain stimulation of the entorhinal area. N Engl J Med 366(6):502–510. doi:10.1056/NEJMoa1107212
61. Hamani C, McAndrews MP, Cohn M, Oh M, Zumsteg D, Shapiro CM et al (2008) Memory enhancement induced by hypothalamic/fornix deep brain stimulation. Ann Neurol 63(1):119–123. doi:10.1002/ana.21295
62. Laxton AW, Tang-Wai DF, McAndrews MP, Zumsteg D, Wennberg R, Keren R et al (2010) A phase I trial of deep brain stimulation of memory circuits in Alzheimer's disease. Ann Neurol 68(4):521–534. doi:10.1002/ana.22089
63. Damasio AR, Fidel J-L (2010) L' autre moi-même les nouvelles cartes du cerveau, de la conscience et des émotions traduit de l'anglais (États-Unis) par Jean-Luc Fidel. O. Jacob, Paris
64. Ansermet F, Magistretti P (2004) À chacun son cerveau plasticité neuronale et inconscient. Collection dirigée par Bertrand Cramer et Bernard Golse. O. Jacob, Paris
65. Hohmann GW (1966) Some effects of spinal cord lesions on experienced emotional feelings. Psychophysiology 3(2):143–156
66. Nicotra A, Critchley HD, Mathias CJ, Dolan RJ (2006) Emotional and autonomic consequences of spinal cord injury explored using functional brain imaging. Brain 129(3):718–728. doi:10.1093/brain/awh699
67. Heller AC, Amar AP, Liu CY, Apuzzo ML (2006) Surgery of the mind and mood: a mosaic of issues in time and evolution. Neurosurgery 59(4):720–733 (discussion 33–9). doi:10.1227/01.NEU.0000240227.72514.27 00006123-200610000-00003 [pii]
68. Torres N, Chabardes S, Benabid AL (2011) Rationale for hypothalamus-deep brain stimulation in food intake disorders and obesity. Adv Tech Stand Neurosurg 36:17–30. doi:10.1007/978-3-7091-0179-7_2

69. Anand BK, Brobeck JR (1951) Localization of a "feeding center" in the hypothalamus of the rat. Proc Soc Exp Biol Med 77(2):323–324
70. Goldney RD (1978) Craniopharyngioma simulating anorexia nervosa. J Nerv Ment Dis 166(2):135–138
71. Heron GB, Johnston DA (1976) Hypothalamic tumor presenting as anorexia nervosa. Am J Psychiatry 133(5):580–582
72. Weller RA, Weller EB (1982) Anorexia nervosa in a patient with an infiltrating tumor of the hypothalamus. Am J Psychiatry 139(6):824–825
73. Anand BK, Dua S, Shoenberg K (1955) Hypothalamic control of food intake in cats and monkeys. J Physiol 127(1):143–152
74. Letter Quaade F (1974) Stereotaxy for obesity. Lancet 1(7851):267
75. Maschke M, Tuite PJ, Pickett K, Wachter T, Konczak J (2005) The effect of subthalamic nucleus stimulation on kinaesthesia in Parkinson's disease. J Neurol Neurosurg Psychiatry 76(4):569–571. doi:10.1136/jnnp.2004.047324
76. Tuite PJ, Maxwell RE, Ikramuddin S, Kotz CM, Billington CJ, Laseski MA et al (2005) Weight and body mass index in Parkinson's disease patients after deep brain stimulation surgery. Parkinsonism Relat Disord 11(4):247–252. doi:10.1016/j.parkreldis.2005.01.006
77. Novakova L, Ruzicka E, Jech R, Serranova T, Dusek P, Urgosik D (2007) Increase in body weight is a non-motor side effect of deep brain stimulation of the subthalamic nucleus in Parkinson's disease. Neuro Endocrinol Lett 28(1):21–25. doi:NEL280107A05
78. Tomycz ND, Whiting DM, Oh MY (2012) Deep brain stimulation for obesity–from theoretical foundations to designing the first human pilot study. Neurosurg Rev 35(1):37–42 (discussion 3). doi:10.1007/s10143-011-0359-9
79. Sano K, Mayanagi Y, Sekino H, Ogashiwa M, Ishijima B (1970) Results of timulation and destruction of the posterior hypothalamus in man. J Neurosurg 33(6):689–707. doi:10.3171/jns.1970.33.6.0689
80. Sano K, Mayanagi Y (1988) Posteromedial hypothalamotomy in the treatment of violent, aggressive behaviour. Acta Neurochir Suppl (Wien) 44:145–151
81. Bejjani BP, Houeto JL, Hariz M, Yelnik J, Mesnage V, Bonnet AM et al (2002) Aggressive behavior induced by intraoperative stimulation in the triangle of Sano. Neurology 59(9):1425–1427
82. May A, Bahra A, Buchel C, Frackowiak RS, Goadsby PJ (1998) Hypothalamic activation in cluster headache attacks. Lancet 352(9124):275–278. doi:10.1016/S0140-6736(98)02470-2
83. Leone M, Franzini A, Bussone G (2001) Stereotactic stimulation of posterior hypothalamic gray matter in a patient with intractable cluster headache. N Engl J Med 345(19):1428–1429. doi:10.1056/NEJM200111083451915
84. Woon FL, Sood S, Hedges DW (2010) Hippocampal volume deficits associated with exposure to psychological trauma and posttraumatic stress disorder in adults: a meta-analysis. Prog Neuropsychopharmacol Biol Psychiatry 34(7):1181–1188. doi:10.1016/j.pnpbp.2010.06.016
85. Brown ES, Rush AJ, McEwen BS (1999) Hippocampal remodeling and damage by corticosteroids: implications for mood disorders. Neuropsychopharmacology 21(4):474–484. doi:10.1016/S0893-133X(99)00054-8
86. Starkman MN, Gebarski SS, Berent S, Schteingart DE (1992) Hippocampal formation volume, memory dysfunction, and cortisol levels in patients with Cushing's syndrome. Biol Psychiatry 32(9):756–765
87. Kosfeld M, Heinrichs M, Zak PJ, Fischbacher U, Fehr E (2005) Oxytocin increases trust in humans. Nature 435(7042):673–676. doi:10.1038/nature03701
88. Andari E, Duhamel JR, Zalla T, Herbrecht E, Leboyer M, Sirigu A (2010) Promoting social behavior with oxytocin in high-functioning autism spectrum disorders. Proc Natl Acad Sci U S A 107(9):4389–4394. doi:10.1073/pnas.0910249107
89. Feifel D, Macdonald K, Nguyen A, Cobb P, Warlan H, Galangue B et al (2010) Adjunctive intranasal oxytocin reduces symptoms in schizophrenia patients. Biol Psychiatry 68(7):678–680. doi:10.1016/j.biopsych.2010.04.039

90. Olds J, Milner P (1954) Positive reinforcement produced by electrical stimulation of septal area and other regions of rat brain. J Comp Physiol Psychol 47(6):419–427
91. Schvarcz JR (1993) Long-term results of stimulation of the septal area for relief of neurogenic pain. Acta Neurochir Suppl (Wien) 58:154–155
92. Schvarcz JR (1985) Chronic stimulation of the septal area for the relief of intractable pain. Appl Neurophysiol 48(1–6):191–194
93. Heath RG (1963) Electrical self-stimulation of the brain in man. Am J Psychiatry 120: 571–577
94. Oshima H, Katayama Y (2010) Neuroethics of deep brain stimulation for mental disorders: brain stimulation reward in humans. Neurol Med Chir (Tokyo) 50(9):845–852. doi:JST. JSTAGE/nmc/50.845 [pii]
95. Heath RM, WA (1960) Evaluation of seven years' experience with depth electrode studies in human patients. In: Hoeber PB, O'Doherty DS (ed) Electrical studies on the unanesthetized human brain. New York, pp 214–247
96. Gol A (1967) Relief of pain by electrical stimulation of the septal area. J Neurol Sci 5(1):115–120
97. Moan CH R (1972) Septal stimulation for the initiation of heterosexual behavior in a homosexual male. Experimental Psychiatry 3(1):23–26
98. Hodaie M, Wennberg RA, Dostrovsky JO, Lozano AM (2002) Chronic anterior thalamus stimulation for intractable epilepsy. Epilepsia. 43(6):603–608
99. Pollo C, Villemure JG (2007) Rationale, mechanisms of efficacy, anatomical targets and future prospects of electrical deep brain stimulation for epilepsy. Acta Neurochir Suppl 97(2):311–320
100. Chabardes S, Minotti L, Chassagnon S, Piallat B, Torres N, Seigneuret E et al (2008) Basal ganglia deep-brain stimulation for treatment of drug-resistant epilepsy: review and current data. Neurochirurgie 54(3):436–440. doi:10.1016/j.neuchi.2008.02.039
101. Alexander GE, DeLong MR, Strick PL (1986) Parallel organization of functionally segregated circuits linking basal ganglia and cortex. Annu Rev Neurosci 9:357–381. doi:10. 1146/annurev.ne.09.030186.002041
102. Llinas RR, Ribary U, Jeanmonod D, Kronberg E, Mitra PP (1999) Thalamocortical dysrhythmia: a neurological and neuropsychiatric syndrome characterized by magnetoencephalography. Proc Natl Acad Sci U S A 96(26):15222–15227
103. Yelnik J (2002) Functional anatomy of the basal ganglia. Mov Disord 17(Suppl 3):S15–S21. doi:10.1002/mds.10138
104. Kumar R, Lozano AM, Kim YJ, Hutchison WD, Sime E, Halket E et al (1998) Double-blind evaluation of subthalamic nucleus deep brain stimulation in advanced Parkinson's disease. Neurology 51(3):850–855
105. Pillon B, Ardouin C, Damier P, Krack P, Houeto JL, Klinger H et al (2000) Neuropsychological changes between "off" and "on" STN or GPi stimulation in Parkinson's disease. Neurology 55(3):411–418
106. Alegret M, Junque C, Valldeoriola F, Vendrell P, Pilleri M, Rumia J et al (2001) Effects of bilateral subthalamic stimulation on cognitive function in Parkinson disease. Arch Neurol 58(8):1223–1227. doi:noc00295
107. Brusa L, Pierantozzi M, Peppe A, Altibrandi MG, Giacomini P, Mazzone P et al (2001) Deep brain stimulation (DBS) attentional effects parallel those of l-dopa treatment. J Neural Transm 108(8–9):1021–1027
108. Dujardin K, Defebvre L, Krystkowiak P, Blond S, Destee A (2001) Influence of chronic bilateral stimulation of the subthalamic nucleus on cognitive function in Parkinson's disease. J Neurol 248(7):603–611
109. Moretti R, Torre P, Antonello RM, Capus L, Gioulis M, Marsala SZ et al (2001) Effects on cognitive abilities following subthalamic nucleus stimulation in Parkinson's disease. Eur J Neurol 8(6):726–727. doi:263

110. Moretti R, Torre P, Antonello RM, Capus L, Gioulis M, Marsala SZ et al (2002) Cognitive changes following subthalamic nucleus stimulation in two patients with Parkinson disease. Percept Mot Skills 95(2):477–486

111. Valldeoriola F, Pilleri M, Tolosa E, Molinuevo JL, Rumia J, Ferrer E (2002) Bilateral subthalamic stimulation monotherapy in advanced Parkinson's disease: long-term follow-up of patients. Mov Disord 17(1):125–132. doi:10.1002/mds.1278

112. Daniele A, Albanese A, Contarino MF, Zinzi P, Barbier A, Gasparini F et al (2003) Cognitive and behavioural effects of chronic stimulation of the subthalamic nucleus in patients with Parkinson's disease. J Neurol Neurosurg Psychiatry 74(2):175–182

113. Gironell A, Kulisevsky J, Rami L, Fortuny N, Garcia-Sanchez C, Pascual-Sedano B (2003) Effects of pallidotomy and bilateral subthalamic stimulation on cognitive function in Parkinson disease A controlled comparative study. J Neurol 250(8):917–923. doi:10.1007/s00415-003-1109-x

114. Saint-Cyr JA, Trepanier LL, Kumar R, Lozano AM, Lang AE (2000) Neuropsychological consequences of chronic bilateral stimulation of the subthalamic nucleus in Parkinson's disease. Brain 123(10):2091–2108

115. Trepanier LL, Kumar R, Lozano AM, Lang AE, Saint-Cyr JA (2000) Neuropsychological outcome of GPi pallidotomy and GPi or STN deep brain stimulation in Parkinson's disease. Brain Cogn 42(3):324–347. doi:10.1006/brcg.1999.1108

116. Kleiner-Fisman G, Fisman DN, Sime E, Saint-Cyr JA, Lozano AM, Lang AE (2003) Long-term follow up of bilateral deep brain stimulation of the subthalamic nucleus in patients with advanced Parkinson disease. J Neurosurg 99(3):489–495. doi:10.3171/jns.2003.99.3.0489

117. Hershey T, Revilla FJ, Wernle A, Gibson PS, Dowling JL, Perlmutter JS (2004) Stimulation of STN impairs aspects of cognitive control in PD. Neurology 62(7):1110–1114

118. Moretti R, Torre P, Antonello RM, Capus L, Marsala SZ, Cattaruzza T et al (2003) Neuropsychological changes after subthalamic nucleus stimulation: a 12 month follow-up in nine patients with Parkinson's disease. Parkinsonism Relat Disord 10(2):73–79. doi:S1353802003000737

119. Temel Y, Visser-Vandewalle V, Aendekerk B, Rutten B, Tan S, Scholtissen B et al (2005) Acute and separate modulation of motor and cognitive performance in parkinsonian rats by bilateral stimulation of the subthalamic nucleus. Exp Neurol 193(1):43–52. doi:10.1016/j.expneurol.2004.12.025

120. Krack P, Kumar R, Ardouin C, Dowsey PL, McVicker JM, Benabid AL et al (2001) Mirthful laughter induced by subthalamic nucleus stimulation. Mov Disord 16(5):867–875. doi:10.1002/mds.1174

121. Kulisevsky J, Berthier ML, Gironell A, Pascual-Sedano B, Molet J, Pares P (2002) Mania following deep brain stimulation for Parkinson's disease. Neurology 59(9):1421–1424

122. Romito LM, Raja M, Daniele A, Contarino MF, Bentivoglio AR, Barbier A et al (2002) Transient mania with hypersexuality after surgery for high frequency stimulation of the subthalamic nucleus in Parkinson's disease. Mov Disord 17(6):1371–1374. doi:10.1002/mds.10265

123. Rodriguez MC, Guridi OJ, Alvarez L, Mewes K, Macias R, Vitek J et al (1998) The subthalamic nucleus and tremor in Parkinson's disease. Mov Disord 13(Suppl 3):111–118

124. Kumar R, Lozano AM, Sime E, Halket E, Lang AE (1999) Comparative effects of unilateral and bilateral subthalamic nucleus deep brain stimulation. Neurology 53(3):561–566

125. Moro E, Scerrati M, Romito LM, Roselli R, Tonali P, Albanese A (1999) Chronic subthalamic nucleus stimulation reduces medication requirements in Parkinson's disease. Neurology 53(1):85–90

126. Molinuevo JL, Valldeoriola F, Tolosa E, Rumia J, Valls-Sole J, Roldan H et al (2000) Levodopa withdrawal after bilateral subthalamic nucleus stimulation in advanced Parkinson disease. Arch Neurol 57(7):983–988. doi:noc90071

127. Berney A, Vingerhoets F, Perrin A, Guex P, Villemure JG, Burkhard PR et al (2002) Effect on mood of subthalamic DBS for Parkinson's disease: a consecutive series of 24 patients. Neurology 59(9):1427–1429

128. Brown RG (2002) Behavioural disorders, Parkinson's disease, and subthalamic stimulation. J Neurol Neurosurg Psychiatry 72(6):689

129. Doshi PK, Chhaya N, Bhatt MH (2002) Depression leading to attempted suicide after bilateral subthalamic nucleus stimulation for Parkinson's disease. Mov Disord 17(5): 1084–1085. doi:10.1002/mds.10198

130. Houeto JL, Mesnage V, Mallet L, Pillon B, Gargiulo M, du Moncel ST et al (2002) Behavioural disorders, Parkinson's disease and subthalamic stimulation. J Neurol Neurosurg Psychiatry 72(6):701–707

131. Martinez-Martin P, Valldeoriola F, Tolosa E, Pilleri M, Molinuevo JL, Rumia J et al (2002) Bilateral subthalamic nucleus stimulation and quality of life in advanced Parkinson's disease. Mov Disord 17(2):372–377. doi:10.1002/mds.10044

132. Ostergaard K, Sunde N, Dupont E (2002) Effects of bilateral stimulation of the subthalamic nucleus in patients with severe Parkinson's disease and motor fluctuations. Mov Disord 17(4):693–700. doi:10.1002/mds.10188

133. Thobois S, Mertens P, Guenot M, Hermier M, Mollion H, Bouvard M et al (2002) Subthalamic nucleus stimulation in Parkinson's disease: clinical evaluation of 18 patients. J Neurol 249(5):529–534. doi:10.1007/s004150200059

134. Iranzo A, Valldeoriola F, Santamaria J, Tolosa E, Rumia J (2002) Sleep symptoms and polysomnographic architecture in advanced Parkinson's disease after chronic bilateral subthalamic stimulation. J Neurol Neurosurg Psychiatry 72(5):661–664

135. Vingerhoets FJ, Villemure JG, Temperli P, Pollo C, Pralong E, Ghika J (2002) Subthalamic DBS replaces levodopa in Parkinson's disease: two-year follow-up. Neurology 58(3): 396–401

136. Volkmann J, Allert N, Voges J, Weiss PH, Freund HJ, Sturm V (2001) Safety and efficacy of pallidal or subthalamic nucleus stimulation in advanced PD. Neurology 56(4):548–551

137. Krack P, Batir A, Van Blercom N, Chabardes S, Fraix V, Ardouin C et al (2003) Five-year follow-up of bilateral stimulation of the subthalamic nucleus in advanced Parkinson's disease. N Engl J Med 349(20):1925–1934. doi:10.1056/NEJMoa035275

138. Krause M, Fogel W, Heck A, Hacke W, Bonsanto M, Trenkwalder C et al (2001) Deep brain stimulation for the treatment of Parkinson's disease: subthalamic nucleus versus globus pallidus internus. J Neurol Neurosurg Psychiatry 70(4):464–470

139. Burn DJ, Troster AI (2004) Neuropsychiatric complications of medical and surgical therapies for Parkinson's disease. J Geriatr Psychiatry Neurol 17(3):172–180. doi:10.1177/0891988704267466

140. Witjas T, Baunez C, Henry JM, Delfini M, Regis J, Cherif AA et al (2005) Addiction in Parkinson's disease: impact of subthalamic nucleus deep brain stimulation. Mov Disord 20(8):1052–1055. doi:10.1002/mds.20501

141. Temel Y, Kessels A, Tan S, Topdag A, Boon P, Visser-Vandewalle V (2006) Behavioural changes after bilateral subthalamic stimulation in advanced Parkinson disease: a systematic review. Parkinsonism Relat Disord 12(5):265–272. doi:10.1016/j.parkreldis.2006.01.004

142. Nowinski WL, Belov D, Pollak P, Benabid AL (2005) Statistical analysis of 168 bilateral subthalamic nucleus implantations by means of the probabilistic functional atlas. Neurosurgery 57(4 Suppl):319–330 (discussion 30). doi:00006123-200510004-00014 [pii]

143. Aouizerate B, Martin-Guehl C, Cuny E, Guehl D, Amieva H, Benazzouz A et al (2005) Deep brain stimulation of the ventral striatum in the treatment of obsessive-compulsive disorder and major depression. Med Sci (Paris) 21(10):811–813. doi:10.1051/medsci/20052110811

144. Jog MS, Kubota Y, Connolly CI, Hillegaart V, Graybiel AM (1999) Building neural representations of habits. Science 286(5445):1745–1749

145. Mogenson GJ, Jones DL, Yim CY (1980) From motivation to action: functional interface between the limbic system and the motor system. Prog Neurobiol 14(2–3):69–97

146. Sturm V, Lenartz D, Koulousakis A, Treuer H, Herholz K, Klein JC et al (2003) The nucleus accumbens: a target for deep brain stimulation in obsessive-compulsive- and anxiety-disorders. J Chem Neuroanat 26(4):293–299

147. Heinze HJH M. Voges J, Hinrichs H, Marco-Pallares J, Hopf JM, Muller UJ, Galazky I, Sturm V, Bogerts B, Munte TF (2009) Counteracting incentive sensitization in severe alcohol dependence using deep brain stimulation of the nucleus accumbens: clinical and basic science aspects. Frontiers Hum Neurosci 3(22)

148. Huff W, Lenartz D, Schormann M, Lee SH, Kuhn J, Koulousakis A et al (2010) Unilateral deep brain stimulation of the nucleus accumbens in patients with treatment-resistant obsessive-compulsive disorder: outcomes after one year. Clin Neurol Neurosurg 112(2):137–143. doi:10.1016/j.clineuro.2009.11.006

149. van Kuyck K, Gabriels L, Cosyns P, Arckens L, Sturm V, Rasmussen S et al (2007) Behavioural and physiological effects of electrical stimulation in the nucleus accumbens: a review. Acta Neurochir Suppl 97(Pt 2):375–391

150. Lopes da Silva FH, Arnolds DE, Neijt HC (1984) A functional link between the limbic cortex and ventral striatum: physiology of the subiculum accumbens pathway. Exp Brain Res 55(2):205–214

151. DeFrance JF, Marchand JF, Sikes RW, Chronister RB, Hubbard JI (1985) Characterization of fimbria input to nucleus accumbens. J Neurophysiol 54(6):1553–1567

152. Yang CR, Mogenson GJ (1984) Electrophysiological responses of neurones in the nucleus accumbens to hippocampal stimulation and the attenuation of the excitatory responses by the mesolimbic dopaminergic system. Brain Res 324(1):69–84

153. Berendse HW, Groenewegen HJ (1990) Organization of the thalamostriatal projections in the rat, with special emphasis on the ventral striatum. J Comp Neurol 299(2):187–228. doi:10.1002/cne.902990206

154. Brog JS, Salyapongse A, Deutch AY, Zahm DS (1993) The patterns of afferent innervation of the core and shell in the "accumbens" part of the rat ventral striatum: immunohistochemical detection of retrogradely transported fluoro-gold. J Comp Neurol 338(2):255–278. doi:10.1002/cne.903380209

155. Montaron MF, Deniau JM, Menetrey A, Glowinski J, Thierry AM (1996) Prefrontal cortex inputs of the nucleus accumbens-nigro-thalamic circuit. Neuroscience 71(2):371–382

156. de Koning PP. van den Munckhof P, Figee M, Schuurman PR, Denys D (2012) Deep bain stimulation in obsessive-compulsive disorder targeted at the nucleus accumbens. In: Denys D, Feenstra M, Schuurman R (eds) Deep Brain Stimulation: a new frontier in psychiatry. Springer, pp 43–51

157. Yang CR, Mogenson GJ (1989) Ventral pallidal neuronal responses to dopamine receptor stimulation in the nucleus accumbens. Brain Res 489(2):237–246

158. Churchill L, Kalivas PW (1994) A topographically organized gamma-aminobutyric acid projection from the ventral pallidum to the nucleus accumbens in the rat. J Comp Neurol 345(4):579–595. doi:10.1002/cne.903450408

159. Zaborszky L, Cullinan WE (1992) Projections from the nucleus accumbens to cholinergic neurons of the ventral pallidum: a correlated light and electron microscopic double-immunolabeling study in rat. Brain Res 570(1–2):92–101

160. Fallon JH, Moore RY (1978) Catecholamine innervation of the basal forebrain. IV. Topography of the dopamine projection to the basal forebrain and neostriatum. J Comp Neurol 180(3):545–580. doi:10.1002/cne.901800310

161. Phillipson OT, Griffiths AC (1985) The topographic order of inputs to nucleus accumbens in the rat. Neuroscience 16(2):275–296

162. Heimer L, Zahm DS, Churchill L, Kalivas PW, Wohltmann C (1991) Specificity in the projection patterns of accumbal core and shell in the rat. Neuroscience 41(1):89–125

163. Mogenson GJ, Takigawa M, Robertson A, Wu M (1979) Self-stimulation of the nucleus accumbens and ventral tegmental area of Tsai attenuated by microinjections of spiroperidol into the nucleus accumbens. Brain Res 171(2):247–259

164. Prado-Alcala R, Wise RA (1984) Brain stimulation reward and dopamine terminal fields. I. Caudate-putamen, nucleus accumbens and amygdala. Brain Res 297(2):265–273. doi:0006-8993(84)90567-5 [pii]
165. Rolls ET, Burton MJ, Mora F (1980) Neurophysiological analysis of brain-stimulation reward in the monkey. Brain Res 194(2):339–357
166. Zacharko RM, Kasian M, Irwin J, Zalcman S, LaLonde G, MacNeil G et al (1990) Behavioral characterization of intracranial self-stimulation from mesolimbic, mesocortical, nigrostriatal, hypothalamic and extra-hypothalamic sites in the non-inbred CD-1 mouse strain. Behav Brain Res 36(3):251–281
167. Van Ree JM, Otte AP (1980) Effects of (Des-Tyr1)-gamma-endorphin and alpha-endorphin as compared to haloperidol and amphetamine on nucleus accumbens self-stimulation. Neuropharmacology 19(5):429–434
168. West TE, Wise RA (1988) Effects of naltrexone on nucleus accumbens, lateral hypothalamic and ventral tegmental self-stimulation rate-frequency functions. Brain Res 462(1):126–133
169. Costentin J (2006) Halte au cannabis. O. Jacob, Paris
170. Pontieri FE, Tanda G, Di Chiara G (1995) Intravenous cocaine, morphine, and amphetamine preferentially increase extracellular dopamine in the "shell" as compared with the "core" of the rat nucleus accumbens. Proc Natl Acad Sci U S A 92(26):12304–12308
171. Di Chiara G, Tanda G, Bassareo V, Pontieri F, Acquas E, Fenu S et al (1999) Drug addiction as a disorder of associative learning. Role of nucleus accumbens shell/extended amygdala dopamine. Ann N Y Acad Sci 877:461–485
172. Costa VD, Lang PJ, Sabatinelli D, Versace F, Bradley MM (2010) Emotional imagery: assessing pleasure and arousal in the brain's reward circuitry. Hum Brain Mapp 31(9):1446–1457. doi:10.1002/hbm.20948
173. Sabatinelli D, Bradley MM, Lang PJ, Costa VD, Versace F (2007) Pleasure rather than salience activates human nucleus accumbens and medial prefrontal cortex. J Neurophysiol 98(3):1374–1379. doi:10.1152/jn.00230.2007
174. Schlaepfer TE, Cohen MX, Frick C, Kosel M, Brodesser D, Axmacher N et al (2008) Deep brain stimulation to reward circuitry alleviates anhedonia in refractory major depression. Neuropsychopharmacology 33(2):368–377. doi:10.1038/sj.npp.1301408
175. Bewernick BH, Hurlemann R, Matusch A, Kayser S, Grubert C, Hadrysiewicz B et al (2010) Nucleus accumbens deep brain stimulation decreases ratings of depression and anxiety in treatment-resistant depression. Biol Psychiatry 67(2):110–116. doi:10.1016/j.biopsych.2009.09.013
176. Abosch A, Cosgrove GR (2008) Biological basis for the surgical treatment of depression. Neurosurg Focus 25(1):E2. doi:10.3171/FOC/2008/25/7/E2
177. Irle E, Exner C, Thielen K, Weniger G, Ruther E (1998) Obsessive-compulsive disorder and ventromedial frontal lesions: clinical and neuropsychological findings. Am J Psychiatry 155(2):255–263
178. Feil J, Zangen A (2010) Brain stimulation in the study and treatment of addiction. Neurosci Biobehav Rev 34(4):559–574. doi:10.1016/j.neubiorev.2009.11.006
179. Carter A, Hall W (2011) Proposals to trial deep brain stimulation to treat addiction are premature. Addiction 106(2):235–237. doi:10.1111/j.1360-0443.2010.03245.x
180. Hall W, Carter A (2011) Is deep brain stimulation a prospective "cure" for addiction? F1000 Med Rep. 3:4. doi:10.3410/M3-4
181. Kuhn J, Moller M, Muller U, Bogerts B, Mann K, Grundler TO (2011) Deep brain stimulation for the treatment of addiction. Addiction 106(8):1536–1537. doi:10.1111/j.1360-0443.2011.03452.x
182. Luigjes J, van den Brink W, Feenstra M, van den Munckhof P, Schuurman PR, Schippers R et al (2011) Deep brain stimulation in addiction: a review of potential brain targets. Mol Psychiatry. doi:10.1038/mp.2011.114
183. Li N, Wang J, Wang XL, Chang CW, Ge SN, Gao L et al (2012) Nucleus accumbens surgery for addiction. World Neurosurg. doi:10.1016/j.wneu.2012.10.007

184. Bard P (1928) A diencephalic mechanism for the expression of rage with special reference to the central nervous system. Am J Physiol 84:490–513
185. Scoville WB, Milner B (1957) Loss of recent memory after bilateral hippocampal lesions. J Neurol Neurosurg Psychiatry 20(1):11–21
186. Dalgleish T (2004) The emotional brain. Nat Rev Neurosci 5(7):583–589. doi:10.1038/nrn1432
187. Kanba S (2004) Brain science in emotional memory: role of the hippocampus. Fukuoka Igaku Zasshi 95(11):281–285
188. Lestienne R (2009) La bonne influence de nos émotions. La recherche (432)
189. Lisman JE, Grace AA (2005) The hippocampal-VTA loop: controlling the entry of information into long-term memory. Neuron 46(5):703–713. doi:10.1016/j.neuron.2005.05.002
190. McGaugh JL (2004) The amygdala modulates the consolidation of memories of emotionally arousing experiences. Annu Rev Neurosci 27:1–28. doi:10.1146/annurev.neuro.27.070203.144157
191. Bremner JD (2006) Traumatic stress: effects on the brain. Dialogues Clin Neurosci 8(4):445–461
192. Pare D, Quirk GJ, Ledoux JE (2004) New vistas on amygdala networks in conditioned fear. J Neurophysiol 92(1):1–9. doi:10.1152/jn.00153.2004
193. Le Jeannerod M (2002) cerveau intime. Odile Jacob, Paris
194. Darwin C (1872) The expression of the emotions in man and animals. London J. Murray
195. MacLean P (1952) Some psychiatric implications of physiological studies on frontotemporal portion of limbic system. Electroencephalogr Clin Neurophysiol 4(4):407–418
196. Le Jouvent R (2009) cerveau magicien de la réalité au plaisir psychique. O. Jacob, Paris
197. Kopell BH, Greenberg BD (2008) Anatomy and physiology of the basal ganglia: implications for DBS in psychiatry. Neurosci Biobehav Rev 32(3):408–422. doi:10.1016/j.neubiorev.2007.07.004
198. Krack P, Hariz MI, Baunez C, Guridi J, Obeso JA (2010) Deep brain stimulation: from neurology to psychiatry? Trends Neurosci 33(10):474–484. doi:10.1016/j.tins.2010.07.002
199. Haber SN, Fudge JL, McFarland NR (2000) Striatonigrostriatal pathways in primates form an ascending spiral from the shell to the dorsolateral striatum. J Neurosci 20(6):2369–2382
200. Levesque J, Eugene F, Joanette Y, Paquette V, Mensour B, Beaudoin G et al (2003) Neural circuitry underlying voluntary suppression of sadness. Biol Psychiatry 53(6):502–510
201. Alexander GE, Crutcher MD, DeLong MR (1990) Basal ganglia-thalamocortical circuits: parallel substrates for motor, oculomotor, "prefrontal" and "limbic" functions. Prog Brain Res 85:119–146
202. Bunney WE, Bunney BG (2000) Evidence for a compromised dorsolateral prefrontal cortical parallel circuit in schizophrenia. Brain Res Brain Res Rev 31(2–3):138–146
203. Daffner KR, Mesulam MM, Holcomb PJ, Calvo V, Acar D, Chabrerie A et al (2000) Disruption of attention to novel events after frontal lobe injury in humans. J Neurol Neurosurg Psychiatry 68(1):18–24
204. Heath RB (1954) Studies in Schyzophrenia (The initial report of findings in 26 patients prepared with depth electrodes was made in 1952 at a meeting in New Orleans, Louisiana). Harvard University Press, Cambridge
205. Pool JL (1954) Psychosurgery in older people. J Am Geriatr Soc 2(7):456–466
206. Burchiel K (2002) Surgical management of pain. Thieme
207. Mega MS, Cummings JL (1994) Frontal-subcortical circuits and neuropsychiatric disorders. J Neuropsychiatry Clin Neurosci 6(4):358–370
208. Duffy JD, Campbell JJ 3rd (1994) The regional prefrontal syndromes: a theoretical and clinical overview. J Neuropsychiatry Clin Neurosci 6(4):379–387
209. Damasio H, Damasio AR (1989) Lesion analysis in neuropsychology. Oxford University Press, New York
210. Magill PJ, Bolam JP, Bevan MD (2000) Relationship of activity in the subthalamic nucleus-globus pallidus network to cortical electroencephalogram. J Neurosci 20(2):820–833

211. Beurrier CGL, Bioulac B (2002) Subthalamic nucleus: a clock inside basal ganglia? Thalamus Related Syst 2:1–8
212. Buzsaki G, Draguhn A (2004) Neuronal oscillations in cortical networks. Science 304(5679):1926–1929. doi:10.1126/science.1099745
213. Bonnet-Brilhault FTF, Petit M (2001) Données biologiques de la schizophrénie. Encycl Méd Chir vol 285 p 11
214. Piacentini S, L. Romito A, Franzini A, Granato G, Broggi, Albanese A (2008) Mood disorder following DBS of the left amygdaloid region in a dystonia patient with a dislodged electrode. Mov Disord 23:147–150
215. Koenigs MED, Huey V, Raymont B, Cheon J, Solomon EM, Wassermann, Grafman J (2008) Focal brain damage protects against post-traumatic stress disorder in combat veterans. Nat Neurosci 11:232–237
216. Langevin JP, De Salles AA, Kosoyan HP, Krahl SE (2010) Deep brain stimulation of the amygdala alleviates post-traumatic stress disorder symptoms in a rat model. J Psychiatr Res 44:1241–1245
217. Bechara AD, Tranel H, Damasio R, Adolphs C, Rockland AR, Damasio (1995) Double dissociation of conditioning and declarative knowledge relative to the amygdala and hippocampus in humans. Science 269:1115–1118
218. Proust M (1913–27). Remembrance of things past. Swann's way: within a budding grove. The definitive French Pleiade. In: Scott Moncrieff CK, Terence Kilmartin (ed) vol 1, Vintage, New York, pp 51
219. Bartholomei F, Barbeau E, Gavaret M, Guye M, McGonigal A, Régis J, Chauvel P (2004) Cortical stimulation study of the role of rhinal cortex in deja vu and reminiscence of memories. Neurology 63:858–864
220. Naqvi NH, Rudrauf D, Damasio H, Bechara A (2007) Damage to the insula disrupts addiction to cigarette smoking. Science 315:531–534
221. Coenen VA, Schlaepfer TE, Maedler B, Panksepp J (2011) Cross-species affective functions of the medial forebrain bundle-implications for the treatment of affective pain and depression in humans. Neurosci Biobehav Rev 35:1971–1981

Chapter 3
Psychosurgical Procedures

Abstract There are two types of psychosurgical interventions. The first consists in creating a lesion via stereotaxy using heat (thermocoagulation) or ionizing radiation (radiosurgery) in one or more precise areas of the brain. The second, more recent type of intervention uses stimulation to target both deep brain structures and the cortex or the vagus nerve. In contrast to previous techniques, the effects of stimulation are reversible and adaptable and make use of implanted devices: electrodes and stimulators.

The development of *stereotaxy* in the early 1950s enabled neurosurgeons to perform much more targeted lesions of brain structures, which led to better results and fewer complications. In 1947, Spiegel and his colleagues, working with patients with severe psychiatric disorders, developed a sophisticated apparatus capable of targeting a precise anatomical target: the dorsomedial nucleus of the thalamus[1] [1]. Many years later when describing the genesis of the technique, Spiegel, described how he *was horrified by the brain damage and personality changes in patient's* [after a frontal lobotomy—Author's note] *and* [he] *was convinced that a reduction in emotional and behavioral complications from lobotomies was possible by a much more targeted procedure in the dorsomedial nucleus of the thalamus connected to this frontal lobe* [2]. His invention marked the birth of a new type of neurosurgery: stereotactic surgery (Fig. 3.1).

Stereotaxy

Today stereotactic surgery is not only used in psychosurgery but also in countless other branches of neurosurgery. It is used to perform biopsies of brain tumors, surgery of movement disorders (Parkinson's disease, essential tremors generalized dystonia), recordings of intracerebral electrical activity in patients with epilepsy and more rarely in the treatment of pain. In psychosurgery, stereotaxy allows for

---

[1] Cf. p. 123.

M. Lévêque, *Psychosurgery*, DOI: 10.1007/978-3-319-01144-8_3,
© Springer International Publishing Switzerland 2014

Fig. 3.1 The different
techniques and diseases
relevant to psychosurgery

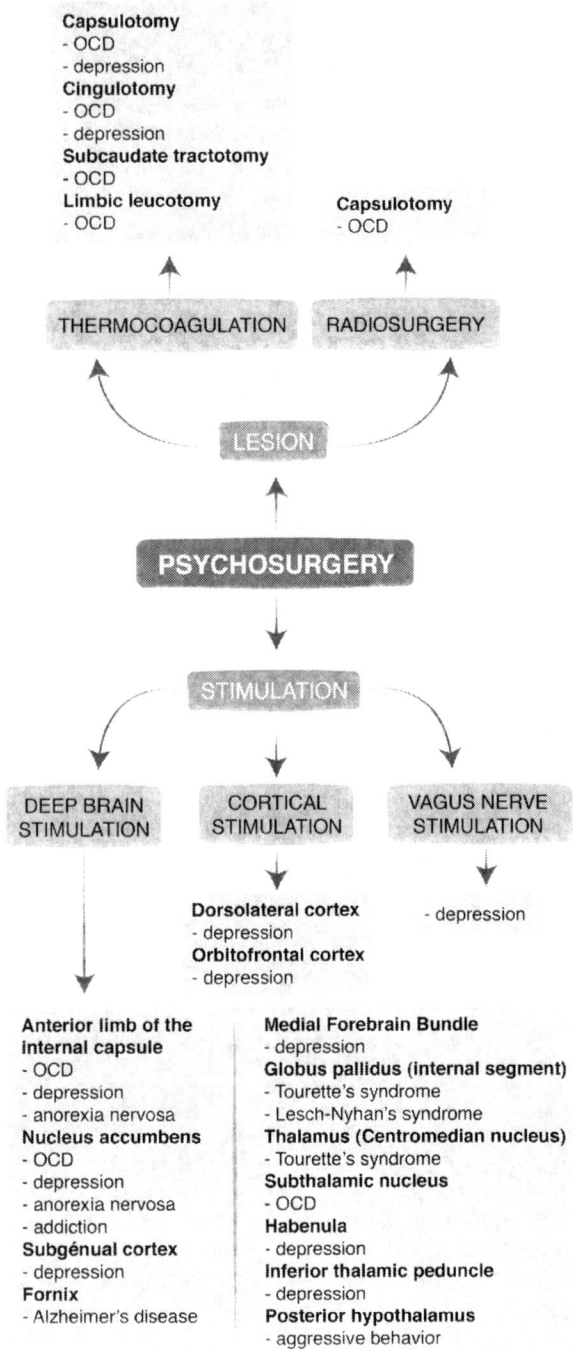

Capsulotomy
- OCD
- depression
Cingulotomy
- OCD
- depression
Subcaudate tractotomy
- OCD
Limbic leucotomy
- OCD

Capsulotomy
- OCD

THERMOCOAGULATION   RADIOSURGERY

LESION

PSYCHOSURGERY

STIMULATION

DEEP BRAIN
STIMULATION

CORTICAL
STIMULATION

VAGUS NERVE
STIMULATION

Dorsolateral cortex
- depression
Orbitofrontal cortex
- depression

- depression

**Anterior limb of the
internal capsule**
- OCD
- depression
- anorexia nervosa
Nucleus accumbens
- OCD
- depression
- anorexia nervosa
- addiction
Subgénual cortex
- depression
Fornix
- Alzheimer's disease

Medial Forebrain Bundle
- depression
Globus pallidus (internal segment)
- Tourette's syndrome
- Lesch-Nyhan's syndrome
Thalamus (Centromedian nucleus)
- Tourette's syndrome
Subthalamic nucleus
- OCD
Habenula
- depression
Inferior thalamic peduncle
- depression
Posterior hypothalamus
- aggressive behavior

the thermocoagulation electrodes to be brought within millimeters of the ana-tomical structure to be lesioned during *lesioning or ablative surgery* or stimulated during *deep brain stimulation* (DBS). Stereotactic surgery can be used to target highly specific points, or regions in the brain. First, an apparatus called a *stereotactic frame* is fitted on the surface of the skull of a patient under local or general anesthesia (Fig. 3.15, p. 137). Stereotaxy views the brain like a geo-graphical map in which all structures can be described using a three-dimensional coordinate system with an x, y, and z axis (Fig. 3.2). The stereotactic frame both immobilizes the patient's head and maps out the workspace. Once the frame is in place, the patient is brought into a radiology department to perform an MRI or CT scan in order to acquire three-dimensional images of the brain.

Next, using these images the coordinates of the target are determined. Identi-fication of the anatomical structure usually requires the use of an *anatomical atlas*, a sort of probabilistic *chart*—now often computerized—developed from dissec-tions (Fig. 3.3).

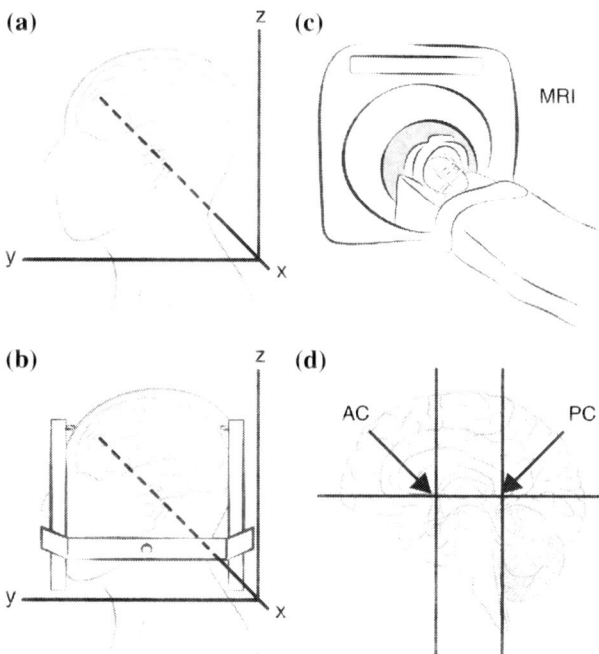

Fig. 3.2 Stereotactic procedure. **a** Three axes defining a volume (*x left* to *right*, *y back* to *front*, *z bottom* to *top*). **b** Stereotactic frame to immobilize the skull and delimit the work space. **c** Performing imaging (usually MRI) with the frame affixed to the patient's skull. **d** Imaging is used to locate easily identifiable anatomical landmarks, constant from one individual to another, such as the line connecting the anterior commissure (*AC*) to the posterior commissure (*PC*)

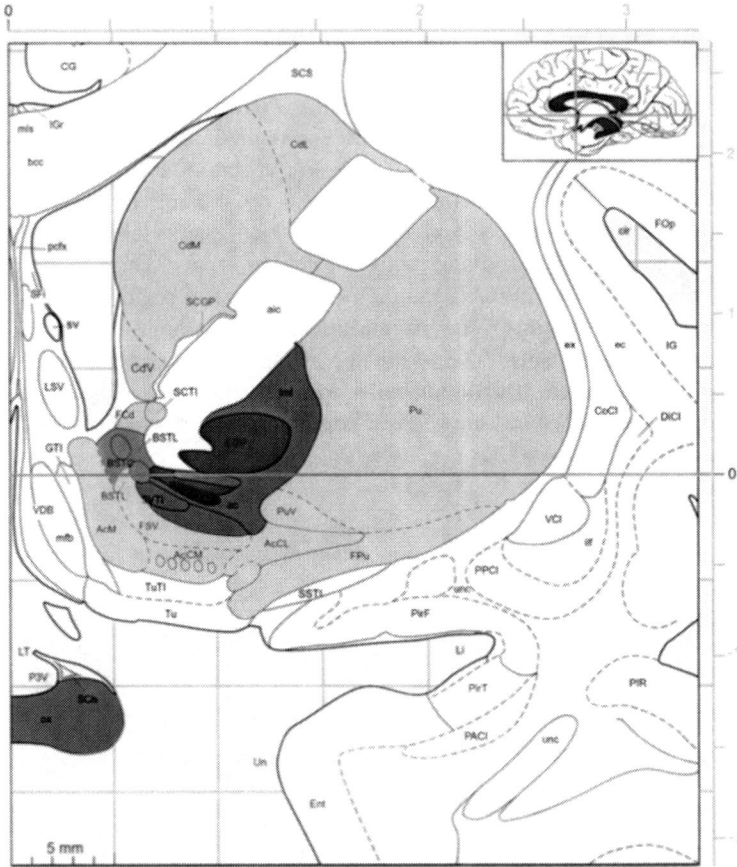

Fig. 3.3 Example of anatomical atlas (Atlas by Mai, Paxinos and Voss.). On this coronal section, the putamen (*Pu*) is recognizable in *gray* separated by the anterior limb of the internal capsule (*ALIC*), the caudate nucleus in *gray* (*CdM*) is also visible, below we distinguish the nucleus accumbens (*MAb, ACCM*) and within the medial forebrain bundle (*MFB*) [3]

These atlases, of which there are many, give the probable location of brain structures based on reference points common to all adult humans. This information can prove crucial given that certain structures can be particularly difficult to identify from MRI images alone. Once the target is identified, the stereotactic frame is fitted with an instrument holder running on an arc which can be positioned according to the x, y, and z coordinates of the target. After a route which avoids veins, arteries, the base of the furrows containing vessels and the ventricles has been planned out, an incision is made in the skin and a burr hole drilled into the cranium. Finally an electrode—for thermocoagulation or stimulation depending on the type of procedure—is inserted millimeter by millimeter into the brain parenchyma (Fig. 3.4). We will return to these steps in more detail in the following paragraphs.[2]

---

[2] Cf. pp. 202–204.

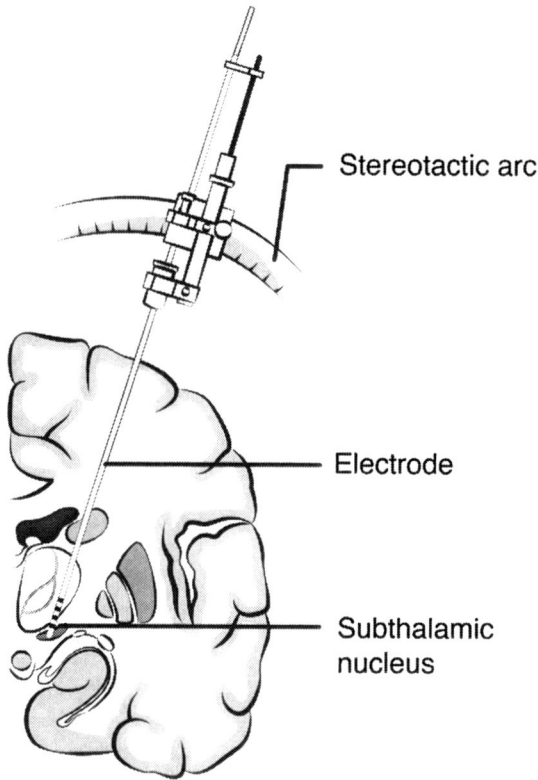

Fig. 3.4 Stereotactic arc equipped with an instrument holder. This package allows the descent of the stimulating electrode or thermocoagulation—depending on whether a stimulation procedure or injury—to the anatomical target. In this example the subthalamic nucleus there is only a stimulation procedure

Technical Lesioning

Procedures Using Thermocoagulation

Abstract Lesional psychosurgery, as it is practiced today using stereotaxy, entails focalized destruction of one or more specific areas of the brain usually through heat or radiation. There are four main types of lesional surgeries: the capsulotomy, which targets the anterior limb of the internal capsule, the cingulotomy, which targets the anterior cingulate cortex, the subcaudate tractotomy, which interrupts the fibers below the head of the caudate nucleus, and the limbic leucotomy, which is a combination of the cingulotomy and sub caudate tractotomy. Most practitioners currently favor the first two types of intervention. The type of pathology as well as the expertise of the team performing the surgery determines whether a capsulotomy or a cingulotomy is performed. Currently, the two primary indications are OCD and severe depression.

In lesional surgery, also known as ablative surgery because in the past brain tissue was resected rather than selectively lesioned through heat, cold or radiation, the changes wrought to the brain tissue are irreversible. This is one of the downsides to the technique: neuropsychological impairment following surgery is often permanent. However, it has the advantage of being comparable in efficacy to deep brain stimulation at a much lower cost (Table 6.1, p. 309) [4]. The surgical procedure uses the stereotactic technique previously described (Fig. 3.2, p. 109). Lesional procedures differ from deep brain stimulation (DBS) in that the electrode is used for thermocoagulation and is only temporarily inserted into the parenchyma. Before a lesion is made by heating the tip of the electrode to a temperature of between 70 and 90 °C, a low frequency electrical stimulation can be performed to ensure there are no adverse clinical effects. The very localized heat source destroys brain parenchyma in a radius of about five 5 mm around the tip of the electrode through a process of electrothermocoagulation. Though more rarely, cold can also be used. In such case, rather than an electrode, a *cryoprobe* [5–10] is used to lower the temperature of the targeted tissue to below −70 °C and create a lesion.

Anatomical Targets

Currently, there are three anatomical targets for lesioning and four types of interventions, though the two main techniques remain the capsulotomy and cingulotomy (Fig. 3.5). It is estimated that only 20 such interventions are performed annually in the United States and Great Britain mostly as part of research studies [11]. Other areas of the brain have also been targeted in recent years for the treatment of addiction[3] [12–14] and some aggressive behavior

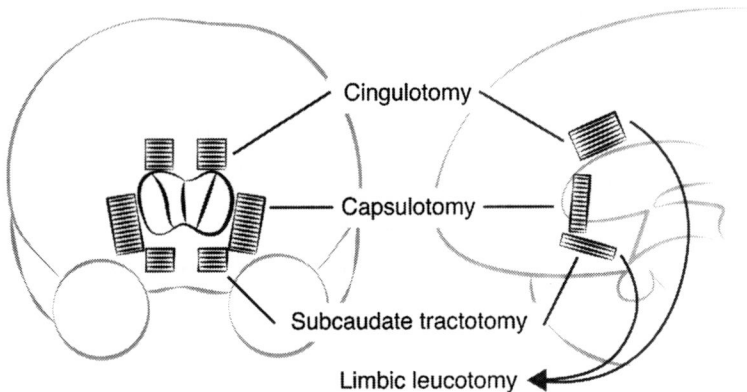

Fig. 3.5 The four types of interventions in lesional psychosurgery

---

[3] Cf. p. 358.

disorders[4] [6, 7, 15, 16] but indication for such diagnoses remains contested, and consequently, are discussed only briefly in this section. We will return to them, however, in the chapters devoted to pathologies[5] and ethics.[6]

Capsulotomy

Abstract The capsulotomy aims to sever some of the fibers running through the anterior limb of the internal capsule connecting the prefrontal cortex to the thalamus. Performed using thermocoagulation or radiosurgery, this procedure is indicated for the treatment of severe forms of OCD, anxiety disorders and, less commonly, depression.

History and Outline of Procedure

In the decade following the WWII, the "open surgery" prefrontal leucotomy was used for diverse psychiatric disorders from depression to schizophrenia. While reviewing his clinical data, Meyer observed that better postoperative results were obtained when the intervention was limited to the anterior limb of the internal capsule (ALIC) [17]. In 1949, the French and Swedish neurosurgeons, Talairach[7] and Leksell, were the first to specifically target this area. They chose it because fibers connecting the prefrontal cortex to the thalamus run though it (Fig. 3.6) [18]. Through their interventions focusing on this area, particularly on its anterior portion, the teams achieved much better results especially in indications of depression, severe anxiety disorders, and OCD [19]. As detailed in the previous chapter,[8] the cortico-thalamic bundles run through the lower portion of the ALIC located between the head of the caudate nucleus and the putamen [20]. They reciprocally link the dorsomedial nucleus of the thalamus to the entire prefrontal cortex[9] and the ventral anterior nucleus,[10] more specifically the dorsolateral and orbitofrontal cortices (Fig. 2.17, p. 76). The anterior limb also contains cortico-striatal connections linking the prefrontal cortex to the striatum.[11] Thus, input (cortico-striatal bundle) and output (cortico-thalamic bundle) information

---

[4] Cf. p. 345.

[5] Chapter 4, p. 271.

[6] Chapter 5, p. 418.

[7] Talairach was the first to discuss the subject while Leksell published the first clinical results and popularized the technique.

[8] Cf. p. 125.

[9] Cf. p. 90.

[10] Cf. p. 124.

[11] Cf. p. 128.

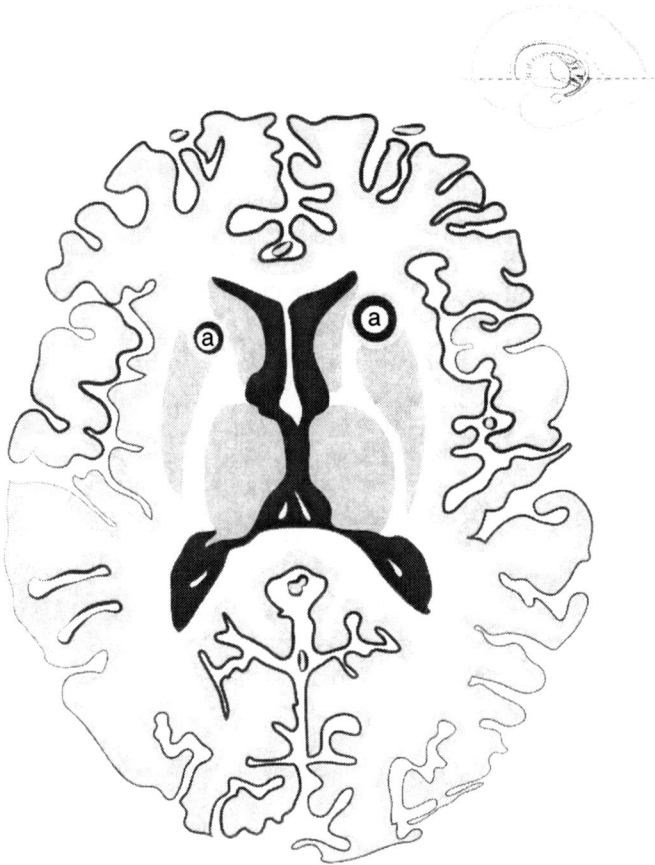

Fig. 3.6 Diagram of an axial MRI showing lesions cockade **a** a bilateral capsulotomy. [Lesion made on both sides, 20 mm from the *midline* and 5 mm behind the front end of the anterior horn of the lateral ventricle in the plane connecting the anterior and posterior commissure named AC-PC (cf. Fig. 3.2)]. According to [32]

along the cortico-striato-thalamo-cortical (CSTC) associative and limbic loops[12] as conceptualized by Alexander passes through this region (Figs. 2.27, p. 89 and 2.28, p. 91) [21]. Additionally, the corticopontine bundle, which connects the prefrontal cortex to the brainstem also passes through this region though its function remains unclear [22–25]. A tractographic study[13] of patients treated by capsulotomy revealed degeneration in all three of these bundles while PET Scan

---

[12] Cf. pp. 141 and 143.

[13] DTI is a technique using MRI to calculate the diffusion of water molecules for each pixel of the image. The water molecule is constrained in its diffusion by its surroundings. This type of imaging enables the position and orientation of fibers such as white matter bundles to be calculated indirectly.

showed decreased activity in the orbitofrontal cortex and striatum following the procedure [26]. Despite this imaging data, the neurophysiological mechanism leading to clinical improvements in patients with OCD[14] or depression is not yet fully understood [27]. Capsulotomies are performed in two different ways, either by thermocoagulation or radiosurgery.[15] Thermocoagulation procedures rely on stereotactic surgical techniques. On each side, the thermocoagulation electrodes are lowered to different depths in the ALIC in order to make two tiered, over-lapping lesions of about 5 mm radius each which are visible on an MRI [28, 29]. Opinions vary significantly on the exact area to target within this region. Lippitz, of the Karolinska Institute in Sweden, advocates the middle third. According to him, patients present greater regression of their OCD symptoms following a lesion in this area. Additionally, he also claims that the right side provides better results than the left [30, 31].

Results

Treating OCD

In patients with OCD, results for capsulotomy procedures range from 70 % clinical improvement in a series of more than a hundred patients published in 1961 by the Karolinska team [33] to 50–57 % improvement in more modern studies [30, 34, 35]. The poorer results obtained in studies from the past 25 years most likely reflect the stricter scales practitioners now use to assess patient progress. Only a decrease of at least 35 % in the Y-BOCS[16] score is now considered clinical improvement. Meanwhile, techniques and indications have been refined.[17]

Treating Severe Anxiety Disorders

Patients suffering from severe debilitating anxiety disorders may also be candidates for a capsulotomy. The Swedish psychiatrist P. Mindus has reported up to 80 % improvement in a cohort of 24 patients treated by capsulotomy [36]. However, this percentage is debatable because the nonhomogeneous group included patients with OCD. The same team at the Karolinska Institute published, in 2003, the results for 26 patients operated between 1975 and 1991. Thirteen suffered from generalized anxiety disorder, eight from panic disorders, and five from social phobias [37].

---

[14] Cf. physiopathology of OCD p. 278.

[15] Cf. p. 187.

[16] Cf. the chapter summarizing the scales used in OCD, p. 273.

[17] Cf. p. 184.

After 1 year, 92 % of patients saw their anxiety symptoms reduced by at least 50 % according to the BSA scale. After long-term monitoring for an average of 3 years, 67 % of patients remained responders with a normalized score on the global functioning[18] (GAF) scale. These satisfactory results must, however, be considered alongside the neuropsychological complications reported: seven patients showed deterioration or apathy, and seven suicide attempts were recorded.

Treating Depression[19]

Only two studies have been published indicating capsulotomies for the treatment of severe depression. The first, published by the Karolinska team in 196, is difficult to interpret because validated scales were not used to make the clinical evaluations [33]. What is clear is that of the 19 patients with severe depression treated, 14 (74 %) saw their condition improve permanently, while for 3 other patients (16 %) improvement was only temporary. The second, a prospective study published in 2011 by a British team from Dundee, reported on 20 patients operated on between 1992 and 1999 [25]. Christmas showed that after a mean period of 7 years, 50 % were responders and 40 % in remission. *Remission* signifies a one half decrease in the depression score on the Hamilton scale (HRSD).[20] *Response* signifies a score below 10. Unlike other studies, no neuropsychological deterioration was reported in the subjects. In fact, they showed improved performance test scores, which according to the authors was due to improved psychomotor function resulting from thymic improvement. In 2003, a second British team reported 60 % improvement in a set of 24 patients suffering from severe depression. But for now the details of these operations performed in Cardiff remain unpublished [20].

Complications

In a little under 1 % of cases, intracranial haemorrhaging, post-operative seizures, or transient hallucinations have been reported. The most common side effects reported were often transitory apathy and confusion (86 % of patients), urinary incontinence lasting a few days (27 %), persistent fatigue (32 %), and significant weight gain (10 %) [33, 38]. Rück reported a 4 % suicide rate among 26 patients being treated and followed long-term for OCD, while no mention is made of autolysis in 22 patients treated for depression by Christmas [25, 37]. The authors

---

[18] Ibid.

[19] See also p. 326.

[20] Cf. p. 310.

remain divided on the subject of neuropsychological loss. As we saw, the Scottish team reported virtually no cognitive deterioration, and neither did Mindus [28, 39, 40]. However Rück, who is a member of the Karolinska Institute team, reported apathy and a decline in executive functions for 7 of the 26 patients operated in 2003 [37, 41, 42]. By pairing the occurrences of cognitive loss with brain scans, the Swedish team discovered that the larger the thermocoagulation lesions and the more they extended toward the back and inside of the anterior limb, particularly on the right side, the greater the risk of complications. In addition, a small study of nine patients showed that, as with those treated by cingulotomy, patients treated by capsulotomy had greater difficulty assessing the emotional states of those around them [43]. A disability, which can make social reintegration more challenging for these patients.

Cingulotomy

Abstract A cingulotomy creates a bilateral lesion in the anterior cingulate cortex. It is comparable to capsulotomies in terms of efficacy when treating OCD but appears more effective in the treatment of depression even if additional procedures may sometimes be necessary. The technique involves stereotactic thermocoagulation and is mainly practiced in the United States. Unlike with capsulotomies, radiosurgery and deep brain stimulation have hardly ever been used on this target. The use of this type of intervention for the treatment of addiction or aggressive behavior disorders remains controversial.

The cingulotomy is and has been for some time the most widespread psychosurgical intervention in the United States for the treatment of depression and severe OCD [44–46].

History and Principle

The cingulate gyrus[21] which is located on the inner surface of each brain hemisphere, is part of the memory loop, the Papez circuit,[22] and more broadly the limbic loop.[23] It is considered indispensable to the formation and expression of emotions [47]. In the early 1950s, the American neurophysiologist Fulton practiced lesions in the cingulate gyrus of monkeys. He did not witness any changes in social behavior or any neurological disorders as a result; but, he did notice that the monkeys had a higher tolerance to frustration [48–50]. A few years prior to his experiments, it had been observed that electrical stimulation of the cortex in

---

[21] Cf. p. 95.

[22] Cf. p. 133.

[23] Cf. p. 137.

humans caused autonomic manifestations similar to those produced during states of stress as well as altering anxiety [51, 52]. At Oxford, Cairns, influenced by the work of his friend Fulton was one of the first to perform an "open" cingulectomy [53], but the American Scoville was the first to publish results of such a procedure. In 1951, he published his (rather mediocre) results for the procedure, which he had performed on 40 patients. His poor results can be attributed to his choice to target a relatively posteriori area of the cingulate gyrus. At Oxford, Whitty, a colleague of Cairns, targeted the anterior portion of the cingulate cortex instead, and his study yielded 75 % good or excellent outcomes in 24 patients suffering from a variety of psychiatric disorders [53, 54]. In 1954, Le Beau neurosurgeon at the Salpêtrière Hospital and father of the cingulectomy[24] (Fig. 1.15, p. 25) noted that the best results were obtained in violent, agitated, and aggressive patients [55]. Subsequent studies confirmed that the anterior area of the cingulate gyrus was indeed the best target, and that patients with OCD were the best candidates for this surgery [56, 57]. In 1967 at *Massachusetts General Hospital*, Ballantine improved outcome rates for the procedure (79 % satisfactory results) by replacing the open surgery technique with one using an electrothermocoagulation needle guided using data obtained through pneumoencephalography[25] (Fig. 3.7) [48].

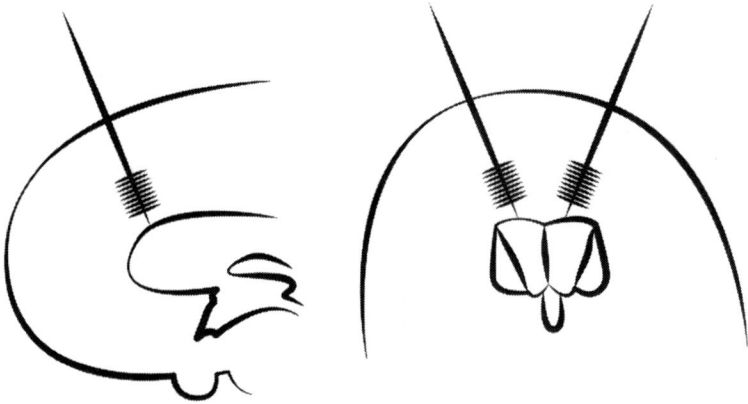

Fig. 3.7 Cingulotomy. Air is injected within the ventricles (pneumoencephalography) so that they become visible on a radiograph (*left*) and side (*right*). Thermocoagulation needles are then lowered toward the roof of the lateral ventricles. Coagulation is induced a few millimeters from the ventricular landmarks, at the anterior part of the cingulate cortex, according to [58]

---

[24] Cf. p. 49.

[25] An old X-ray imaging technique using a gas as a contrast medium to obtain images of ventricles in the brain (Fig. 3.7). The gas was injected by lumbar puncture, suboccipitally or even by direct puncture of the ventricles after trepanning. This test was replaced by MRI or brain scans used today.

The new technique had first been used 5 years earlier in the treatment of cancer pain, which could not be dulled even through large amounts of morphine [59]. It was soon noticed that in addition to relieving the pain, the procedure severed the patient's dependency to morphine. Consequently, the intervention was put to use treating addiction[26] to opiates [9, 60–62]. Despite all the empirical clinical data showing that the procedure effectively counters depression and OCD, how exactly it does so is still misunderstood. The only certainty, which has been revealed through functional imaging, is that the cingulate and orbitofrontal cortices present increased metabolisms in severe depression [27] and OCD[28] [63–69]. The effectiveness of cingulotomies, as well as of subcaudate tractotomies, discussed below,[29] may be a result of a reorganization of the neural network and activation of certain structures to compensate. This hypothesis would account for the delayed nature of the clinical improvement, which can occur up to 6 months after surgery [70] (Fig 3.8).

Fig. 3.8 Sagittal section showing the rosette **b** resulting from an earlier cingulotomy (Lesions performed on either side and 7 mm from the *midline* and 20–25 mm behind the *front end* of the anterior horn of the lateral ventricle) [32]

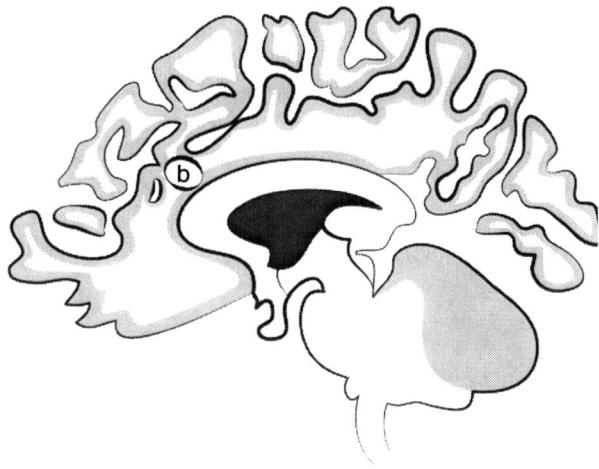

---

[26] Cf. p. 358.

[27] Hyperactivity in the temporal cortex is witnessed, in particular of the hippocampus and of the amygdala.

[28] Hyperactivity of the central gray nuclei and of the thalamus can also be seen.

[29] Cf. p. 180.

Results

Scoville was the first to observe that with the exception of a rapid decrease in anxiety clinical improvement did not occur immediately [71]. In fact, symptoms of OCD and depression, usually take 6 to 12 weeks to diminish; and as Cosgrove has noted, in patients suffering from both obsession and depression, the symptoms of depression are the first to disappear [72].

Treating OCD

The largest retrospective study ever conducted, which was led by Ballantine and included nearly a quarter of the 800 patients operated on over the last 40 years at *Massachusetts General Hospital* (MGH), showed that over an average follow-up period of 8 years 56 % of OCD patients saw their symptoms lessened [73]. However, 40 % of them required additional cingulotomy lesions [74]. Later, the same team reevaluated the data using stricter criteria (Y-BOCS, CGI, BDI) and found 25–30 % remission and 10–15 % response rates [75]. The first long-term prospective study at MGH, conducted among 18 patients, showed 28 % remission and 17 % response rates. Also working in Boston, Dougherty, presented slightly better prospective results. He recorded 32 % remission and 14 % response rates for a cohort of 44 patients [76]. Two recent Korean publications, which had examined the same group of 14 and subsequently 17 patients, reported response or remission rates between 43 and 47 % after 1 to 2 years [77, 78]. In 2004, Lozano's team in Toronto published less promising results with only a 27 % response or remission rate among 21 patients with OCD [79, 80]. The Canadian team explained the discrepancy by pointing out that unlike the MGH team they only performed supplementary follow-up cingulotomies in 2 of the 21 patients [76].

Treating Depression

The number of patients treated for severe depression is significantly lower than the number treated for OCD. However, the procedure seems slightly more effective in the first group. In 1996, Ballantine's team in Boston treating a set of five patients with refractory depression succeeded in halving the BDI for 60 % and achieving a partial response in 12 % of them [74]. In 2008, a prospective study of 33 patients by the same institution confirmed the encouraging results with a one-third response rate and 43 % partial response, according to the BDI and CGI scales [70]. It must be noted however that if after 6 months no clinical improvement was recorded, a supplementary more anterior cingulotomy or a subcaudate tractotomy[30] was performed. Of the 16 patients who received a second operation, a quarter responded and 50 % responded partially.

---

[30] Ibid.

Treating Other Indications: Addiction and Violent Behavior

In the 1970s, the Indian neurosurgeon Balasubramaniam performed cingulotomies on 73 patients suffering from addiction to alcohol or opiates [62]. Within 1 to 6 years, 80 % of the morphine addicts and 68 % of the alcoholics were reportedly cured. This highly controversial indication for the procedure was abandoned until the end of 1990s, when the Russian Medvedev again used the procedure on nearly 350 heroin addicted subjects. The interventions were conducted using a cryoprobe, and after 2 years 45 % of subjects had been fully weaned and 17 % partially weaned (presenting one or two relapses) off heroin [9]. Cingulotomy treatment of patients with aggressive behavior disorders raises similarly uncomfortable ethical questions, addressed in Chap. 5.[31] In 1970 at the Second Congress of Psychosurgery in Copenhagen, Turner, of the Queen Elizabeth Hospital in Birmingham, reported that in a study of 30 patients treated with a posterior cingulectomy 80 % of the subjects no longer presented aggressive behavior after the procedure [81]. However, Turner did not explain his reasons for selecting a posterior target and gave no information on the complications that may have arisen. A Mexican team has recently published two studies supporting a new procedure which combines the cingulotomy and capsulotomy, for the treatment of aggressive behavior disorders for which drug treatment is ineffective [82, 83]. The authors reported an "improvement" in over half of the 12 and 10 subjects, respectively. Complications such as somnolence, hyperphagia, disinhibition, hypersexuality, infection, and paraparesis were reported for five of the subjects.

Complications

Infection, intracranial hemorrhaging, or postoperative epileptic seizures have been reported in 1–2 % of cases and episodes of transient urinary incontinence in 5–12 % of cases [48, 70, 75, 76, 84]. Cosgrove notes that no deaths resulted from the nearly one thousand procedures performed in Boston [72]. Only four patients suffered subdural hematoma (SDH), and only one suffered any lasting neurological affects. It should nonetheless be noted that among the nearly 200 patients who received a cingulotomy at MGH the suicide rate was 9 % for the average 9-year follow-up period [73]. This elevated number is nevertheless an improvement on the high suicide rate (15–30 %) for patients with severe depression [10, 85]. Neuropsychological tests conducted during long-term follow-up, when they have been done, do not seem to reveal any personality change, cognitive impairment or, significantly, memory loss [60, 78, 86]. This contrasts with capsulotomies, for which the occurrence of transient apathy is not uncommon.

---

[31] Cf. p. 418.

Subcaudate Tractotomy

Abstract The subcaudate tractotomy, a rarely used procedure, aims to sever the connections between the amygdala, hypothalamus, and prefrontal cortex. Initially, pellets of radioactive yttrium were used, but this approach has now been replaced by the thermocoagulation technique. Most of the studies into the effects of the subcaudate tractotomy have taken place in Great Britain, and it has been suggested for the treatment of depression, anxiety disorders, and OCD.

Less practiced than the capsulotomy or cingulotomy, the subcaudate tractotomy has few indications but is often relied upon in cases of a failed cingulotomy. It is then referred to as a limbic leucotomy, which aims to interrupt the bundles connecting the orbitofrontal cortex[32] to the thalamus, the amygdala, the hypothalamus, and the striatum. Thermocoagulation lesions the white matter bundles just below the head of the caudate nucleus, in what, oddly enough, is named the unnamed substance (*substantia innominata*). Preclinical trials in monkeys showed that stimulation of Brodmann area 13, a region located just below the unnamed substance could provoke violent emotions. Knight, a neurosurgeon at Brook Hospital in the south of London concluded that lesioning of the unnamed substance might influence the intensity of emotional responses [87]. The technique he devised in 1955 was based on the orbital leucotomy[33] practiced by Scoville in Connecticut but was less invasive [88]. The new tractotomy technique reduced the risk of complications by, among other things, replacing open surgery with radioactive yttrium (Y^{90}) pellets inserted into the ventral part of the *substantia innominata* using a stereotactically guided cannula (Fig. 3.9).

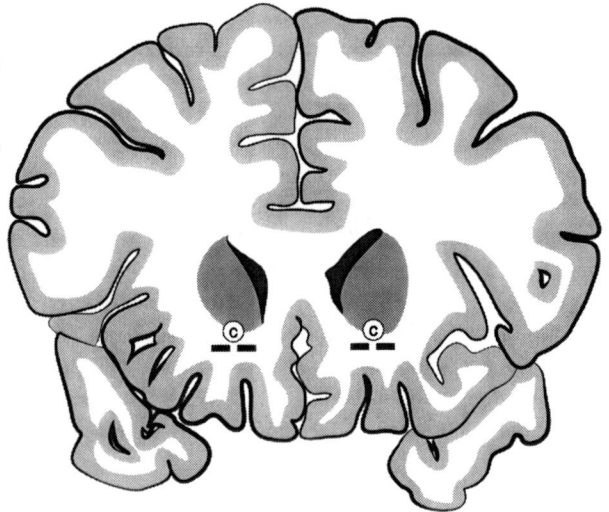

Fig. 3.9 Coronal section of the brain showing the four pellets of radioactive Yttrium c for the realization of a subcaudate tractotomy (Lesions made at 15 mm from the *midline* and 10–11 mm behind the sella) [32]

---

[32] Cf. p. 93.

[33] Cf. p. 47.

In 1990, his successor, Bartlett and the psychiatrist Bridges began performing the procedure with thermocoagulation. Over 1,300 patients, nearly one-third of all patients treated by psychosurgery in the United Kingdom from the 1960s to the 1980s, received tractotomies [10]. The procedures were most effective in patients suffering from depression, and as with the cingulotomy, the effects could begin up to a year after. Some reports have claimed a nearly 70 % success rate across all pathologies and low complication rates [89–93]. Bridges and Goktepe found that for a sample of 134 patients the procedure had yielded good results in 68 % of cases of depression, 62 % of anxiety disorders, and 50 % of OCD [93]. However, results were disappointing in patients with schizophrenia, personality disorders, or addiction. Complications—aside from the risk of epilepsy (2.2 %), hemorrhage and infection—such as weight gain and transient states of disinhibition, delirium (10 %), and memory loss were reported [89, 90, 94]. One percent of 300 post-operative patients followed for a period of 3–13 years committed suicide.

Limbic Leucotomy

Abstract The combination of a cingulotomy and a subcaudate tractotomy is called a limbic leucotomy. When the clinical results of a cingulotomy are not considered sufficient, a subcaudate tractotomy is sometimes performed.

Introduced in 1973 by the psychiatrist Kelly and neurosurgeon Richardson, the procedure is the combination of a subcaudate tractotomy and a cingulotomy (Fig. 3.5) [95]. These two British practitioners thought to sever, on the one hand, the bundles connecting the orbitofrontal cortex[34] to the thalamus, the amygdala, and the striato-pallidal complex, and on the other hand, the limbic circuit by interrupting it in the cingulate gyrus. In 1976, the team from *St George's Hospital* in London reported that for 66 patients who had received a limbic leucotomy, 89 % of those with OCD, 66 % of those with anxiety disorders, and 78 % of those with depression had improved [96]. Since then, only one prospective study of 21 patients was published in 2002 by Cosgrove's team in Boston. Only 5 of the 21 patients had not received any prior surgery (cingulotomy or subcaudate tractotomy). Of these patients, one-fifth of the 12 suffering from OCD (42 %) responded to the leucotomy surgery (Y-BOCS score decreased by more than a third), while three of the six patients with depression (50 %) also responded favorably (BDI score halved) [97]. Two patients, one suffering from depression and the other from OCD, committed suicide. The authors did not know that these patients complained of marked suicidal ideation before the interventions. Possible complications, from this technique are,

---

[34] Cf. p. 93.

of course, similar to those from cingulotomy and subcaudate tractotomy procedures: often transient urinary incontinence (24 %), delirium, or drowsiness lasting a few weeks (25–30 %), and complaints of persistent lethargy (12 %) [32].

The Debatable Results of Clinical Studies

The four types of interventions mentioned above are used almost exclusively to treat patients with OCD or severe depression, but several factors make it difficult to determine which is best suited to each pathology. The first two are methodological. Indeed, virtually no study has been conducted with the explicit design of comparing two or more of the techniques. The only such study, comparing *cingulotomy* and *capsulotomy*, though randomized only included four patients with OCD: two for each procedure [98]. As for the older studies, though they do include larger patient sets, they present several drawbacks. First, they were all conducted retrospectively and included multiple pathologies. Second, they did not call for either pre-surgical or post-surgical evaluations using validated scales, which would have allowed for reliable cross-study comparisons. Furthermore, many studies are marred by another methodological bias: until the late 1980s, the team that made the diagnosis was often the same team that assessed the clinical outcome of the surgery. The practice, now prohibited by ethical guidelines and, more importantly, the peer review committees of scientific journals—compromises the objectivity of these older studies and the modern meta-analyses which draw on them [10]. Finally, another bias in older studies is related to how the authors define the notion of *treatment resistance*. The concept—when specified at all—varies greatly among the various teams. Again, this makes comparing the results of different studies problematic. Recent studies, in contrast, are not affected by these biases, but they have the disadvantage of examining relatively small sets of subjects. One methodological flaw common to all the studies, old or new, is the lack of randomization with prospective, double-blind evaluation. This is currently a requirement in any study of a new molecule and is intended to eliminate the placebo effect. Such a study would require that a control group of patients be given *sham surgery*.[35] However, such a practice would most probably be unethical [99–102]. Consequently, it is impossible to rule out involvement of the placebo effect in clinical improvement.[36] Additionally, assessment of the results by a psychiatrist cannot be "blind" because she knows that the patient underwent/benefited from (depending on the physician's own views of this kind of treatment) a psychosurgical intervention.

---

[35] This sort of operation is unthinkable with invasive surgical procedures such as stereotactic thermocoagulation. However, it would be conceivable in operations done with radiosurgery. In such a "sham" procedure, a stereotaxic frame is placed on the patient's skull, the imaging is done but no radiation is released when the patient is inside the radiosurgery device. A team from São Paulo performed this procedure on an OCD patient. Over a year later, the same procedure was done, but this time releasing gamma rays. Thus, the patient was his own witness [115].

[36] This lacuna must however be nuanced in cases of severely depressed patients: this effect is considered marginal [338].

Table 3.1 Clinical results by pathology, the four acts of stereotactic psychosurgery

Results (%)	Depression (n = 727)	OCD (n = 478)	GAD (n = 290)
Marked improvement	63	58	52
Partial improvement	22	27	25
No response	14	14	21
Aggravation	1	1	1

Meta-analysis published in 2000 of the most recent data available in publications [104]
GAD generalized anxiety disorder, *n* number of patients

Conclusion

Stereotactic thermocoagulation surgery as well as radiosurgery, discussed below, have become relatively safe. The perioperative mortality rate is below 1 %, and morbidity rates, including neuropsychological deficits, are also low. Success rates meanwhile, ranging from 30 to 70 % [103] depending on the methodology and pathology, are non-negligible for a patient population presenting severe psychiatric symptoms refractory to treatment (Table 3.1).

Radiosurgery

Abstract Radiosurgery involves administering a dose of energy, usually gamma radiation, to an anatomical structure in order to create a localized lesion. This technique is similar in effect to stereotactic thermocoagulation and is also irreversible. But unlike thermocoagulation, it does not require trepanning and, therefore, presents virtually no surgical risk. In psychosurgery, radiosurgery is used for capsulotomies, lesioning of the anterior limb of the internal capsule. A small number of teams, including ones in Sweden and the United States, use "Gamma Knife" radiosurgery for the treatment of severe OCD.

Psychosurgery probably gave rise to radiosurgery. In the early 1950s, concerned with the hemorrhagic and infectious complications of capsulotomy procedures in patients with severe anxiety disorders, the Swedish neurosurgeon Lars Leksell, began creating focused lesions by means of ionizing radiation without having to open the skull [105]. In "Gamma Knife" surgery gamma rays replace the surgeon's knife [106, 107].

Principle and Technique

A Gamma-Knife is a device which focuses photons emitted by some 200 Cobalt-60 sources through a single point (Fig. 3.10). In order to spare surrounding brain tissue as much as possible, the target which will receive this single dose of high-energy radiation must be located with great accuracy. Over the last 20 years,

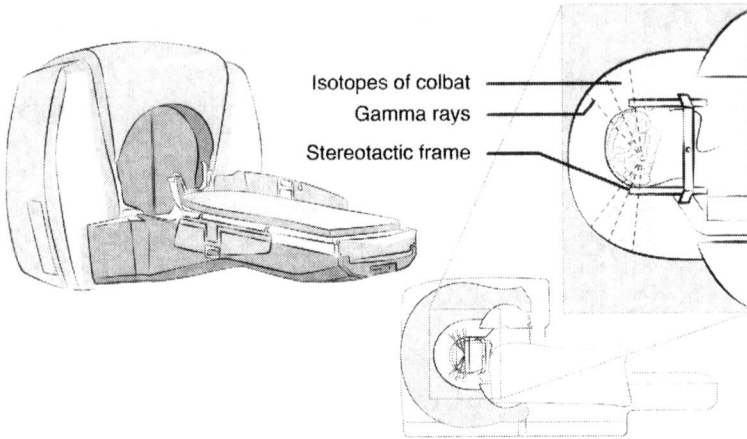

Isotopes of colbat
Gamma rays
Stereotactic frame

Fig. 3.10 Apparatus for Gamma Knife Perfexion radiosurgery

this effective technique has spread to the treatment of benign intracranial tumors, such as acoustic neuromas, meningiomas, pituitary adenomas, as well as brain metastases, arteriovenous malformations, facial neuralgia, and even some rare forms of epilepsy. In the procedure, which is usually performed on an outpatient basis and under local anesthesia only, a metal frame is affixed with four screws to the surface of the patient's skull. The frame both delimits the stereotactic space for calculating the coordinates of the target and immobilizes the subject's head. The dose of radiation is administered in a single session lasting a few hours.

Indications and Anatomical Targets

In psychiatry, except for a very small number of patients with severe anxiety disorders radiosurgery is mainly indicated for patients with OCD. For now, the anterior limb of the internal capsule is the only anatomical structure to have been targeted. Generally, "shots" of radiation ranging from 140 to 200 Gy[37] create two 4 mm lesions bilaterally. Necrosis of the brain parenchyma resulting from the radiation typically occurs within 2–4 months, which explains why symptoms begin to improve only after a few weeks. Although there is limited information on the first series of patients treated in 1978 at the Karolinska Institute, Leksell reported a decrease in symptoms in 70 % of the subjects [30, 108–110]. Following these encouraging results, 30 other Swedish patients were treated. Toward the end of the 1990s, teams at *Brown University* and in Pittsburgh also began administering the procedure, which became known as a *gamma capsulotomy*. Including patients

---

[37] Gy is the symbol for Gray, a unit that measures the amount of energy released.

treated in Sao Paulo and Mexico City, to date about 60 patients have been treated for their psychiatric condition with Gamma Knife surgery.

Results and Complications

The Swedish and American teams reported that 55–70 % of patients saw a significant decrease in their OCD symptoms according to the Y-BOCS[38] scale. These results remain stable over the years [30, 108–111]. Side effects such as fatigue, weight gain, or apathy were recorded primarily in patients who received doses exceeding 180 Gy [42]. Recently, a team in Pittsburgh demonstrated comparable efficacy with no side effects in three patients given a dose of 140 Gy [112]. Only one publication has made a thorough assessment of neuropsychological functioning before and after this type of intervention for a small number of patients [113, 114]. The authors reported no cognitive impairment or personality changes following surgery. They did find increased memory performance, attention, and capacity for abstraction probably related to patients' clinical improvement.

Future Applications

Even though the damage it causes is irreversible, radiosurgery is superior to thermocoagulation in that there is absolutely no risk infection or hemorrhage. The noninvasive nature of the procedure makes it permissible to perform randomized double-blind studies to objectively assess effectiveness. It also allows "sham surgery" to be used as a control for the actual procedure in order to eliminate any potential placebo effect [115]. These rigorous evaluation methods, unprecedented in the field, will help evaluate the effectiveness of radiosurgery alongside that of deep brain stimulation. Contiguous lesions are at less risk than with thermocoagulation. Consequently a more cautious, step-by-step approach could be envisioned. One in which a first series of "shots" may be extended the following month if necessary. New tractography imaging techniques now make it possible to assess the number of interrupted bundles and thus quantify the anatomical efficacy of an intervention. It must also be remembered that only a single target has been tried: the anterior limb of the internal capsule. Thanks to the reversibility of its effects, deep brain stimulation enables the exploration of an increasing number of targets. It is likely that in the wake of this exploration, new anatomical targets will be identified and become candidates for radiosurgery. However, it is possible that in the future radiosurgery will gradually be replaced by High Intensity Focused Ultrasound (HIFU).[39] The energy delivered by the ultrasound can coagulate tissue at the focal point through a highly focused and controlled increase in temperature (Fig. 3.11). Like radiosurgery

---

[38] Scale of OCD severity (cf. p. 273).
[39] Details of this technique cf. p. 457.

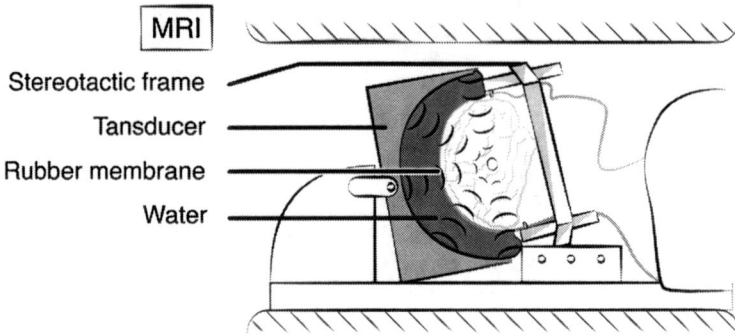

Fig. 3.11 Ultrasound lesioning: high intensity focused ultrasound (*HIFU*) apparatus

this technique is noninvasive; but unlike radiosurgery, its effect is immediate. This allows the intensity of the thermocoagulation to be modulated in real-time according to the patient's clinical response. For now, it has only been used to perform tha-lamotomies in the treatment of tremors and neuropathic pain [116].

Stimulation Techniques

– "*Here, professor, I need to give you some background information,*" *Captain Nemo said. So kindly hear me out.*

He fell silent for some moments, then he said:

– *There's a powerful, obedient, swift, and effortless force that can be bent to any use and which reigns supreme aboard my vessel. It does everything. It lights me, it warms me, it's the soul of my mechanical equipment. This force is electricity.*

Jules Verne's *Twenty Thousand Leagues Under the Sea*. Vol 1. Paris, 1870, p. 83. Translated from the original French by F.P. Walter.

The increasing accuracy of stereotactic techniques coupled with advances in brain imaging allow thermocoagulation and radiosurgery to make more targeted, millimeter-sized lesions in brain tissue. Though highly localized, these lesions are no less permanent; consequently, complications, including neuropsychological alterations, from the surgeries are also often permanent. Additionally, if the results of the procedure are unsatisfactory, the treatment area can be extended but only at the cost of a new intervention. These two shortcomings of lesional surgery have encouraged research into reversible and adaptable techniques, such as deep brain stimulation, stimulation of the vagus nerve and, more recently, cortical stimulation. Stimulation techniques, including deep brain stimulation, have undoubtedly reinvigorated the once controversial field of psychosurgery. The medical use of electricity dates back to antiquity. The Roman physician Scribonius Largus used electric rays and eels to treat gouty arthritis and headaches: the fish was placed on the headache patient's forehead until it discharged its curative electric jolt [117]. Around the same time that Jules Verne praised electricity as a powerful, obedient agent suited to all purposes, psychiatrists were enthusiastically developing thera-peutic applications for electricity. As the philosopher E. Fournier wrote, *electri-fying is animating with sudden energy, driving towards action. Not only can electricity give organs back their strength, but it can also remove what blocks them and help the patient regain the use of a lost pathway.* Guillaume Duchenne de Boulogne developed *faradization* in the mid-nineteenth century, and as the industrial and scientific revolutions spread, many hospital were equipped with *electrical machines* or *healing machines*. After this era of over-abundant, even fraudulent, electrotherapies, enthusiasm waned on the eve of WWI.[40] Although therapeutic gains were meager, this era did lead to advances in the field of elec-trophysiology and, above all, a new diagnostic tool, electroencephalography (EEG). This technique for recording cortical electrical activity really began to be used in the early 1950s in the field of epileptology. Meanwhile, neurosurgeons began to use electrical stimulation, sometimes routinely, to identify functional areas of the brain. In Montreal, W. Penfield relied predominantly on cortical stimulation to map the human cortex for his interventions [118, 119]. In Philadelphia, the inventors of stereotaxy, Spiegel and Wycis, also performed stimulation, but of the deep brain parenchyma. Brief electrical impulses were sent through the anatomical structure to be lesioned and the clinical manifestations recorded to be used in confirming the position of the target and the absence of adverse effects. Today, psychosurgery uses three types of stimulation: deep brain stimulation (DBS) which is used on many targets and for an increasing number of indication, cortical stimulation (CS), in which stimulation is limited to the prefrontal cortex and vagus nerve stimulation (VNS) (Fig. 3.12).

---

[40] We have evoked p. 33 the memory of Clovis Vincent, who along with Thierry de Martel was one of the pioneers of neurosurgery in France. Vincent was a war surgeon during WWI. He was known for his "torpillage" technique: he used electrical stimulations to distinguish traumatised soldiers from those only pretending to be traumatized.

This French expression came from one of his patients who stated that "it turns you upside down like a torpedo ("torpille" in French)." Military staff and then the Undersecretary for Health, J. Godart became aware of this dubious practice and stated, "the emotion that it would arouse in Tours and in that region the procedure implemented by the head-physician of the neurology centre, Clovis Vincent [...]. This procedure called "torpillage" was actually adopted and its therapeutic value shown at the meeting of neurologic physicians gathered under my initiative and who defined treatment methods for nervous system functional disorders [...]. Do not take into account the emotions of the public, which gets easily impressed when not well informed. Nau, J. Y. 2011. When Dr. Clovis Vincent "torpedoed" his patients. Rev Med Suisse 7:630–631.

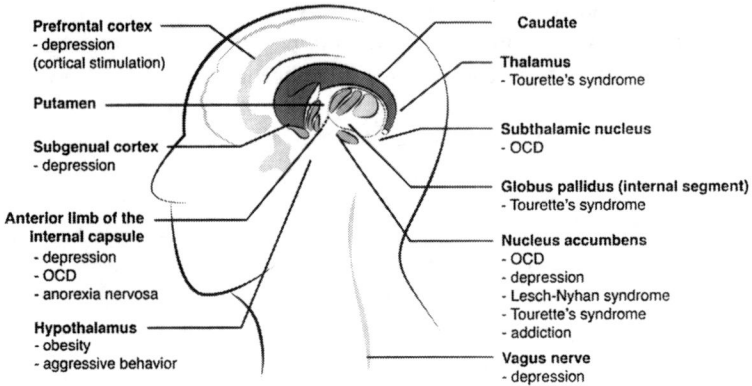

Prefrontal cortex
- depression
(cortical stimulation)

Putamen

Subgenual cortex
- depression

**Anterior limb of the
internal capsule**
- depression
- OCD
- anorexia nervosa

Hypothalamus
- obesity
- aggressive behavior

Caudate

Thalamus
- Tourette's syndrome

Subthalamic nucleus
- OCD

Globus pallidus (internal segment)
- Tourette's syndrome

Nucleus accumbens
- OCD
- depression
- Lesch-Nyhan syndrome
- Tourette's syndrome
- addiction

Vagus nerve
- depression

Fig. 3.12 The different stimulation targets in psychosurgery

Deep Brain Stimulation

In 1948, Pool, a neurosurgeon at Columbia University, was the first to implant electrodes intended not for diagnosis but for treatment. The electrode was implanted in the right caudate nucleus, of an elderly woman suffering from anorexia and depression [120]. Stimulation lasted 8 weeks and, apparently, gave favorable results. In a well-documented history of brain stimulation [121], the London neurosurgeon Hariz writes that in 1952 the neurophysiologist Delgado suggested using a recording and stimulation technique to assess treatment options for psychotic patients [122]. Delgado reported:*stimulation of the dorsolateral nucleus of the thalamus provoked exactly the same type of attack with symptoms directly proportional to the current. It was possible to identify the electrical threshold for mild anxiety and increase it to very high levels simply by turning the knob on the stimulator. Sitting with a hand on the knob of the stimulator one could control his level of anxiety"* [123]. A few years later, and under dubiously ethical conditions [124], a team from New Orleans led by the psychiatrist Heath performed some 100 brain stimulations of psychotic patients among others [125–127]. In a few scattered Scandinavian [128–130] and American [131] publications can be found reports of deep brain stimulation of the septal area having been used to treat the symptoms of depression. These patients, some of whom were indeed helped by the procedure, remained dependent on bulky external devices which were both a source of discomfort and, over time, infection. These hard to reproduce and often ethically questionable studies remained few up until the end of the 1980s. In 1987, a French team led by the neurosurgeon Benabid and neurologist Pollack began to successfully treat patients with Parkinson's disease by implanting electrodes in the thalamic nuclei[41] [132]. The same team, using the same

---

[41] Cf. p. 123.

technique, also successfully treated debilitating essential tremors [133, 134]. In Montpellier, a team led by Coubes adapted the procedure for the treatment of generalized dystonia, an abnormal movement disorder manifested by debilitating muscle contractions, by stimulating the internal globus pallidum [135].

The Contribution of Deep Brain Stimulation to the Treatment of Parkinson's Disease

Since 1987, nearly 80,000 patients, mostly with Parkinson's disease, have benefited from this technique worldwide with most interventions targeting the subthalamic nucleus. This large set of patient data has shown that certain electrode placements and stimulation parameters lead to emotional or behavioral modifications. Emotional changes can vary from simple euphoria [136–138] to manic or hypersexual states [139, 140] sadness [141], severe depression, or suicidal acts [142–144]. Aggressive behavior [136, 145], pathological gambling, emotional indifference or blunting of emotions, and apathy are among the behavioral modifications also observed [146]. Two prospective studies have also shown [138, 147] that the anxiety disorders, OCD among them, affecting nearly 60 % of patients regressed in 30–65 % of cases [148]. Both teams led by the psychiatrist Mallet in Paris and the neurosurgeon Fontaine in Nice observed that stimulation alleviated some of the compulsions of Parkinson's patients who had OCD as well [149, 150].

First Successes and the Favorable Opinion of the French National Ethics Advisory Council

In 1999, the *Lancet* published two landmark articles [151]. That year, Nuttin, a neurosurgeon in Leuven, Belgium, announced encouraging results from brain stimulation in three patients with OCD. The Belgian team implanted electrodes in the anterior limb of the internal capsule (ALIC), an area commonly targeted by lesional surgery to treat OCD. The authors reported that one patient, *a 39-year-old woman suffering from extremely severe OCD for more than 20 years, reported when stimulation was on, an almost instantaneous feeling of being relieved of anxiety and obsessive thinking, which disappeared after turning the stimulation off. She was continuously stimulated for 2 weeks and her parents reported that about 90 % of her compulsive behavior and rituals had vanished.* The same year, a neighboring Benelux team led by Visser-Vandewalle reported similar success with a patient suffering from Gilles de la Tourette syndrome after thalamic stimulation.

In an editorial published in 2002, Nuttin and 12 other signatories[42] insisted on the
need for strict oversight of research into *deep brain stimulation for psychiatric
disorders* and laid out the ethical prerequisites for this research[43] [152]. In France
the same year, at the behest of Benabid, the *Comité National Consultatif d'Ethique*
(national ethics advisory council) approved of the use of functional neurosurgery
for severe psychiatric disorders. The council considered that "given their
encouraging results, the development of promising new brain neurostimulation
techniques for certain diseases such as Parkinson's disease raises the question of
whether they could be extended to other conditions, in particular psychiatric
conditions. Advances in imaging and the a priori reversible nature of these techniques justifies reexamining the technical issue of brain surgery for psychiatric
illness. The issue had, in fact, been entirely barred since the tragic legacy of
destructive surgery, especially frontal surgery, of the 1950s. A number of clinical
observations have indeed shown the effectiveness of these new methods, especially
for OCD (debilitating obsessive psychoses are a real source of moral pain for
patients because an important part of their lives becomes devoted to their rituals).
It is therefore appropriate to reconsider anew this therapeutic modality while
asking a number of questions" [153, 154]. In the first decade of the new millen-
nium, clinical studies were conducted to evaluate the effectiveness of deep brain
stimulation in the treatment of psychiatric disorders, OCD, and depression first and
foremost, but also to a lesser extent addiction, aggressive behavior, and eating
disorders.

Principle

The mechanism of action of deep brain stimulation remains unclear. High frequency
electrical stimulation, greater than 100 Hz, has a similar clinical effect on lesions,
i.e., inhibition of the anatomical region targeted. The target structure is generally in
a state of hyperactivity related to the psychiatric disorder. Several hypotheses have
been put forward to explain the blocking effect of stimulation: inhibition of neuronal
discharge, changes in oscillation rate, or release of inhibitory neurotransmitters.
Depending on the structure targeted and the type of tissue it contains—axons are
located in the white matter and cell bodies in the gray matter—the mechanisms
leading to inhibition may differ or be intertwined [155].

---

[42] The ethicists J. Gybels, Jan and J. Fins (President of the American BioEthics Society), the
psychiatrists L. Gabriel, P. Cosyns, D. Malone, B. Greenberg, S. Rasmunsen, the neurosurgeons
A. Rezai, G. Friehs, B. Meryerson and the neurologist E. Montgomery.

[43] Cf. ethical safe-guards p. 443.

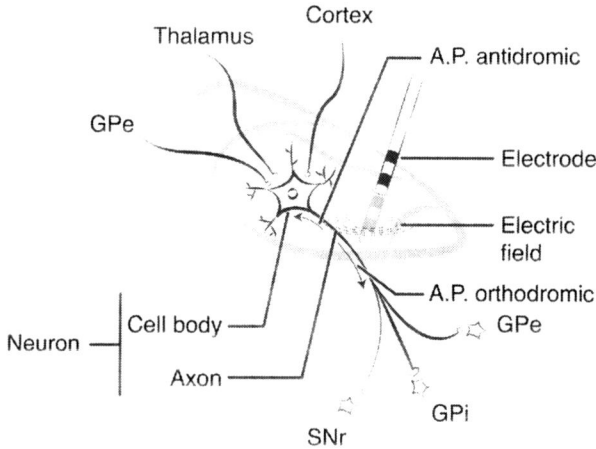

Fig. 3.13 Deep brain stimulation in the subthalamic nucleus. The *arrow* show the orthodromic action potentials (*AP*) travelling away from the neuron cell body and the antidromic AP, caused by electrical stimulation, travelling in the opposite direction toward the cell body *Gpe* external globus pallidus. *Gpi* internal globus pallidus. *SNr* substantia nigra reticulata, according to [156]

Neural Tissue

Brain tissue consists of neurons and surrounding cells called glia. Neurons communicate with each other through projections called axons (Fig. 3.13). These neurons, close to 100 billion in humans, and the axons linking them together in a network give rise to our brain functions. The information traveling along the axons, the *action potential* (AP), referred to as *orthodromic*, from the body of the neuron to the projecting axon. At the end of the axon is a gap called a synapse which enables communication with other neurons. Communication across the synapse is accomplished biochemically by molecules called neurotransmitters.

Stimulation and Its Enigmas

An electric field forms between the positive terminal of the electrode, the anode and the negative terminal, the cathode. When applied to the nerve tissue, this field triggers APs, i.e., electrical waves propagating along the axons. To accomplish this, the electrical current must have an amplitude high enough to reach the "electric field threshold" and trigger an AP (Fig. 3.19, p. 140). The axons targeted for stimulation must neither be too close to the electrode, in the "toxicity zone," nor too far from it, in the "loss of efficacy zone." They must be located between these two areas in the *threshold zone* (Fig. 3.14). It should be noted that the threshold for efficacy is lower near the cathode than the anode.

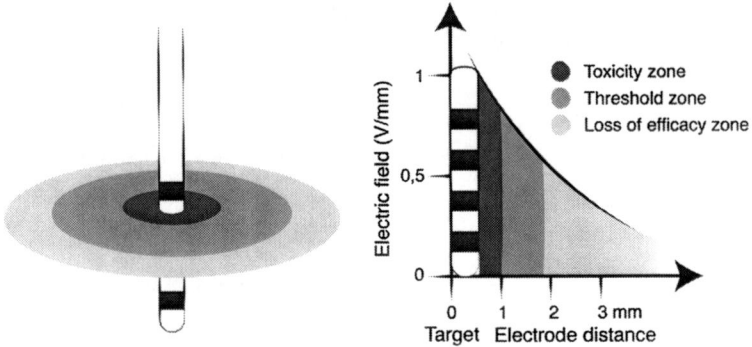

Fig. 3.14 Window of effective stimulation. According to [157]

The electrode triggers *orthodromic* action potentials, which move along the axon toward the synapse, as well as *antidromic* action potentials, which flow "against the current" toward the body of the neuron (Fig. 3.13). Orthodromic electrical signals flowing out from the cell may be blocked by these antidromic action potentials. Neurophysiologists suspect that a high frequency of orthodromic APs, i.e., electrical signals flowing outwards from the cell body toward the synapse, may eventually exhaust a neurons supply of neurotransmitters and thus block synaptic function. Researchers also suspect that steady stimulation may "smooth" pathological and erratic electrical activity. These two effects, whether orthodromic or antidromic, of electrical stimulation lead to the same outcome: inhibition of pathological activity in the nervous tissue surrounding the electrode terminals [156, 158, 159]. This schematic explanation is of limited use because the nature of the tissue surrounding the electrode also affects the response. High frequency stimulation of nuclei leads to inhibition, while stimulation of white-matter bundles leads to activation [160]. The situation is further complicated by the fact that nuclei and bundles can be in close proximity or even entangled. Additionally, an electric field of greater intensity may broaden the range of the stimulation and "recruit" neighboring regions. As Nuttin indicated concerning stimulation of the anterior limb of the internal capsule (ALIC), "it is unclear whether the effects obtained are a consequence of the activation or inhibition of fibers or cell bodies" [161]. It would be expected, for example, that high-frequency stimulation of white matter in the ALIC would cause activation yet the opposite is true. The clinical effect is similar to those of a lesion (capsulotomy). Nuclei adjacent to the ALIC white matter[44] such as the nucleus accumbens[45] and the bed nucleus of the stria terminalis may therefore also be receiving some form of stimulation. Conversely, high-frequency stimulation of a nucleus can lead to phenomena that resemble activation more than inhibition. It has been observed, for example, that stimulation

---

[44] Cf. pp. 210 and 290.

[45] Cf. p. 129.

of the subthalamic nucleus may cause symptoms of hypomania. This may indicate that the medial forebrain bundle[46] (MFB) a bundle of white matter which passes nearby, may be activated by the stimulation (Fig. 3.3, p. 110) [162]. Along with the local effects of this "deep" stimulation, it is possible that the oscillatory rhythm of cortical, or surface, areas of the brain are also being modulated [155, 163, 164]. Recent developments in optogenetics[47] should help us better understand some of the phenomena involved (Fig. 6.2, p. 313) [165].

Plasticity and Neurogenesis

In addition to the acute phenomena of neuronal activation and inhibition mentioned above, it is likely that other mechanisms also contribute to clinical effects observed. These other processes could account for the delayed, sometimes by several weeks, effects of stimulation. Over time, stimulation may lead to the formation of new neural connection and thus changes in the pathological functioning of the entire network. Neurogenesis, the process in question, has been demonstrated in the hippocampus of animals after stimulation of the anterior nucleus of the thalamus[48] [166, 167] or the entorhinal cortex[49] [167–169]. More recently, Lozano's team in Toronto demonstrated, this time in humans, an increase in the volume of the hippocampus[50] after several months of stimulation of the fornix[51] in patients with Alzheimer's. This disease normally causes degeneration of the hippocampus reducing its volume by about 5 % per year [170–172]; but after 1 year of stimulation, two of the six subjects presented, respectively, a 4.5 and 9.8 % increase in volume coupled with improved memory faculties [173].

The Benefits and Limits of Stimulation

The reversibility and adaptability of electrical stimulation, made possible by adjusting parameters such as frequency and intensity, are among the obvious advantages of this technique (Fig. 3.19, p. 140). It is also possible to move the loca to different points along the electrode (Fig. 3.18, p. 140). The electrode is a rigid cable covered by insulation with metal terminals at the tip. There are generally four terminals spaced a few millimeters apart[52] thereby allowing the site of the stimulation to

---

[46] Cf. p. 146.

[47] Cf. p. 463.

[48] Cf. p. 123.

[49] Cf. p. 103.

[50] Ibid.

[51] Ibid.

[52] This distance can change depending on the type of electrode. Electrodes destined to stimulate "small" structures like the subthalamic nucleus, have more closely spaced contacts than those conceived for the stimulation of larger structures like the globus pallidus. The types of electrodes change depending on the area of stimulation.

be varied depending on which terminals are positively or negatively energized. In case of adverse reaction or in the absence of therapeutic benefits, it is possible to stop the stimulation, modulate the settings, or change the site of the stimulation, options unavailable in lesional surgery. In terms of methodological advantages, it is possible to undertake double-blinded studies with deep brain stimulation. Since stimulation is imperceptible to the patient, it is possible to alternate periods of stimulation with periods of no stimulation, and neither the patient nor his psychiatrist can know whether the stimulator is switched on or off. Only the neurosurgeon, neurologist, or psychiatrist tasked with setting the electrical parameters knows. This type of study, in which the patient is his own witness, allows the impact of the placebo effect on the clinical response to be evaluated and the true impact of the treatment better understood (Fig. 4.2, p. 201). However, the placebo effect tends to diminish as the severity of symptoms increases, such as with severe depression [174, 175]. The stimulation electrodes also offer the possibility of making electrophysiological recordings of deep anatomical structures[53] and increase our understanding of the pathophysiology of neuropsychiatric disorders. These recordings can be made during the few days between implantation of the electrodes and implantation of the neurostimulation control box and are invaluable clinical and scientific research tools [176]. Deep brain stimulation does also have some disadvantages compared to other lesional techniques such as the high cost of the implantable device. Installation of the electrodes and stimulator can cost up to 15,000 euros, and the stimulator must be replaced every 5–6 years at a cost of 10,000 euros [177]. Additionally, the large sums of money involved are likely to foster conflicts of interest[54] or introduce biases in the publication of results of clinical studies. Lesional radiosurgery techniques[55] in comparison are less costly and require a period of hospitalization of no more than 2 or 3 days. The dangers inherent to intracranial surgery and the presence of implanted devices, such as hemorrhage, infection, disconnected wires, and failure of the pacemaker are among the disadvantages of deep brain stimulation (Table 6.1, p. 309).

Technique

Today, functional neurosurgery departments are well practiced at implanting deep brain stimulation electrodes, which require a multidisciplinary team of psychiatrists, neurologists, neuroradiologists, and neurosurgeons adept at stereotaxy. Although there are some differences in the techniques used at different hospitals, particularly with regard to anesthesia, the general principle[56] of stereotactic implantation remains the same. The intervention is accomplished in several stages in a little over 12 h.

---

[53] Other noninvasive brain recording techniques are those performed on the surface of the cortex like electroencephalograms (EEG). DBS electrode recording offers the advantage of having a very good temporal and spatial resolution and a good sound-to-noise ratio (SNR).

[54] Cf. Conflicts of interest p. 432.

[55] Cf. p. 187.

[56] Cf. 164.

Fig. 3.15 Stereotactic frame
being affixed to the skull

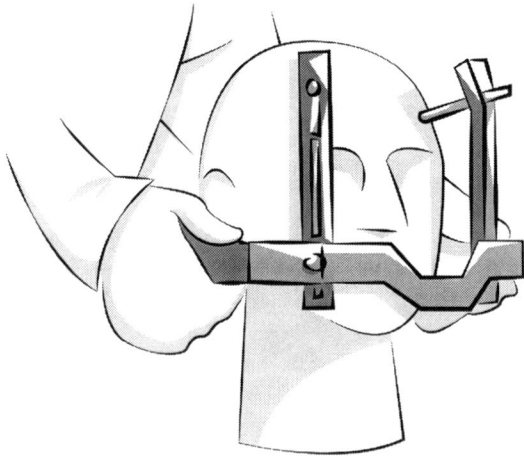

Image Acquisition

In the operating room under general or local anesthesia, a metal, stereotactic frame
is affixed to the surface of the skull by four screws (Fig. 3.15). The patient is then
transported to the radiology department to undergo an MRI and sometimes a CT
scan[57] as well. Some centers also perform a *ventriculography*, a radiography of the
skull after injection of a contrast agent into the ventricles, in order to better
visualize the anatomical landmarks.

Determining the Anatomical Target

After returning to the operating room, the neurosurgeon and neuroradiologist
determine the anatomical target to be stimulated. Two complementary methods are
used. The first, *statistical*, method determines the coordinates of the target based
on an anatomical atlas (Fig. 3.3, p. 110). The neurosurgeon locates a number of
clearly visible reference anatomical structures in the patient's imaging results and
then identifies these same structures in an atlas where the chosen target appears.
Through simple math, the coordinates of the target site are calculated with respect
to the position of the reference structures (Fig. 3.2 p.109) and overlaid onto the
MRI. This method can be likened in aviation to making an instrument landing
when the runway, i.e., the target, is hard to discern. Whenever the target is clearly
identifiable on the MRI, its coordinates are directly calculated from the image.

---

[57] This test can be associated with the previous one to correct image distortions seen on MRI
related to the magnetic field.

This second, *direct targeting* method is equivalent to making a visual landing. Once the coordinates for the target have been determined, a route to the target bypassing all vessels and cavities is planned out.

Descent of the Electrode

Once the coordinates and the resulting trajectory have been calculated for the target, the neurosurgeon adjusts the instrument holder mounted on the stereotactic frame (Fig. 3.16). A small incision is made in the skin in order to reveal the skull and perform a *craniotomy*, the drilling of a burr hole a few millimeters in diameter into the cranium. The surgeon then pierces the membrane—the dura mater— enveloping the brain. The electrode, guided by the instrument holder, is then lowered millimeter by millimeter toward the target (Fig. 3.4, p. 111).

Electrophysiological recordings are sometimes made before placing the final electrode by inserting very thin recording needles instead. The recorded electrical brain activity gives information about the brain structures being traversed, and so, serves to confirm that the electrode will follow the correct trajectory to the target. If the aviation metaphor is extended, these recordings can be likened to a pilot's radar. Throughout the procedure, radiographies of the patient's skull are performed to ensure that the electrode is following the planned trajectory. Once the electrode is in place, the cable is attached to the skull and the burr hole is filled with biological cement or covered by a small plate.

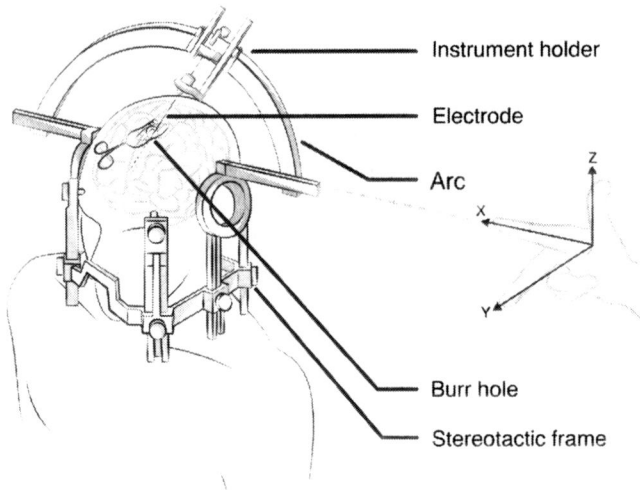

Fig. 3.16 *Arc* and *instrument holder* attached to *the stereotactic frame. The stereotactic arc* system uses *x, y* and *z* coordinates to locate the target. *The electrode* can descend at different angles to avoid fragile structures (arteries or veins) or alter the trajectory

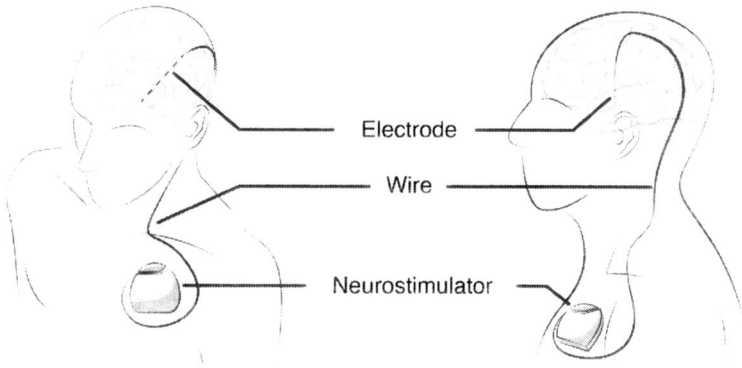

Fig. 3.17 Complete implanted system

Connecting the Neurostimulation Box

In general, this procedure is performed bilaterally with the same anatomical structure being targeted in each hemisphere. Both electrodes where they exit the brain are then connected subcutaneously to the neurostimulator by means of a cable. The neurostimulator is generally located under the skin in the chest or abdomen (Fig. 3.17).

Post-surgical Follow-up and Adjustments

Immediately following the surgery, a CT scan is performed in order to ensure that there are no complications and to check the positioning of the electrodes. The settings on the neurostimulator are then adjusted by the team using a remote control (Fig. 3.18).

Depending on the clinical response obtained, the amplitude, frequency, and duration of the stimulation pulses are adjusted (Fig. 3.19). The choice of which electrode terminals, the metal contacts spaced every 2–4 mm along the length of the electrode, to activate modifies the depth of the stimulation. These parameters combine to offer a wide range of possible settings.

The fact that several weeks can sometimes elapse[58] between changes in these settings and corresponding clinical changes adds another level of complexity. As the psychiatrist Goodman explains: *This delay between the start of the*

---

[58] This delay can vary depending on the chosen target. A clinical effect may occur in a matter of seconds which is the case of subgenual cortex DBS. Mayberg observes in the first five patients: "They all mentioned spontaneously acute effects like 'sudden calm or lightness,' 'disappearance of the void,' 'a feeling of growing awareness' [...] in response to this electrical stimulation" [240].

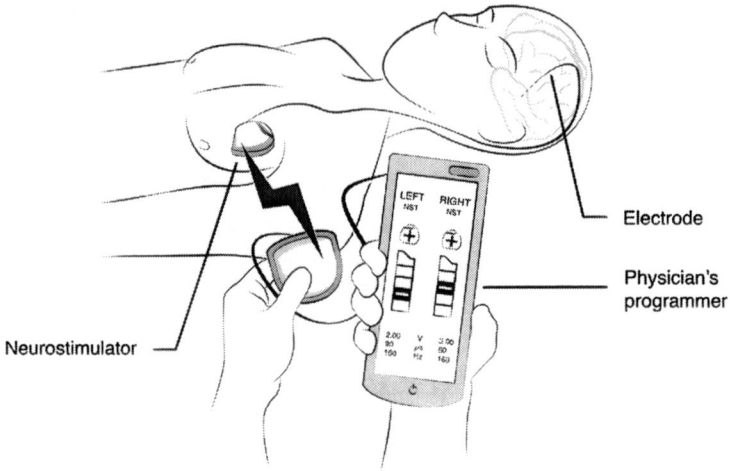

Fig. 3.18 Remote programming and neurostimulation

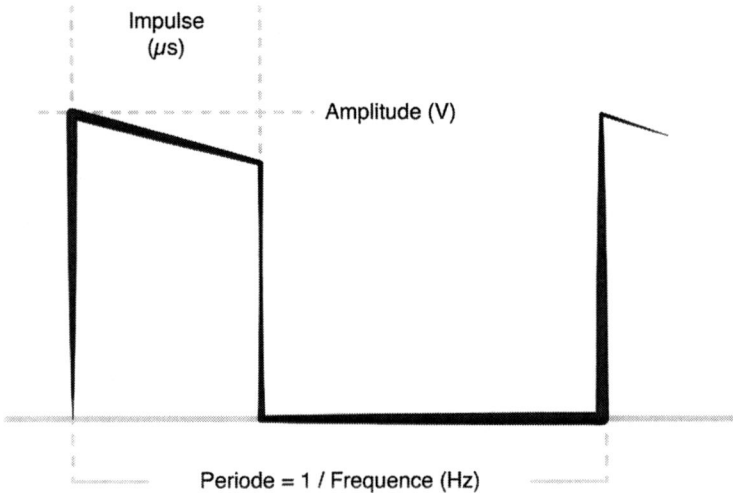

Fig. 3.19 Different adjustable pulse stimulation parameters

stimulation and the clinical response makes programming laborious.... For these reasons, optimization of the deep brain stimulation parameters in the treatment of psychiatric disorders is more art than science and requires a lot of patience from the patient as well as from the clinician [178].

Surgical Complications

This invasive surgical procedure can result in potentially severe complications with incidence rates varying from one team to another. A distinction is made between complications arising from the surgical procedures and those inherent to the stimulation tools or the stimulation itself. Only the first two sources of complications are discussed here. Those related to stimulation itself are discussed in a later section describing each anatomical target individually. According to a meta-analysis conducted in 2006 of nearly 1000 patients treated for Parkinson's disease, the surgical procedure can lead to intracerebral hematoma in 4 % of patients [179]. The percentage however varied significantly, between 0 and 10 %, in the various publications the researchers analyzed [180]. Postoperative epileptic seizures and postoperative delirium were also reported in 1 and 15 % of patients, respectively. The latter percentage also varied between 24.5 % [136] and 40 % [181] depending on the type of anesthesia [182]. Complications resulting directly from the devices included secondary displacement of the electrode in 1.5 % patients and malfunction of the implanted system in 3 % of patients [179]. In 4.4 % of patients these complications made new surgical procedures necessary. Surgery led to infection in 3.6 % of cases, but again, this rate varied significantly, ranging from 0 to 15 %, among the publications [179, 180]. These infections often required removal of all or part of the device for at least the duration of the antibiotic treatment. A period of several months must elapse before reimplantation can be considered. Curiously, this complication was more common in patients who suffered from OCD and had cleaning rituals. As has been noted, serious complications can result from this type of procedure. But for the most part, these can be treated or are temporary, as with delirium. However, these figures should be received with caution given that they come from a series of patients operated during the course of their treatment for Parkinson's disease and not from a cohort of patients treated for a psychiatric disorder. Such patients remain too few to draw any specific conclusions. It is nonetheless foreseeable, that the younger the psychiatric patient the lower the risk of complications.

Anatomical Targets for Given Indications

Abstract Knowledge about which anatomical site to target during deep brain stimulation comes from lesional surgery, results of stimulation in the treatment of certain neurological diseases, and more recently, functional brain imaging data. The internal capsule was initially chosen because good results had been obtained with lesional surgery in the treatment of OCD and depression. Observations made during treatment of Parkinson's disease have led the subthalamic nucleus to be targeted for the treatment of OCD. The subgenus area was targeted after imaging revealed hyperactivity in this area in patients with depression. Many more

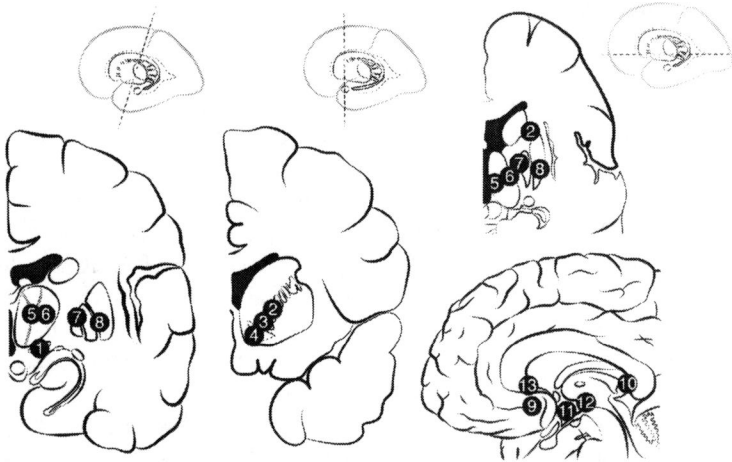

Fig. 3.20 Targets of deep brain stimulation (*DBS*) for the treatment of psychiatric disorders. (1) Subthalamic nucleus DBS: OCD, (2) anterior limb of the internal capsule DBS: OCD, depression, anorexia nervosa, (3) ventral striatum DBS: OCD, (4) nucleus accumbens DBS: depression, ODC, addiction, (5) inferior thalamic peduncle DBS: depression, (6) thalamus infralaminar nucleus DBS: Gilles de la Tourette syndrome (*GTS*), (7) internal globus pallidus DBS: GTS, Lesch-Nyhan syndrome, (8) external globus pallidus DBS, (10) habenula DBS: depression, (11) posterior hypothalamus: aggressive behavior disorder, (12) ventromedial hypothalamus DBS: obesity, (13) medial forebrain bundle DBS: depression

anatomical targets are still under investigation in a growing number of psychiatric disorders.

As much as the choice of anatomical sites for deep brain stimulation (Fig. 3.20) explored by psychosurgery over the past 10 years has been informed by empirical results of lesional psychosurgery interventions and a better understanding of functional anatomy, it has also been due to serendipity.

The Internal Capsule in the Treatment of OCD, Depression, and Other Pathologies

Abstract The anterior limb of the internal capsule is a band of white matter located between the caudate nucleus and the putamen through which pass the associative and limbic thalamocortical fibers connecting the prefrontal cortex to the thalamus. Since the 1950s, lesional surgery of this target has successfully been used in the treatment of OCD and depression. Today, deep brain stimulation of this area is being used to treat these same pathologies. The possibility of reversing the effects of stimulation eliminates some of the neuropsychological complications, such as apathy, which can result from a capsulotomy. Recently, this area has also been targeted to treat anorexia nervosa and addiction. Given this structure's proximity to other key regions involved in emotions—such as the nucleus accumbens and the bed of the stria terminalis—it is likely that stimulation of these areas also contributes to clinical efficacy.

In 1999, the anterior limb of the internal capsule (ALIC) was the first structure, along with the thalamus, to be targeted by deep brain stimulation in order to treat a psychiatric disorder [151, 183]. Ever since the work conducted by Talairach and Leksell in 1949 [18], in Europe this has been one of lesional surgery's favored targets for the treatment of both OCD and depression.

Anatomy

This anatomical area is composed of a band of white matter containing bundles of axons which reciprocally connects the dorsomedial nucleus[59] of the thalamus to the orbitofrontal,[60] cingulate[61] (Fig. 2.18, p. 77) and dorsolateral[62] cortices. It also contains fibers linking the ventral anterior nucleus[63] of the thalamus to these same prefrontal regions, with the exception of the cingulate cortex and cortico-striatal fibers linking the prefrontal cortex to the striatum. Finally, it is located near the nucleus accumbens[64]—involved in the *reward circuit*—and the bed nucleus of the stria terminalis, which is involved in regulating anxiety and stress, and their proximity suggests that they are also affected during deep brain stimulation. It should be noted that although capsulotomies have been performed successfully for over 60 years, knowledge of how these CSTC[65] loops function is more recent, dating back only to 1986 when Alexander conceptualized them [21].

Results of the Treatment for OCD

In 1999, DBS of the anterior limb of the internal capsule in the treatment of OCD was reported for the first time. In a report published in *The Lancet*, Nuttin presented favorable results for three of the four patients who had received the operation [151]. Other teams in the United States, including one led by Greenberg at Brown University, have targeted a more ventral area of the anterior limb of the internal capsule where it meets a neighboring region, the ventral striatum. The reason his team selected this more posterior and medial site is that at this point the bundle of thalamocortical fibers is more compact thus allowing a more targeted modulation of the famous CSTC loop [184, 185]. This area, known as Ventral

---

[59] Cf. p. 123.
[60] Cf. p. 93.
[61] Cf. p. 95.
[62] Cf. p. 92.
[63] Cf. p. 124.
[64] Cf. p. 129.
[65] Cf. pp.142 and 143.

Capsule/Ventral Striatum (for VC/VS), astride two structures and close to the nucleus accumbens and the nucleus of the stria terminalis would appear to be a critical junction. By varying the parameters and depth of stimulation, clinicians can focus on one or more of these structures. A prospective, multicenter international study by Greenberg and Nuttin of 26 patients with severe OCD reported a 28 % response rate (defined by a Y-BOCS score reduced by at least 35 %) 1 month after surgery and 61.5 % after an average follow-up period of 31 months. The authors also observed at the end of 36 months of stimulation a significant reduction in the symptoms of depression initially present for 22 patients whose HAM-D depression score was reduced by 43.2 %. A significant improvement in quality of life and a significant reduction in non-specific anxiety of OCD was also recorded [185]. Other studies, all prospective but sometimes also including patients from previous studies, have given comparable results [161, 186, 187].

Results of the Treatment for Depression

Again, based on the results of lesional surgery, indication of this target for the treatment of drug-resistant depression has also been explored. This is supported by data from functional imaging, which as with OCD, points to a probable malfunction of the CSTC loops [188–192]. When treating patients with OCD who also suffered from depression, the teams reported a net regression in the symptoms of depression following stimulation of the capsule [151, 185–187, 193]. In 2008, the American teams of Malone, Dougherty and Greenberg showed that in five patients with drug-resistant depression 40 % responded after 6 months and 53.3 % after an average of a little under 2 years, while 20 % were in remission after 6 months and 40 % long-term [188].

Results of the Treatment for Anorexia Nervosa[66] and Addiction

The existence of obsessional personality traits [194, 195], obsessive fear of weight gain, and recurrent or intrusive thoughts about body image in patients with anorexia nervosa allows some parallels to be drawn between anorexia nervosa and OCD. As mentioned earlier, Nuttin's team in Leuven, Belgium, repeatedly observed that in patients with both OCD and anorexia nervosa brain stimulation of the ALIC resulted in regression of all symptoms [161, 196]. Recently, a Dutch team observed that stimulation of this region in a patient with a heroin addiction resulted in a marked decrease in opioid consumption. Initially, the neurosurgeons intended to target the nucleus accumbens, a key structure in the reward circuit.

---

[66] Cf. also p. 358 about anorexia nervosa and p. 366 about the treatment of addiction using deep brain stimulation.

But to reach this region they decided to have the electrode pass through the ALIC), and ultimately, stimulation of the dorsal part of the ALIC is what allowed the daily consumption 0.68–0.1 g of heroin to be reduced. Once again, the compulsive behavior associated with drug abuse indicates some clinical similarities between addictive behaviors and OCD. However, successes in these two indications remain anecdotal and must be confirmed by larger studies.

Complications Specifically Linked to Stimulation

The large-scale prospective study conducted by Greenberg reported no cognitive impairments due to DBS of the ALIC, contrary to what has been observed for the capsulotomy, which contains a certain risk of postoperative apathy.[67] Three of the 26 patients (11 %) had episodes of depression during stimulation similar to ones they had before stimulation. In two other patients a recurrence of suicidal ideation was recorded after the neurostimulation control box was accidentally shut off. When the stimulator was turned back on the two patients suffered from transient insomnia [185]. Mood elevation was observed in 9 of the 26 patients leading to an episode of hypomania, resolved by decreasing the stimulation parameters, in 1 patient. A similar case, associated with hypersexuality, was also reported by a Chinese team. In that study, a decrease in stimulation intensity also normalized the situation but at the cost of a recurrence of the OCD symptoms [197]. Finally, Manole's study identified no complications linked specifically to stimulation [188].

The Nucleus Accumbens in the Treatment of Depression, OCD, and Addiction

Abstract Near the anterior limb of the internal capsule, the nucleus accumbens, consisting of a heart and a shell, is a primary relay in the reward circuit. While the heart is involved in motor control, the shell is connected to the amygdala and the rest of the limbic system and is thus involved in the regulation of emotions. It functions as an interface between the various emotion circuits, which makes it a preferred target in the treatment of depression as well as OCD and addictions.

Functional imaging studies suggest a functional impairment of the nucleusac-cumbens[68] in patients with depression. When these patients are given pleasant stimuli, activity in their nucleus accumbens differs from that of control subjects [198, 199]. The participation of the nucleus accumbens in the reward circuit—i.e., pleasure—as well as in motivation is now well established. Loss of pleasure, "anhedonia," of motivation, or even of the will to live, key symptoms of

---

[67] Cf. the complications of capsulotomy, p. 179.

[68] Cf. p. 129.

depression, have logically attracted the attention of researchers to the possible links between this nucleus and depression (Fig. 4.4, p. 216) [200, 201]. In 2004, a Bordeaux team led by Aouizerate and Cuny, observed mood improvement in a patient with concomitant OCD and depression following stimulation of the nucleus. The electrodes, originally intended to treat OCD, were placed in the ventral part of the caudate nucleus, but some of the terminals were in contact with the nucleus accumbens [193, 202].

As will be shown[69] one of the prevailing explanations for OCD is "overheating" of the CSCT loop[70] involving the orbitofrontal cortex[71] and an excess of activity along the direct pathway through the striatum,[72] particularly the ventromedial part of the caudate nucleus. The nucleus accumbens, located at the base of the ventral striatum, is also implicated in this modulation. The reader will recall that the dorsal part of the nucleus borders the ventral part of the anterior limb of the internal capsule[73] (ALIC) (p. 120 and Fig. 3.3), a structure targeted in both ablative surgery[74] and deep brain stimulation.[75] High voltages of up to 10 v may be necessary to obtain a therapeutic effect during stimulation of the capsule. Some authors, such as Nuttin, wonder if this high voltage may not also be stimulating the nucleus accumbens, the bed nucleus of the stria terminalis, or even the medial forebrain bundle[76] (FMT) [203]. Secondary stimulation of the nucleus accumbens rather than of the ALIC itself could be the source of the clinical effect [151]. A similar observation was made by the Karolinska Institute team in MRI followups to radiosurgery[77] of the anterior capsule: Meyerson found that satisfactory clinical outcomes required the target site to be located near the nucleus accumbens. Sturm and his colleagues at the University of Cologne have also obtained regression in OCD symptoms through stimulation applied unilaterally on the right side in three of four patients whose electrodes were in contact with the shell of the nucleus accumbens [204].

Results for Depression

In 2010, a team from Bonn published its results for a series of ten patients with severe drug-resistant depression [205]. Bewernick and Schlaepfer found that five

---

[69] Cf. p. 278.

[70] Cf. p. 139.

[71] Cf. p. 93.

[72] Cf. p. 128.

[73] Cf. p. 125.

[74] Cf. p. 167.

[75] Cf. p. 193.

[76] Cf. p. 146.

[77] Cf. p. 187.

of their ten patients had HDRS scores reduced by one-half a year after surgery. They also noted diminished anxiety in all the subjects, including those who did not feel their mood improve. Functional imaging by PET scan showed less metabolism in area 25 and in the orbitofrontal cortex following stimulation.

Results for OCD

Also in 2010, the Germans Huff and Sturm published the results for a series of ten patients implanted unilaterally. The Cologne team reported that after 1 year five patients had Y-BOCS scores decreased by at least 25 % and one patient by 35 % [206].

Results of the Treatment for Addictions

The nucleus accumbens plays a central part in the dopaminergic reward circuit.[78] High levels of dopamine in the nucleus are systematically observed in cases of addiction.[79] In 2012, a team at the Chinese military hospital in Xi'an published the results of 272 heroin addicts treated by having their nucleus accumbens removed [207]. The same year, the German team from Magdeburg presented the results of stimulation of the nucleus accumbens in a series of five chronic severe alcoholic patients [208]. These patients aged 36–65 had been addicted a minimum of 18 years, and all their attempts to quit had ended in failure. Four years after the intervention, two patients had achieved complete abstinence and had been able to resume working. The other three patients were also able to stop drinking but suffered three to four relapses. Two of these patients also began working again but the third remained incarcerated. The literature also mentions three addicts, two in China and another in the Netherlands, who were weaned from their opiate addiction following implantation of electrodes at this site [209–211].

Specific Complications

In Bewernick's study, changing the parameters of stimulation (2–4 V, 130 Hz, 90 μs) led to increased anxiety and sweating in three patients and agitation or hypomania in two others [205]. These symptoms disappeared after the settings were changed. Of the five non-responder patients, one committed suicide and another attempted suicide. The authors noted that no changes had been made to the stimulation parameters, but that the patient who committed suicide was having difficulties in his personal life as he was undergoing a separation [205]. One of the patients had a history of suicidal ideation prior to implantation and presented a

---

[78] Cf. p. 146.
[79] Cf. p. 359.

new episode requiring hospitalization and renewed antidepressant treatment [206]. Two patients developed self-limited hypomania and two others gained 5 kg in the year following the intervention. One patient complained of increased insomnia and another presented memory loss and decreased concentration which resolved itself after the parameters were changed. The Cologne team identified four states of agitation and anxiety which occurred when the voltage was increased and subsided when it was decreased.

The Subthalamic Nucleus in the Treatment of OCD

Abstract The subthalamic nucleus has been a target for Parkinson's disease treatments for the past two decades. Observations made among the tens of thousands of patients operated in this indication have shown that high-frequency stimulation of the subthalamic nucleus could also reduce the symptoms of OCD in patients suffering from both. Studies have subsequently confirmed the effectiveness of high-frequency stimulation of this structure, particularly its cognitive and limbic area, for the treatment of patients with refractory OCD.

Unlike the previous target, which owes much to findings in lesional surgery, the choice of the subthalamic nucleus (STN) comes primarily from research with deep brain stimulationin Parkinson's disease. Beyond its success in treating this neurological disease, many clinical observations have highlighted its potential for modulating behavior like, for example, reducing repetitive behaviors or anxiety [147, 150, 212]. In British neurosurgeon Hariz's words, *the marriage of deep brain stimulation and the subthalamic nucleus has been very fruitful.* Two reports relate the case of three patients who, along with Parkinson's disease, suffered from OCD. After 6 months of stimulation of the STN, these three patients presented a 58, 64, and 94 % reduction in the intensity of their symptoms [149, 150].

Anatomy

As described in the previous chapter, the STN is where motor, cognitive, and emotional components traveling via the CSTC loop circuits[80] are integrated into our behavior [213, 214]. Studies with retrograde testing in animals have shown mirroring between motor, cognitive, and emotional functions of the cortex and territories of the basal ganglia [213, 215, 216]. The STN has the following *somatotopic*[81] arrangement: the dorsolateral area, targeted in the treatment of Parkinson's disease, processes motor information while the anteroventral part of the nucleus processes limbic and associative information. Several hypotheses

---

[80] Cf. p. 139.

[81] It is the detailed representation of the body or functions within a nerve structure.

attempting to explain the importance of the STN in the pathophysiology of OCD characterize it as a filter tasked with detecting errors. A pathologically high threshold level in the STN would lead to the production of repeated iterations within the CSTC loop in order to erase the doubt [217]. In monkeys, the injection of *bicuculline,* an antagonist of GABA receptors, into the limbic region of the STN, produces stereotypies[82] which are negated by high frequency stimulation of the area. These laboratory results along with the clinical experience of deep brain stimulation of the STN in Parkinson's disease led French researchers to target the cognitive-limbic junction of this nucleus [218].

Results for OCD

In 2008, a study published in the *New England Journal of Medicine* presented the results of a French multicenter prospective double-blinded study conducted coordinated by Mallet of 16 patients with severe drug-resistant OCD. Seventy-five percent of the subjects present decreased Y-BOCS scores during the periods of stimulation. The average Y-BOCS score for all patients was 28 ± 7 during non-stimulation versus 19 ± 8 when the device was running, which equals a 32 % reduction in symptoms. In terms of *overall functioning* measured on the Global Assessment of Functioning scale, patients improved significantly from 43 to 56. However, no improvement was recorded on the scales measuring depression [219]. Recently, a team in Grenoble led by Chabardes and Benabid succeeded in reducing the Y-BOCS scores of three patients by 71–78 % and by 34 % in a fourth after 6 months of subthalamic stimulation [218]. All the patients cited above received bilateral stimulation; however, unilateral stimulation may also be effective. Indeed, it has been observed that even when an electrode has missed the STN due to a trajectory error [149] or had to be removed due to infection, the beneficial effects of the stimulation have persisted. A French study now underway is attempting to compare the effects of bilateral and unilateral subthalamic stimulation.

Complications Specifically Linked to Neurostimulation

The *New England Journal of Medicine* account of the French study included seven patients who suffered motor or psychiatric disorders during the first month of stimulation which either resolved themselves or were eliminated by changes in the stimulation parameters. Of these patients, three (18 %) suffered self-limiting hypomanic episodes and one (6 %) showed symptoms of depression and transient suicidal ideation. This seems in line with the tens of thousands of observations

---

[82] However, certain authors have questioned the validity of this animal-based model which compares these behavior iterations in monkeys with the rituals of an obsessive–compulsive disorder subject [220].

made during stimulation of the subthalamic nucleus in the treatment of Parkinson's disease. However, various studies have reported contradictory results. While some have reported thymic damage caused by the surgery [143, 221–223], others have shown no lasting effect on the mood of patients, 40 % of whom suffer from a depressive disorder in addition to Parkinson's disease [182, 224–226]. Other studies still have found a beneficial effect on mood in the short [138, 227–231] or long term [138, 232]. Because of these wide variances, it is difficult to fully assess the positive and negative impacts of stimulation on mood. Especially when external factors, as with Parkinson's disease, may also be altering mood. These variable include improvements in patient's quality of life as a result of increased motor function, the effects of dopaminergic medications, and conversely, the degenerative effects of the disease which after attacking the dopamine system can affect the serotonergic and noradrenergic systems. The *New England Journal of Medicine* article reported no neuropsychological deterioration. If we continue the comparison with subthalamic stimulation in Parkinson's disease, some data might lead us to believe that this stimulation would be responsible for alterations in some executive functions such as reduction of verbal fluency [138, 226, 227, 229, 233, 234], inhibition [226, 235], working memory [234, 235], and even the ability to form long-term verbal memory and ecode visuospatial information [234]. But again, it is difficult to ascertain whether these are due to cognitive impairment related to progression of the degenerative disease or deleterious effects of the stimulation of the associative CSTC loop. Studies incorporating long-term neuropsychological evaluation of patients with OCD but without Parkinson's disease are expected to shed some light on this question.

The Subgenual Area in the Treatment of Depression

Abstract Located in front of the cingulate cortex in the corpus callosum, the subgenual cortex (Brodmann area 25, GC25) is a mass of gray matter. Functional imaging has revealed that it is hyperactive in depressed patients. High frequency stimulation of the structure can slow this activity, thereby reducing the symptoms of depression. At present, it seems the most promising target for DBS in the treatment of refractory depression.

In 2005, Mayberg and Lozano working in Toronto pioneered the exploration of the subgenual area in the treatment of depression. Unlike other areas known from ablative surgery techniques or deep brain stimulation used in neurology, their interest derived from observations made using functional imaging techniques.

Anatomy

Depressed patients were seen to have increased metabolic activity in area 25, the most anterior part of the cingulate gyrus located just below the genu of the corpus callosum (hence the term subgenual) and decreased activity in the neighboring area 46/9 [68, 236, 237]. Meanwhile, when depression is successfully treated, whether by antidepressants [68], ECT[83] [238] or transcranial magnetic stimulation[84] (rTMS) [239], area 25 becomes less active [68, 236, 237, 240]. It has also been observed that hyperactivity in this region in patients being treated for cancer could be predictive of a reactive depression [241, 242]. The subgenual area is closely connected to the ventral striatum,[85] the shell of the nucleus accumbens[86], and the rest of the limbic CSTC loop.[87] It has numerous additional reciprocal connections to the amygdala,[88] the bed nucleus of the stria terminalis[89], hypothalamus[90] the bed nucleus of the stria terminalis[91] which make it crucial to the modulation of mood. It is also involved in vegetative phenomena [192, 202, 243–245]. The next step seems logical: reduce the activity in this region through DBS in order to alleviate the symptoms of depression in patients suffering treatment failure. When this was attempted, high frequency stimulation did indeed result in decreased activity coupled with a decline in depression symptoms (Fig. 4.4, p. 216) [240].

Results

The process of implanting the electrodes for deep brain stimulation is usually performed under local anesthesia with the subject conscious. During placement of the electrodes, electrophysiological recordings can be used to determine when the electrode has reached the junction of the white and gray matters. Following the recording phase, patients undergo stimulation (3–4 V, 130 Hz, 60 μs) and according to Hamani, nearly 70 % report decreased symptomology [246]. He conducted a study of 20 patients suffering from severe depression for 6 years on average who had been given no less than four different antidepressants. He and his co-authors related that after 1 year, eleven patients (55 %) were classified as responders and eight in remission (less than eight on the $HAMD_{17}$ scale). Improvement plateaued after 6 months [240, 247].

---

[83] Cf. p. 321.

[84] Cf. p. 232.

[85] Cf. p. 128.

[86] Cf. p. 129.

[87] Cf. p. 143.

[88] Cf. p. 98.

[89] Cf. p. 129.

[90] Cf. p. 112.

[91] Cf. p. 149.

Complications Specifically Linked to Stimulation

No specific neurological or psychological complications were reported by the pioneering Toronto team. In fact, performance on neuropsychological tests improved, as is frequently observed when the symptoms of depression subside [248]. Complications inherent to all deep brain stimulation techniques can of course arise[92] [240, 247].

The Middle Forebrain Bundle in the Treatment of Depression

When Schlaepfer and his team from Bonn reviewed treatments for depression targeting the anterior limb of the internal capsule, the subgenual area or the nucleus accumbens, they found that high intensity stimulation was generally required to obtain a clinical effect. Consequently, they hypothesized that the targeted structures were not necessarily the ones responsible for the clinical effect [203]. The German researchers then modeled the electric fields produced by the arrangement of the electrodes during the different procedures. Based on their calculations, they conclude that it is probably stimulation of the medial forebrain bundle (MFB), which passes close to all three target sites that induce the antidepressant effect (Fig. 2.30, p. 93). Evidencing the same model, they suggest that symptoms of hypomania observed in some Parkinson's patients during stimulation of the subthalamic nucleus could be caused by excitation of the nearby MFB[93] [162, 203]. Based on their clinico-pathological data, Coenen and his colleagues placed electrodes in seven patients suffering from severe depression in the superolateral branch of the right and left MFBs. The preliminary results released in 2012 [249] are encouraging: six out of the seven patients met the criteria for therapeutic response after only a few days of stimulation, including three with MADRS scores under 11 who were considered to be in remission. As the German researcher's model suggested, the interventions used low amplitude stimulation. At this stage, results are only available for 12–23 weeks of stimulation and follow-up, which remains too short a period to evaluate clinical outcomes.

The Inferior Thalamic Peduncle in the Treatment of Depression and OCD

Inferior thalamic peduncle was considered by Velasco and Jiménez's team as a potential target in the treatment of refractory depression on essentially anatomical

---

[92] In Lozano's study, two infections at the implant sites in the scalp and the thorax and a cutaneous erosion were recorded. The complications of this DBS technique and its frequencies are detailed on p. 206.

[93] This hypothesis implies that high frequency stimulation (100–180 Hz) would have an excitatory effect, and not an inhibitory effect, when it is applied to axons. The inhibitory effect concerns neuron and not axons [160].

arguments. Within the stem travel beams connecting the orbitofrontal cortex to intralaminar nuclei of the thalamus. One patient suffering from depression underwent deep brain stimulation targeting the inferior thalamic peduncle with immediate effect. His HAD score increased by 43 even before the neurostimulator was attached [250]. Symptoms quickly returned, stimulation then started with a positive effect: the HAD score fell below eight for 8 months. A double-blind protocol was then established. The results of five patients with OCD were published in 2009 by the same South American team. Over the first year, the average Y-BOCS score was halved and the average score assessing global functioning (GAF) increased from 20 to 70 % [251]. No complications or neuropsychological deterioration were reported.

The Habenula in the Treatment of Depression

The term *habenula* comes from the Latin *Habena*, "rein," and means "little reins" because of the elongated shape of this paired structure that connects on each side, the epiphysis with the two thalamus. These lateral parts receive multiple informations coming from the lateral hypothalamus and, via the pallidum, coming from the nucleus accumbens and the thalamus [252]. It seems, at least in animals that unpleasant and unexpected stimuli are part of the information processed by the structure [253]. The habenula, in turn, sends connections on three circuit neurotransmitters: it inhibits dopamine production[94] in the substantia nigra and the ventral tegmental area (VTA), inhibits the secretion of locus coeruleus noradrenergic[95], and slows the serotonergic pathway of the raphe nuclei[96] [254, 255]. In contrast, activation of the hypothalamic-pituitary axis[97] was observed. This inhibitory action of neurotransmitters such as dopamine, which is involved in the reward system has also led some neurobiologists to describe this way as the "circuit disappointment" [256]. Increased activity in this region is observed in depressed patients [257]. Sartorius and his team of Mannheim proposed this target in the treatment of depression [258]. For now, only one patient was treated according to this target with an encouraging result: HAMD score increased from 45 to 3, after a year of stimulation [259].

Conclusion

A review of the literature pertaining to DBS treatments for OCD reveals an average response rate of 50 % among the close to 100 patients treated [260].

---

[94] Cf. p. 146.
[95] Cf. p. 150.
[96] Ibid.
[97] Cf. p. 112.

The response rate rises to 68 % and the remission rate to 26 % among patients who underwent the treatment for severe depression [261]. Among the 99 patients given DBS treatments for Tourette's syndrome, tics decreased by an estimated 40 % [262]. These results are particularly encouraging given that these patients were in treatment failure for many years prior to the intervention. The intervention have been shown to be relatively safe with few irreversible complications including neuropsychological ones [263]. Nonetheless, these overall results must be taken with caution. Few studies have exceeded 20 subjects and methodology remains haphazard. Very few double-blinded studies, when neither the patient nor the medical know whether stimulation is switched on or off, have been completed [219, 264, 265]. Moreover, it is curious given the multiplicity of targets that the same anatomical structures (ALIC for OCD, depression and anorexia; nucleus accumbens for OCD, depression and addiction) can give positive therapeutic outcomes for different indications. Is this indicative of neurobiological similarities between these different pathologies with diverse clinical expressions? Or rather, is this a result of the stimulation affecting a wide area and modulating different circuits and structures functions involved in various unrelated pathologies? For example, the ALIC is surrounded by a number of structures that may be feeling the effects of stimulation: the nucleus accumbens, the medial forebrain bundle, the putamen, the head of the caudate nucleus, the bed nucleus of the stria terminalis, and others. The situation becomes complicated by the fact that high-frequency stimulation may have different effects on white matter (activation) and gray matter (inhibition). Developments in nanotechnology and optogenetics should lead to more precise anatomical targeting and improved understanding of the neurobiological mechanisms underlying mental disorders. The current boom in therapeutic uses for DBS will also lead to exploration of normal and pathological brain function. Such functional mapping of the brain will ultimately give clinicians knowledge about which sets of anatomical targets are relevant to given diseases or symptoms. Once the efficacy and safety of some of these targets have been verified, some lesional techniques such as radiosurgery[98] and soon HIFU,[99] may be used alongside stimulation.[100]

Cortical Stimulation

Abstract Repeated transcranial magnetic stimulation (rTMS) has been available for the past decade to patients with drug resistant depression. It is equivalent in terms of efficacy to electroconvulsive therapy (ECT) but functions according to very different principles. The prefrontal cortex can be activated by stimulation of

---

[98] Cf. p. 187.

[99] Cf. p. 189.

[100] Cf. "Lesion or stimulation" p. 457 for more on this debate.

the left side or slowed by stimulation on the right side. Functional imaging studies have revealed decreased activity in the left dorsolateral prefrontal cortex and increased activity in the right equivalent area. These disturbances in the functioning of the prefrontal lobe may cause the cognitive disorders encountered in patients treated for depression. Although advantageous because of its noninvasive nature and few side effects, rTMS must unfortunately be repeated because its effects are generally only temporary. To sustain the effect, some teams have implanted electrodes opposite the relevant brain regions to provide continuous stimulation. This cortical stimulation technique is already accepted in the routine treatment of certain forms of chronic intractable pain and tinnitus and is currently being evaluated in the treatment of treatment resistant depression.

Transcranial magnetic stimulation (rTMS) is a fast growing discipline. Several hundred articles devoted to the technique are published in scientific journals each year. It is used in the treatment of depression [266–270], chronic pain [271], tinnitus [272], auditory hallucinations in schizophrenic patients [273], obsessive–compulsive disorder[101] [274, 275], epilepsy [276], Parkinson's disease [277], rehabilitation following ischemic strokes, and even fibromyalgia [278]. While the mechanisms of electroconvulsive therapy (ECT) and rTMS remain largely unknown, their efficacy in the treatment of depression has been established. ECT, the inducing of generalized seizures in the patient, is about 85 % effective in the short term [279], but its mechanism of action on depression remains unknown. The intervention, which requires general anesthesia and curarization, is not without side effects and may cause transient confusion, muscle aches, hypomanic excitement, headaches, and transient or even permanent anterograde[102] amnesia. rTMS has similar efficacy [280–283], but unlike ECT, implementation is easier virtually free of side effects. The mechanism of action does not involve inducing seizures. Rather a magnetic pulse is discharged at the surface of the brain. Its weakness compared to ECT resides in its delayed effect which makes it unsuitable for life-and-death emergency treatments such as preventing suicide. The other, more common drawback in the long run is the transient nature of its effect on mood. Regular sessions are required to consolidate positive gains. The installation of cortical stimulation electrodes within the dorsolateral prefrontal regions targeted by rTMS could be a solution to this drawback. These permanent electrodes seem to have a similar effect to rTMS while maintaining the antidepressant effect over the long term. Though such implanted cortical stimulation seems a likely future for rTMS, only two teams

---

[101] Many of the rTMS targets were assessed in the treatment of OCD. The studies targeting the dorsolateral prefrontal cortex were inconclusive. However, the supplementary motor area and the orbifrontal cortex seem promising.

[102] Anterograde amnesia is partial or even complete loss of memory posterior to the disease, the accident, or the operation. The individual becomes incapable of building new memories. We could compare this situation to a computer in which the hard drive could read all the data but a defective writing mechanism would prevent new information from being recorded.

around the world have published on the subject, and additional clinical data is
sorely needed.

Repeated Transcranial Magnetic Stimulation

Arsène d'Arsonval first described the effects of magnetic stimulation on the
cerebral cortex in 1896 [284]. In 1914, Magnuson and Stevens triggered phos-
phenes[103] in a subject whose head was placed inside a coil connected to a capacitor
[285]. In 1980, Merton and Morton stimulated the motor cortex obtaining a motor
response, but the technique was painful. Five years later, Barker [271] by changing
the stimulation parameters was able to render the procedure painless making the
use of stimulation in diagnostic and therapeutic settings possible. The noninvasive
technique uses a coil to create a magnetic field around the brain through the scalp.
As Faraday's law predicts, a rapidly changing magnetic field will induce an
electrical current (Fig. 3.21) which can alter the activity of neurons in the target
region and activate or inhibit cortical areas depending on the stimulation

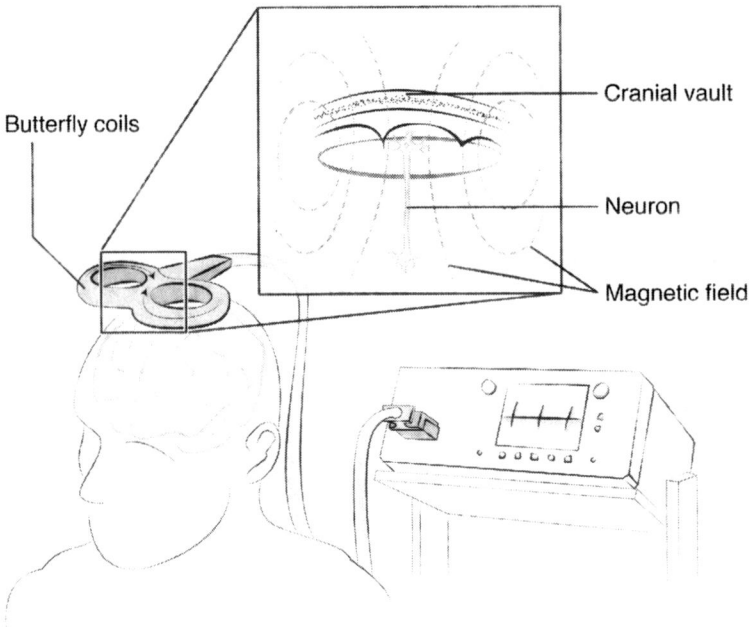

Fig. 3.21 Magnetic field modulating cortical activity during rTMS

---

[103] Phosphene phenomena are flashes or lights appearing in the visual field. They can be caused
by mechanical, electrical, or magnetic stimulation of the retina or the visual cortex, but also by a
cellular destruction in the visual system.

parameters. At frequencies below 1 Hz the field has an inhibitory effect on neuronal activity, and an excitatory effect at frequencies ranging from 5 to 20 Hz.

Hypotheses on the Functioning of rTMS

Functional imaging studies reveal low activity in the dorsolateral prefrontal cortex l in cases of severe depression which is manifested in psychomotor retardation r and symptoms such as apathy and memory, or attention deficit disorders. This region of the cortex is connected to the anterior cingulate gyrus which is also hypoactive, the orbitofrontal cortex and the amygdala. The latter two structures have altered metabolisms. The changes in the amygdala may cause increased sensitivity to pain, and increased anxiety and a loss of motivation related to orbitofrontal cortex. In addition to having different affects in different cortical areas, depression also manifests differently in the two hemispheres with the dorsolateral cortex being more active on the right side than on the left [239, 286]. Therapeutically, this means that *excitatory* rTMS with a high frequency of electric discharges between 5 and 20 Hz is needed to "wake" the left dorsolateral prefrontal cortex l. The right dorsolateral cortex which in opposition to the left is hyperactive, must receive *inhibitory* rTMS with low frequency discharges between 0.5 and 1 Hz. Clinical improvement is always visible in functional imaging as a normalization of activity in the dorsolateral cortex but also in the subgenual and anterior cingulate cortices [287, 288].

A Noninvasive Technique

This technique is noninvasive and involves the application of an electromagnetic coil in the shape as in Fig. 1.8, supplied with an electric current, which will create a magnetic field of 1–2.5 T according to the principles of electromagnetism. However, the intensity of the magnetic field is rather expressed as a percentage: 100 % corresponds to the intensity required for the occurrence of involuntary movement when the coil is applied next to the primary motor area or the cortex, within the *motor threshold*.[104] In general, teams practicing rTMS in the treatment of depression are more willing to target the left dorsolateral prefrontal cortex.[105] to which they apply fast frequency activation, with an intensity ranging from 80 to 110 % of motor threshold [289, 290].

---

[104] Cf. anatomy p. 90.

[105] Usually this area, which corresponds to area 46 and to a lesser extent area 9, is situated 5 cm in front of the point of scalp at which the right thumb can be made to contract using a coil.

Satisfactory Results

The clinical results are published, usually on the fast stimulation of left dorsolateral prefrontal cortex and more rarely on the slow pacing, right, or a combination of both [289]. Nine meta-analyses were performed from publications
comparing rTMS stimulation to placebo. For eight of them the results were in
favor of rTMS [291–295]. This significant difference confirms the efficacy of
rTMS in the treatment of intractable depression medication. It appears from various publications that advanced age or drug resistance count among the negative
factors, while the existence of a marked psychomotor retardation, a recent illness,
or disorders associated with sleep are auspicious. It is assumed that about 20
sessions are required for clinical improvement. However, this efficiency appears to
be transient, with a median duration of remission being around 120 days [288].
The return of depressive symptoms requires regular maintenance sessions. These
results should be taken to improve over the years, with on one hand, the increasing
use of neuronavigation that allows more precise targeting of the dorsolateral
prefrontal cortex and, on the other hand, the optimization stimulation parameters
such as total number of stimuli, the frequency of sessions and adjusting the frequency and intensity. It will also be necessary to better identify patients likely to
respond favorably, functional imaging could help. Finally, if the protocols fast left
and slow right stimulation appear with comparable efficiency, it is possible that
one or the other is selected according to the clinical symptoms or functional
imaging data that also requires new work. The existence of comorbidities, such as
smoking, may also come into play, rTMS may contribute to weaning.[106]

Intracranial Cortical Stimulation

Intracranial cortical stimulation is the application of electrodes on the dura mater
to electrically stimulate the cortex. This technique was evaluated in the treatment
of certain intractable pain of neuropathic [296], tinnitus [297], certain conditions
of motion [298], or to improve motor recovery after stroke [299]. In most of these
diseases, the success observed during rTMS sessions that preceded the act of
surgical implantation has been a good indicator of the effectiveness or otherwise of
this cortical stimulation. Its application in the treatment of severe depression drug
is very recent and still confidential as only two studies recently published on the
subject [301, 302]. It is very likely that in the wake of the increasing success of
rTMS, this technique is made to be much more widely investigated, because, in
theory, this should sustain implanted cortical stimulation results of rTMS. It is also
hoped that its anatomical accuracy coupled with power increased action—the

---

[106] In 2009, Amiaz and et al. reported on a randomized, double-blinded study of a series of 48
smoking patients used to consuming at least 20 cigarettes every day. They received ten sessions
of transcranial magnetic stimulation every day for 10 days. Results showed an objective decrease
in tobacco use in the patients who were actually being stimulated [300].

electrode is separated from the cortex of only a few millimeters—gives it greater efficiency. This technique has the disadvantage of being more invasive than rTMS, because it requires a mini-trepanation. However, there is no opening of the dural envelope, which protects the cortex, or through the brain parenchyma, as may be the case in deep brain stimulation involved in the treatment of depression. A French clinical study, at the national level, has been launched to assess the benefits and risks of this technique in the treatment of severe depression.

Prolonging the Effects of rTMS

As we have seen, the sessions of rTMS, at high frequency, the left dorsolateral prefrontal cortex can induce a reduction in depressive symptoms. The effectiveness of this treatment is associated with the functional imaging of renewed metabolism of the area before hypo-active, and a closely connected region, the cingulate gyrus [287]. An equivalent "rebalancing" is observed at a slow stimulation right [303]. However, this technique has the disadvantage of requiring many sessions and sees its effects fade with time. It is from these functional imaging data that U.S. teams B. Koppel and Z. Nahas speculated that direct and continuous electrical stimulation of the cerebral cortex would result in a permanent reduction in depressive symptoms. We know through experience acquired in the treatment of neuropathic pain and more anecdotal in tinnitus, patients relieved temporarily by rTMS sessions are likely to be permanently relieved after implantation of cortical stimulation electrodes compared to the same anatomical regions [304–307].

An Extracerebral Surgical Technique

After the dorsolateral prefrontal cortex has been located by MRI, the intervention is performed under general anesthesia and lasts about 2 h. A small craniotomy or a burr hole 1 inch in diameter is made; then, using a neuronavigation[107] device and radiography, the neurosurgeon inserts one or more neurostimulation electrodes between the skull and the dura mater next to the target site (Fig. 3.22). The electrode is then connected via a subcutaneous cable to the neurostimulator located in the upper chest area.

---

[107] During the operation, the neuronavigation system allows a patient's MRI images to be superimposed over her actual brain, the way a GPS superimposes a map over the actual route. It is then possible, with control panels, to precisely guide the progression of the electrode at the surface of the cortex.

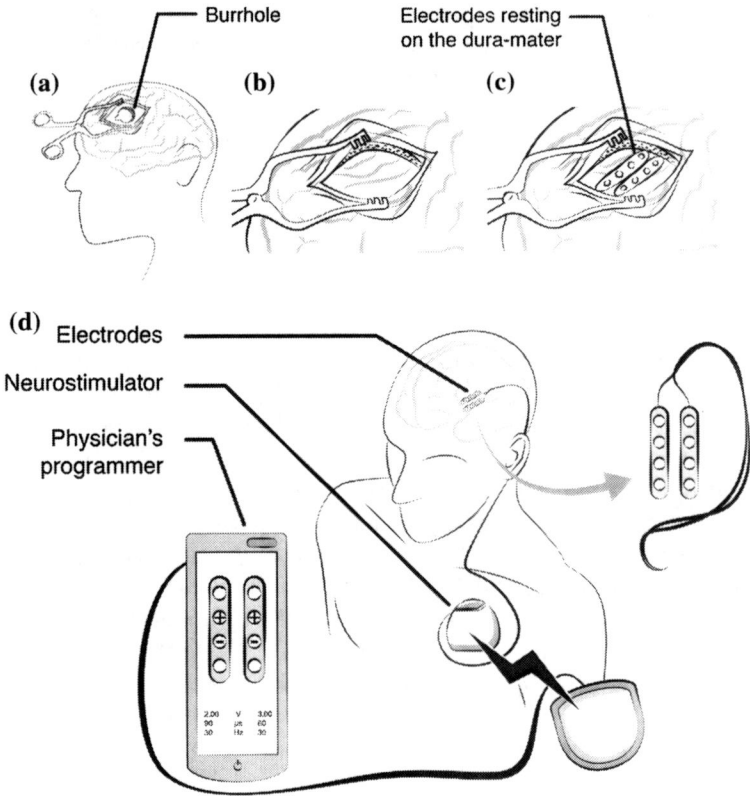

Fig. 3.22 Cortical stimulation

Preliminary Results from a Very Limited Number of Studies

Few scientific articles have been published. Only two very recent U.S. studies in 2008 and 2010 have reported on results for cortical stimulation in the treatment of depression. The first, directed by B. Kopell, D. Kondziolka, and D. Dougherty from the Universities of Milwaukee, Boston and Pittsburgh involved a dozen patients who were each implanted with an electrode at the surface of the dorsolateral pre-frontal cortex 1 (areas 9 and 46) [308–310]. For the first 2 months following the procedure, patients were randomly divided into two groups. One group was given stimulation and the other was not and none of the patients knew which group they belonged to. The researchers found no difference between the groups. However during a second, "open" phase lasting 21 months in which all patients received continuous stimulation, five patients were responders including four in remission. Unfortunately, after 21 months the company which produced the implantable device went bankrupt and all neurostimulators had to be removed. Regrettably, one suicide was reported among the 12 patients. That particular patient had been excluded from the cohort at an early stage after having mistakenly been given rTMS sessions. According to the authors, the patient was undergoing a divorce at the time of his intentional suicide. Nonetheless, they could not discount the possibility that the announcement of the removal of the devices encouraged this patient, whose clinical condition had improved following stimulation, to act [310]. No neuropsychological losses were recorded following stimulation. The second study by a team from South Carolina led by Z. Nahas is more questionable in terms of methodology [302]. His research included five patients with severe depression resistant to drugs. Each patient was implanted with four cortical stimulation electrodes: an electrode at the anterior pole of the dorsolateral cortex (area 10) and another at the posterior pole (area 46), on the left and right sides. On average, patients' HRSD24 scores decreased from 28 before the operation to 25 two weeks after the start of intermittent stimulation, 19 after 4 months, and 13 after 7 months. At that time, four of the five patients were responders including three in clinical remission. Neither team sought to include patients who responded well to rTMS and who thus might be good candidates for cortical stimulation. Future studies will undoubtedly explore this option. More research is also needed to determine the optimal target and parameter settings.

Questions Remaining

Following these two studies on a limited number of patients, 16 in all, many questions remain unanswered. The first is the optimal location of the electrodes, which differs significantly between the teams B. Kopell and Z. Nahas. The prefrontal cortex is a vast area of the brain and the effects of transcranial magnetic stimulation are much less targeted than those achieved using electrodes. From one rTMS session to another, the positioning of the device varies and it is ultimately a relatively wide area that is exposed to this stimulation. Probably well beyond areas 9 and 46 targeted. Should we, with the electrodes, widely cover the whole area affected by rTMS or should we stick to the areas showing the metabolic imaging, a hypo? If this is the case, could we not also consider targeting other hypoactive regions such as the cingulate cortex, inaccessible to rTMS given its depth, but that could be due to the electrodes? Should this coverage be one side or bilateral? This difficulty in identifying an optimal area is considerably enhanced by the delayed nature of the clinical outcome of stimulation. The attenuation of depressive symptoms generally occurs a few days or weeks after an effective stimulation. Other variables are a little more complicated in this equation, such as adjusting the intensity and frequency of the electrical current, or the choice of—permanent or alternating—this stimulation. It took many studies prior to the effectiveness of the established rTMS in depression and the technique is adopted in routine. Nevertheless, many parameters are to be refined in order to optimize clinical outcomes. On cortical stimulation, with less than 20 patients, the technique is still in a preliminary phase compared to the tens of thousands of patients in the rTMS. It will take many more studies to clarify the anatomical targets, the pacing mode, and indications. Because of its invasive nature, cortical stimulation is likely to remain restricted to patients difficult to wean the rTMS or whose sessions get too close.

Stimulation of the Vagus Nerve in the Treatment of Depression

Abstract Stimulation of the vagus nerve, located in the neck, has been used for 20 years to treat otherwise hard to treat forms of epilepsy. This stimulation would also seem to have antidepressant qualities, but this mechanism of action is still poorly understood. Studies in the United States have presented early evidence of its effectiveness in the treatment of drug resistant depression.

The effectiveness of vagus nerve stimulation in the treatment of certain refractory forms of epilepsy was established in the 1990s. It reduces the intensity and frequency of seizures [311, 312]. Over the past 10 years, neurologists have reported beneficial effects on the mood of some of their epileptic patients [313–316]. Once again, chance led researchers to discover the antidepressant effect of vagal stimulation in nonepileptic patients also suffering from depression.

Anatomy

The vagus nerve is the primary nerve of the parasympathetic system. It originates in the brainstem and innervates many organs including those in the thoracic and abdominal cavities. It is a mixed nerve and contains a motor portion responsible for, among other things, swallowing and phonation and a sensory portion, representing 80 %, with afferents from the lungs, heart, and the digestive system [317]. These afferents project to various brain structures via the solitary nucleus (SN) located in the brainstem. Thus, it is anatomically and functionally connected with structures known to induce epileptic discharges, such as the amygdala[108], the hippocampus[109], and the insula[110], also involved in mood regulation (Fig. 3.23) [317]. Moreover, the hypothalamus receives inputs[111], from several limbic structures including the amygdala which projects onto the dorsal nucleus of the vagus nerve, establishing another link between the vagus nerve and the limbic system. The SN also projects

---

[108] Cf. p. 98.

[109] Cf. p. 103.

[110] Cf. p. 107.

[111] Cf. p. 112.

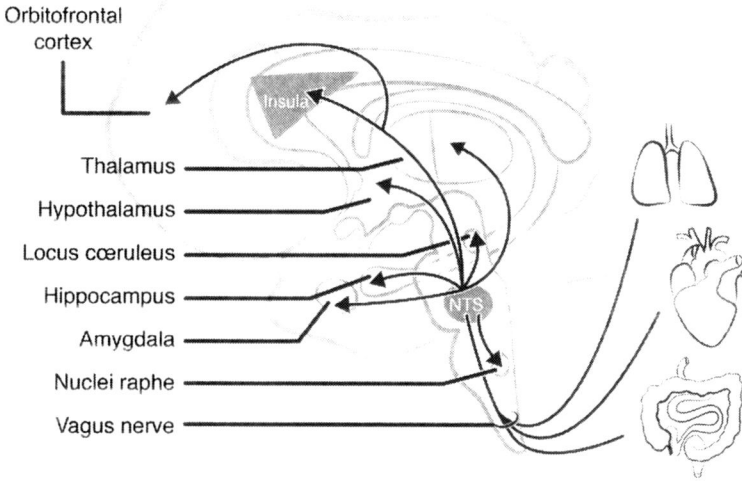

Orbitofrontal
cortex

Thalamus
Hypothalamus
Locus cœruleus
Hippocampus
Amygdala
Nuclei raphe
Vagus nerve

Fig. 3.23 Projections of the vagus nerve to the brain

connections to the thalamus, the orbitofrontal cortex[112], the raphe nuclei[113], and locus coeruleus[114] known to contribute to the regulation of mood.

Principle

The mechanism underlying the stimulation's antidepressant and antiepileptic effects remain unclear [317]. It would appear that these two effects are linked. This is also suggested by the fact that some anticonvulsants such as carbamazepine, lamotrigine, and valproic acid have mood stabilizing properties in addition to their antiepileptic ones [318]. These molecules are thought to increase the concentration of the inhibitory neurotransmitter GABA, while stimulation of the vagus nerve also increases [319]. Models for the affect of vagal stimulation on mood are based in part on data from metabolic imaging[115] of the brain. Decreased blood flow in brain structures involved in the regulation of mood (the cingulate cortex[116], the amygdala[117], and the hippocampus[118]) was observed 4 weeks after implantation of the stimulation device [320, 321]. Functional imaging of depressed patients treated with antidepressants or electroconvulsive therapy showed increased activity in these

---

[112] Cf. p. 93.

[113] Cf. p. 149.

[114] Ibid.

[115] SPECT and O-PET Scan.

[116] Cf. p. 95.

[117] Cf. p. 98.

[118] Cf. p. 103.

same regions [238, 322, 323]. Activity in the left dorsolateral cortex, meanwhile, often hypoactive in depressive disorder [239, 286], is increased after vagal stimulation [324]. As with cortical stimulation[119], normalization of the activity of the dorsolateral cortex is associated with improved mood. Additionally, vagal stimulation has been shown to increase the concentration of serotonin (raphe nuclei) in the brain and promote the release of norepinephrine (locus cœruleus) [320, 325–328]. Increased concentration of one or both of these neurotransmitters, particularly in the cerebrospinal fluid, is known to have an antidepressive effect. The efficacy of some types of antidepressants such as the selective inhibitors of serotonin (*Prozac*®) or norepinephrine (*Effexor*®) re-uptake is derived from this effect.

Procedure

This surgery lasting 1–2 h is performed under general anesthesia. Two incisions of about 4 inches each are made: one in the upper chest about the size of a pocket watch to accommodate the stimulator, and the other on the left side of the neck (Fig. 3.24). This is followed by dissection of the vagus nerve that runs between the carotid artery and jugular vein, in order to twist in the spiral electrode, which resembles a corkscrew. Once the contact is made, the electrode cable is tunneled under the skin and connected to the stimulator in the chest. Ten days after hospitalization, rarely exceeding 72 h, the pacemaker is programmed through the skin, by the physician according to standard parameters: a similar intensity from 0.75 to 2 mA, a frequency of 30 Hz, a signal width of 250–500 s. Discharges occur every 5 min and last 30 s [329]. During follow-up visits, the parameters are adjusted according to measured clinical outcome.

Results

In the United States, vagus nerve stimulation was approved by the *Food and Drug Administration* (FDA) for the treatment of depression in July 2005. The favorable decision was based on the encouraging results of studies by A. J. Rush and M. George of the Universities of Texas and South Carolina [330–332]. The authors conducted a multicenter nonblinded study (D01) and observed that a third of their 59 patients saw their symptoms decrease significantly 3 months after the start of stimulation. They noted that improvements occurred more readily in patients with only mild resistance to traditional antidepressant treatments. In 2007, however *Medicare* and *Medicaid* stopped reimbursing vagal stimulation for the treatment of depression. Aside from the high cost of the stimulator and procedure, totaling nearly $25,000, the review faulted insufficient proof of efficacy and questionable

---

[119] Cf. p. 236.

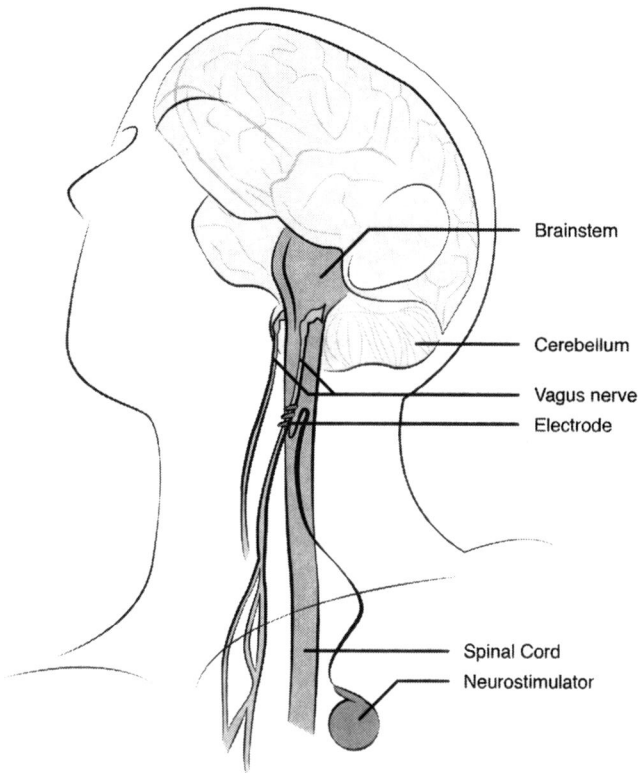

Fig. 3.24 Stimulation of the vagus nerve

methodology in prior studies [333]. It should be mentioned that in the meantime, Rush had published the results of a new series called "D02," double-blind, active-control this time, 112 patients with major depression treated by vagal stimulation. Three months after implantation, only 15 % of these patients had an improvement against 10 % for the control group without stimulation [334]. Nevertheless, it is clear that these poor results in the short term, have improved over the months and change stimulation parameters. Finally, a year later, nearly 30 % of patients had a response while 17.1 % were in remission[120] [335]. In 2008, a first European multicenter study, called "D03" on 74 patients, reported 37 % response and 17 % remission after 3 months of stimulation. After 1 year, the response rate was 53–44 % remission [336]. Since then, only one new study was conducted in the United States, with fewer patients—12 patients—and this time with 28.6 % of responses and 7.1 % remission [337]. These studies were conducted in patients with depression, with a score greater than or equal to 20 on the HRSD and evolving for more than 2 years.

---

[120] Remission signifies a decrease by more than half of the score on the Hamilton scale (HRSD) cf. p. 313, and response signifies a score below 10.

For each of these patients, two families of antidepressants at least were tested. It must also be noted that these studies have been funded in part by Cyberonics™ a laboratory marketing pacemaker. Among the criticisms leveled against this work we always retain the possible influence of the placebo effect in patients considered "responders." This effect is difficult to dismiss in so far as it would be ethically objectionable to use ghost interventions. It is recognized, however, that this effect rarely occurs in cases of severe depression [338]. Unlike deep brain stimulation in which the patient feels no physical sensation when stimulated, the patient can perceive a slight "tingling" in the throat during each cycle of the vagal stimulation. A second methodological reservation with regard to these studies is the lack of control group with the exception of George Rush and sets [334, 339]. Among the patients with thymic improvement through vagal stimulation we cannot, either, exclude the participation of independent spontaneous improvement of stimulation.

Complications

Two types of complications can occur. Infection (3 %) which in a third of cases makes removal of the device necessary, or temporary paralysis in one of the vocal cords (0.7–1.1 %) leading to severe loss of voice, are complications inherent to this type of surgery [340]. Complications from the action of the stimulation are slowed heart rate, inherent to parasympathetic hyperactivity (0.1 %), and the risk of sleep apnea (8–15 %). Special care must be taken with patients already suffering from this condition [341, 342]. Less serious but more frequent occurrences include subtle change in the voice which grows hoarse during the first few months, coughing, and neck pain [330]. No cognitive decline was reported in any of the thorough neuropsychological assessments carried out [343].

Future Applications

Well tolerated with few serious complications, vagus nerve stimulation remains under evaluation in the treatment of depression. This contrast with its routine use in the treatment of refractory epilepsy with over 30,000 patients having benefited from the technique. The encouraging results, a roughly 50 % response and remission rate, need to be confirmed by clinical as well as economic studies given the cost of the device. These studies should also specify indications and predictive criteria (severity of depression, bipolar depression…) for a satisfactory response and refine the parameters of stimulation. Research protocols addressing these issues must be available in Europe soon.

References

1. Spiegel EA, Wycis HT, Marks M, Lee AJ (1947) Stereotaxic apparatus for operations on the human brain. Science 106(2754):349–350. doi:10.1126/science.106.2754.349 106/2754/349 [pii]
2. Schaltenbrand G, Walker AE (1982) Stereotaxy of the human brain : anatomical, physiological, and clinical applications, 2nd (revised and enlarged edition) Thieme, Stratton; Thieme-Stratton, New York
3. Mai JK, Paxinos G, Voss T (2008) Atlas of the human brain. Academic Press, San Diego
4. Leiphart JW, Valone III FH (2010) Stereotactic lesions for the treatment of psychiatric disorders. J Neurosurg 113(6):1204–1211. doi:10.3171/2010.5.JNS091277
5. Lipsman N, McIntyre RS, Giacobbe P, Torres C, Kennedy SH, Lozano AM (2010) Neurosurgical treatment of bipolar depression: defining treatment resistance and identifying surgical targets. Bipolar Disord 12(7):691–701. doi:10.1111/j.1399-5618.2010.00868.x
6. Mpakopoulou M, Gatos H, Brotis A, Paterakis KN, Fountas KN (2008) Stereotactic amygdalotomy in the management of severe aggressive behavioral disorders. Neurosurg Focus 25(1):E6. doi:10.3171/FOC/2008/25/7/E6
7. Fountas KN, Smith JR (2007) Historical evolution of stereotactic amygdalotomy for the management of severe aggression. J Neurosurg 106(4):710–713. doi:10.3171/jns.2007.106.4.710
8. Velasco F, Velasco M, Jimenez F, Velasco AL, Salin-Pascual R (2005) Neurobiological background for performing surgical intervention in the inferior thalamic peduncle for treatment of major depression disorders. Neurosurgery 57(3):439–448; discussion-48. doi:00006123-200509000-00001 [pii]
9. Medvedev SV, Anichkov AD, Poliakov II (2003) Physiological mechanisms of the effectiveness of bilateral stereotactic cingulotomy in treatment of strong psychological dependence in drug addiction. Fiziol Cheloveka 29(4):117–123
10. Binder DK, Iskandar BJ (2000) Modern neurosurgery for psychiatric disorders. Neurosurgery 47(1):9–21 (discussion 3)
11. Lozano A, Gildenberg P, Tasker R, Lozano AM, Gildenberg PL, Tasker RR (2009) Textbook of stereotactic and functional neurosurgery, 2nd edn. Springer, New York, p 2861
12. Lu L, Wang X, Kosten TR (2009) Stereotactic neurosurgical treatment of drug addiction. Am J Drug Alcohol Abuse 35(6):391–393. doi:10.3109/00952990903312478
13. Stelten BM, Noblesse LH, Ackermans L, Temel Y, Visser-Vandewalle V (2008) The neurosurgical treatment of addiction. Neurosurg Focus 25(1):E5. doi:10.3171/FOC/2008/25/7/E5
14. Gao G, Wang X, He S, Li W, Wang Q, Liang Q et al (2003) Clinical study for alleviating opiate drug psychological dependence by a method of ablating the nucleus accumbens with stereotactic surgery. Stereotact Funct Neurosurg 81(1–4):96–104. doi:10.1159/000075111 75111 [pii]
15. Fountas KN, Smith JR, Lee GP (2007) Bilateral stereotactic amygdalotomy for self-mutilation disorder. Case report and review of the literature. Stereotact Funct Neurosurg 85(2–3):121–128. doi:10.1159/000098527 000098527 [pii]
16. Kim MC, Lee TK (2008) Stereotactic lesioning for mental illness. Acta Neurochir Suppl 101:39–43
17. Meyer A (1954) Prefrontal leucotomy and related operations. Oliver & Boyd, London
18. Talairach J, Hecaen H, David M (1949) Lobotomies prefrontal limitee par electrocoagulation des fibres thalamo-frontales à leur emergence du bras anterieur de la capsule interne. In: Proceedings IV congres neurologique international, Paris
19. Bingley T, Leksell L, Meyerson BA et al (1973) Stereotactic anterior capsulotomy in anxiety and obsessive-compulsive states. Surgical approaches in psychiatry. Medical and Technical Publishing, Lancaster

20. Simpson BJ, Thomas RP (ed) (2003) Stereotactic anterior capsulotomy for intractable depression and obsessive compulsive disorder [Abstract]. In: Proceedings of the 143rd meeting of the society of British neurological surgeons. Br J Neurosurg, Cardiff

21. Alexander GE, DeLong MR, Strick PL (1986) Parallel organization of functionally segregated circuits linking basal ganglia and cortex. Annu Rev Neurosci 9:357–381. doi:10.1146/annurev.ne.09.030186.002041

22. Cavada C, Company T, Tejedor J, Cruz-Rizzolo RJ, Reinoso-Suarez F (2000) The anatomical connections of the macaque monkey orbitofrontal cortex. Rev Cereb Cortex 10(3):220–242

23. Axer H, Lippitz BE, von Keyserlingk DG (1999) Morphological asymmetry in anterior limb of human internal capsule revealed by confocal laser and polarized light microscopy. Psychiatry Res 91(3):141–154

24. Spiegelmann R, Faibel M, Zohar Y (1994) CT target selection in stereotactic anterior capsulotomy: anatomical considerations. Stereotact Funct Neurosurg 63(1–4):160–167

25. Christmas D, Eljamel MS, Butler S, Hazari H, MacVicar R, Steele JD et al (2011) Long term outcome of thermal anterior capsulotomy for chronic, treatment refractory depression. J Neurol Neurosurg Psychiatry 82(6):594–600. doi:10.1136/jnnp.2010.217901 jnnp.2010.217901 [pii]

26. Mindus P, Nyman H, Mogard J (1990) Frontal lobe and basal ganglia metabolism studies in patients with incapacitating obsessive-compulsive disorder undergoing capsulotomy. Nord J Psychiatry 44:309–312

27. Hurwitz TA, Mandat T, Forster B, Honey C (2006) Tract identification by novel MRI signal changes following stereotactic anterior capsulotomy. Stereotact Funct Neurosurg 84(5–6):228–235. doi:10.1159/000096496 96496 [pii]

28. Mindus P, Jenike MA (1992) Neurosurgical treatment of malignant obsessive compulsive disorder. Psychiatr Clin N Am 15(4):921–938

29. Mindus P, Meyerson BA (1982) Anterior capsulotomy for intractable anxiety disorders. In: Schmidek H, Sweeney JA (eds) Operative neurosurgical techniques. WB Saunders, Philadelphia

30. Lippitz BE, Mindus P, Meyerson BA, Kihlstrom L, Lindquist C (1999) Lesion topography and outcome after thermocapsulotomy or gamma knife capsulotomy for obsessive-compulsive disorder: relevance of the right hemisphere. Neurosurgery 44(3):452–458; discussion 8–60

31. Lippitz B, Mindus P, Meyerson BA, Kihlstrom L, Lindquist C (1997) Obsessive compulsive disorder and the right hemisphere: topographic analysis of lesions after anterior capsulotomy performed with thermocoagulation. Acta Neurochir Suppl 68:61–63

32. Cosgrove GR, Rauch SL (1995) Psychosurgery. Neurosurg Clin N Am 6(1):167–176

33. Herner T (1961) Treatment of mental disorders with frontal stereotaxic thermo-lesions. Acta Psychiatr Scand 36(158):1–140

34. Liu K, Zhang H, Liu C, Guan Y, Lang L, Cheng Y et al (2008) Stereotactic treatment of refractory obsessive compulsive disorder by bilateral capsulotomy with 3 years follow-up. J Clin Neurosci 15(6):622–629. doi:10.1016/j.jocn.2007.07.086 S0967-5868(07)00497-3 [pii]

35. Oliver B, Gascon J, Aparicio A, Ayats E, Rodriguez R, Maestro De Leon JL et al (2003) Bilateral anterior capsulotomy for refractory obsessive-compulsive disorders. Stereotact Funct Neurosurg 81(1–4):90–95. doi:10.1159/000075110 75110 [pii]

36. Mindus P, Nyman H (1991) Normalization of personality characteristics in patients with incapacitating anxiety disorders after capsulotomy. Acta Psychiatr Scand 83(4):283–291

37. Ruck C, Andreewitch S, Flyckt K, Edman G, Nyman H, Meyerson BA et al (2003) Capsulotomy for refractory anxiety disorders: long-term follow-up of 26 patients. Am J Psychiatry 160(3):513–521

38. Lozano A, Gildenberg P, Tasker R, Lozano AM, Gildenberg PL, Tasker RR (2009) Textbook of stereotactic and functional neurosurgery, 2nd edn. Springer, New York

39. Mindus P, Edman G, Andreewitch S (1999) A prospective, long-term study of personality traits in patients with intractable obsessional illness treated by capsulotomy. Acta Psychiatr Scand 99(1):40–50

40. Mindus P, Nyman H, Rosenquist A, Rydin E, Meyerson BA (1988) Aspects of personality in patients with anxiety disorders undergoing capsulotomy. Acta Neurochir Suppl (Wien) 44:138–144

41. Ruck C, Edman G, Asberg M, Svanborg P (2006) Long-term changes in self-reported personality following capsulotomy in anxiety patients. Nord J Psychiatry 60(6):486–491. doi:10.1080/08039480601022116 Q90002X766K344J8 [pii]

42. Ruck C, Karlsson A, Steele JD, Edman G, Meyerson BA, Ericson K et al (2008) Capsulotomy for obsessive-compulsive disorder: long-term follow-up of 25 patients. Arch Gen Psychiatry 65(8):914–921. doi:10.1001/archpsyc.65.8.914 65/8/914 [pii]

43. Ridout N, O'Carroll RE, Dritschel B, Christmas D, Eljamel M, Matthews K (2007) Emotion recognition from dynamic emotional displays following anterior cingulotomy and anterior capsulotomy for chronic depression. Neuropsychologia 45(8):1735–1743. doi:10.1016/j.neuropsychologia.2006.12.022 S0028-3932(07)00011-5 [pii]

44. Cosgrove GR, Rauch SL (2003) Stereotactic cingulotomy. Neurosurg Clin N Am 14(2):225–235

45. Winn HR, Youmans JR (2011) Youmans' neurological surgery, 6th edn. Saunders, Philadelphia, London

46. Schmidek HH, Roberts DW (2006) Schmidek and Sweet operative neurosurgical techniques: indications, methods, and results, 5th edn. Saunders Elsevier, Philadelphia

47. Vertes RP, Albo Z, Viana Di Prisco G (2001) Theta-rhythmically firing neurons in the anterior thalamus: implications for mnemonic functions of Papez's circuit. Neuroscience 104(3):619–625. doi:S0306-4522(01)00131-2 [pii]

48. Ballantine HT Jr, Cassidy WL, Flanagan NB, Marino R Jr (1967) Stereotaxic anterior cingulotomy for neuropsychiatric illness and intractable pain. J Neurosurg 26(5):488–495. doi:10.3171/jns.1967.26.5.0488

49. Pribram KH, Fulton JF (1954) An experimental critique of the effects of anterior cingulate ablations in monkey. Brain 77(1):34–44

50. Fulton JF (1951) Lobotomy in man. Wis Med J 50(5):387; passim

51. Ward AA Jr (1948) The anterior cingulate gyrus and personality. Res Publ Assoc Res Nerv Ment Dis 27:438–445

52. Pool JL, Ransohoff J (1949) Autonomic effects on stimulating rostral portion of cingulate gyri in man. J Neurophysiol 12(6):385–392

53. Whitty CW, Duffield JE, Tov PM, Cairns H (1952) Anterior cingulectomy in the treatment of mental disease. Lancet 1(6706):475–481

54. Scoville W (1951) Research project of undercut- ting of the medial-cingulate gyrus Brodmann's area 24 and 32. Trans Am Neurol Assoc 56:226–227

55. Le Beau J (1954) Anterior cingulectomy in man. J Neurosurg 11(3):268–276. doi:10.3171/jns.1954.11.3.0268

56. Tow PM, Armstrong RW, Oxon MA (1954) Anterior cingulectomy in schizophrenia and other psychotic disorders; clinical results. J Ment Sci 100(418):46–61

57. Whitty CW, Lewin W (1957) Vivid daydreaming: an unusual form of confusion following anterior cingulectomy. Brain 80(1):72–76

58. Ballantine HT, Cassidy WL, Brodeur J, Giriunas I (eds) (1970) Frontal cingulotomy for mood disturbance. International conference on psychosurgery, Copenhagen, Denmark, Springfield, Ill

59. Foltz EL, White LE Jr (1962) Pain "relief" by frontal cingulotomy. J Neurosurg 19:89–100. doi:10.3171/jns.1962.19.2.0089

60. Brotis AG, Kapsalaki EZ, Paterakis K, Smith JR, Fountas KN (2009) Historic evolution of open cingulectomy and stereotactic cingulotomy in the management of medically intractable psychiatric disorders, pain and drug addiction. Stereotact Funct Neurosurg 87(5):271–291. doi:10.1159/000226669 000226669 [pii]

61. Balasubramaniam V, Kanaka TS, Ramanujam PB (1973) Stereotaxic cingulumotomy for drug addiction. Neurol India 21(2):63–66
62. Kanaka TS, Balasubramaniam V (1978) Stereotactic cingulumotomy for drug addiction. Appl Neurophysiol 41(1–4):86–92
63. Soares JC, Mann JJ (1997) The functional neuroanatomy of mood disorders. J Psychiatr Res 31(4):393–432 S0022-3956(97)00016-2[pii]
64. Frewen PA, Dozois DJ, Lanius RA (2008) Neuroimaging studies of psychological interventions for mood and anxiety disorders: empirical and methodological review. Clin Psychol Rev 28(2):228–246. doi:10.1016/j.cpr.2007.05.002 S0272-7358(07)00102-X [pii]
65. Drevets WC (2001) Neuroimaging and neuropathological studies of depression: implications for the cognitive-emotional features of mood disorders. Curr Opin Neurobiol 11(2):240–249 S0959-4388(00)00203-8[pii]
66. Soares JC, Mann JJ (1997) The anatomy of mood disorders–review of structural neuroimaging studies. Biol Psychiatry 41(1):86–106 S0006322396000066[pii]
67. Drevets WC, Price JL, Simpson JR Jr, Todd RD, Reich T, Vannier M et al (1997) Subgenual prefrontal cortex abnormalities in mood disorders. Nature 386(6627):824–827. doi:10.1038/386824a0
68. Mayberg HS, Liotti M, Brannan SK, McGinnis S, Mahurin RK, Jerabek PA et al (1999) Reciprocal limbic-cortical function and negative mood: converging PET findings in depression and normal sadness. Am J Psychiatry 156(5):675–682
69. Sheline YI, Barch DM, Donnelly JM, Ollinger JM, Snyder AZ, Mintun MA (2001) Increased amygdala response to masked emotional faces in depressed subjects resolves with antidepressant treatment: an fMRI study. Biol Psychiatry 50(9):651–658 S000632230101263X[pii]
70. Shields DC, Asaad W, Eskandar EN, Jain FA, Cosgrove GR, Flaherty AW et al (2008) Prospective assessment of stereotactic ablative surgery for intractable major depression. Biol Psychiatry 64(6):449–454. doi:10.1016/j.biopsych.2008.04.009 S0006-3223(08)00431-9 [pii]
71. Scoville WB, Wilk EK, Pepe AJ (1951) Selective cortical undercutting; results in new method of fractional lobotomy. Am J Psychiatry 107(10):730–738
72. Cosgrove GR (2009) Cingulotomy for depression and OCD. In: Lozano A (ed) Textbook of stereotactic and functional neurosurgery, vol 1, 2nd edn. Springer, New York, pp 2887–2896
73. Ballantine HT Jr, Bouckoms AJ, Thomas EK, Giriunas IE (1987) Treatment of psychiatric illness by stereotactic cingulotomy. Biol Psychiatry 22(7):807–819 0006-3223(87)90080-1 [pii]
74. Spangler WJ, Cosgrove GR, Ballantine HT Jr, Cassem EH, Rauch SL, Nierenberg A et al (1996) Magnetic resonance image-guided stereotactic cingulotomy for intractable psychiatric disease. Neurosurgery 38(6):1071–1076; discussion 6–8
75. Jenike MA, Baer L, Ballantine T, Martuza RL, Tynes S, Giriunas I et al (1991) Cingulotomy for refractory obsessive-compulsive disorder. A long-term follow-up of 33 patients. Arch Gen Psychiatry 48(6):548–555
76. Dougherty DD, Baer L, Cosgrove GR, Cassem EH, Price BH, Nierenberg AA et al (2002) Prospective long-term follow-up of 44 patients who received cingulotomy for treatment-refractory obsessive-compulsive disorder. Am J Psychiatry 159(2):269–275
77. Kim CH, Chang JW, Koo MS, Kim JW, Suh HS, Park IH et al (2003) Anterior cingulotomy for refractory obsessive-compulsive disorder. Acta Psychiatr Scand 107(4):283–290 087 [pii]
78. Jung HH, Kim CH, Chang JH, Park YG, Chung SS, Chang JW (2006) Bilateral anterior cingulotomy for refractory obsessive-compulsive disorder: long-term follow-up results. Stereotact Funct Neurosurg 84(4):184–189. doi:10.1159/000095031 95031 [pii]
79. Richter EO, Davis KD, Hamani C, Hutchison WD, Dostrovsky JO, Lozano AM (2008) Cingulotomy for psychiatric disease: microelectrode guidance, a callosal reference system

for documenting lesion location, and clinical results. Neurosurgery 62(6 Suppl 3):957–965. doi:10.1227/01.neu.0000333763.20575.18 00006123-200806001-00005 [pii]

80. Richter EO, Davis KD, Hamani C, Hutchison WD, Dostrovsky JO, Lozano AM (2004) Cingulotomy for psychiatric disease: microelectrode guidance, a callosal reference system for documenting lesion location, and clinical results. Neurosurgery 54(3):622–28; discussion 8–30

81. Turner E (ed) (1970) Operations for aggression: bilateral temporal lobotomy and posterior cingulectomy. International conference on psychosurgery, Copenhagen, Denmark, Springfield, Ill

82. Jimenez-Ponce F, Soto-Abraham JE, Ramirez-Tapia Y, Velasco-Campos F, Carrillo-Ruiz JD, Gomez-Zenteno P (2011) Evaluation of bilateral cingulotomy and anterior capsulotomy for the treatment of aggressive behavior. Cir Cir 79(2):107–113

83. Jimenez F, Soto JE, Velasco F, Andrade P, Bustamante JJ, Gomez P et al (2012) Bilateral cingulotomy and anterior capsulotomy applied to patients with aggressiveness. Stereotact Funct Neurosurg 90(3):151–160. doi:10.1159/000336746 000336746 [pii]

84. Baer L, Rauch SL, Ballantine HT Jr, Martuza R, Cosgrove R, Cassem E et al (1995) Cingulotomy for intractable obsessive-compulsive disorder. Prospective long-term follow-up of 18 patients. Arch Gen Psychiatry 52(5):384–392

85. Pokorny AD (1983) Prediction of suicide in psychiatric patients. Report of a prospective study. Arch Gen Psychiatry 40(3):249–257

86. Lozano A, Gildenberg P, Tasker R, Lozano AM, Gildenberg PL, Tasker RR (2009) Cingulotomy for depression and OCD, textbook of stereotactic and functional neurosurgery, 2nd edn. Springer, New York, pp 2887–2896

87. Andrade P, Noblesse LH, Temel Y, Ackermans L, Lim LW, Steinbusch HW et al (2010) Neurostimulatory and ablative treatment options in major depressive disorder: a systematic review. Acta Neurochir (Wien) 152(4):565–577. doi:10.1007/s00701-009-0589-6

88. Knight GC, Tredgold RF (1955) Orbital leucotomy: a review of 52 cases. Lancet 268(6872):981–986

89. Bridges PK, Bartlett JR, Hale AS, Poynton AM, Malizia AL, Hodgkiss AD (1994) Psychosurgery: stereotactic subcaudate tractomy. An indispensable treatment. Br J Psychiatry 165(5):599–611; discussion 2–3

90. Hodgkiss AD, Malizia AL, Bartlett JR, Bridges PK (1995) Outcome after the psychosurgical operation of stereotactic subcaudate tractotomy, 1979–1991. J Neuropsychiatry Clin Neurosci 7(2):230–234

91. Knight G (1964) The orbital cortex as an objective in the surgical treatment of mental illness. The results of 450 cases of open operation and the development of the stereotactic approach. Br J Surg 51:114–124

92. Poynton AM, Kartsounis LD, Bridges PK (1995) A prospective clinical study of stereotactic subcaudate tractotomy. Psychol Med 25(4):763–770

93. Goktepe EO, Young LB, Bridges PK (1975) A further review of the results of stereotactic subcaudate tractotomy. Br J Psychiatry 126:270–280

94. Kartsounis LD, Poynton A, Bridges PK, Bartlett JR (1991) Neuropsychological correlates of stereotactic subcaudate tractotomy. A prospective study. Brain 114(Pt 6):2657–2673

95. Kelly D, Richardson A, Mitchell-Heggs N, Greenup J, Chen C, Hafner RJ (1973) Stereotactic limbic leucotomy: a preliminary report on forty patients. Br J Psychiatry 123(573):141–148

96. Mitchell-Heggs N, Kelly D, Richardson A (1976) Stereotactic limbic leucotomy–a follow-up at 16 months. Br J Psychiatry 128:226–240

97. Montoya A, Weiss AP, Price BH, Cassem EH, Dougherty DD, Nierenberg AA et al (2002) Magnetic resonance imaging-guided stereotactic limbic leukotomy for treatment of intractable psychiatric disease. Neurosurgery 50(5):1043–1049 (discussion 9–52)

98. Fodstad H, Strandman E, Karlsson B, West KA (1982) Treatment of chronic obsessive compulsive states with stereotactic anterior capsulotomy or cingulotomy. Acta Neurochir (Wien) 62(1–2):1–23

99. Macklin R (1999) The ethical problems with sham surgery in clinical research. N Engl J Med 341(13):992–996. doi:10.1056/NEJM199909233411312

100. Mehta S, Myers TG, Lonner JH, Huffman GR, Sennett BJ (2007) The ethics of sham surgery in clinical orthopaedic research. J Bone Joint Surg Am 89(7):1650–1653. doi:10.2106/JBJS.F.00563

101. Dekkers W, Boer G (2001) Sham neurosurgery in patients with Parkinson's disease: is it morally acceptable? J Med Ethics 27(3):151–156

102. Means KR Jr (2008) The ethics of sham surgery in clinical orthopaedic research. J Bone Joint Surg Am 90(2):444; author reply 5

103. Juckel G, Uhl I, Padberg F, Brune M, Winter C (2009) Psychosurgery and deep brain stimulation as ultima ratio treatment for refractory depression. Eur Arch Psychiatry Clin Neurosci 259(1):1–7. doi:10.1007/s00406-008-0826-7

104. Christmas D, Morrison C, Eljamel MS, Matthews K (2004) Neurosurgery for mental disorder. Adv Psy chiatr Treat 10:189–199

105. Leksell L (1951) The stereotaxic method and radiosurgery of the brain. Acta Chirurgica Scandinavica 102:316–319

106. Leksell LH, Liden T (1955) Stereotaxic radiosurgery of the brain: report of a case. Kungl Fysiogr Sallsk Lund Forhandl 25:1–10

107. Leksell L, Backlund EO (1979) Stereotactic gammacapsulotomy. In: Hitchcock ER, Ballantine HT, Meyerson BA (eds) Modern concepts in psychiatric surgery. Elsevier, Amsterdam, pp 213–216

108. Mindus P, Bergstrom K, Levander SE, Noren G, Hindmarsh T, Thuomas KA (1987) Magnetic resonance images related to clinical outcome after psychosurgical intervention in severe anxiety disorder. J Neurol Neurosurg Psychiatry 50(10):1288–1293

109. Kihlstrom L, Guo WY, Lindquist C, Mindus P (1995) Radiobiology of radiosurgery for refractory anxiety disorders. Neurosurgery 36(2):294–302

110. Kihlstrom L, Hindmarsh T, Lax I, Lippitz B, Mindus P, Lindquist C (1997) Radiosurgical lesions in the normal human brain 17 years after gamma knife capsulotomy. Neurosurgery 41(2):396–401 (discussion 2)

111. Leksell L, Leksell D, Schwebel J (1985) Stereotaxis and nuclear magnetic resonance. J Neurol Neurosurg Psychiatry 48(1):14–18

112. Kondziolka D, Flickinger JC, Hudak R (2011) Results following gamma knife radiosurgical anterior capsulotomies for obsessive compulsive disorder. Neurosurgery 68(1):28–32; discussion 23–33. doi:10.1227/NEU.0b013e3181fc5c8b 00006123-201101000-00005 [pii]

113. Taub A, Lopes AC, Fuentes D, D'Alcante CC, de Mathis ME, Canteras MM et al (2009) Neuropsychological outcome of ventral capsular/ventral striatal gamma capsulotomy for refractory obsessive-compulsive disorder: a pilot study. J Neuropsychiatry Clin Neurosci 21(4):393–397. doi:10.1176/appi.neuropsych.21.4.393 21/4/393 [pii]

114. Lopes AC, Greenberg BD, Noren G, Canteras MM, Busatto GF, de Mathis ME et al (2009) Treatment of resistant obsessive-compulsive disorder with ventral capsular/ventral striatal gamma capsulotomy: a pilot prospective study. J Neuropsychiatry Clin Neurosci 21(4):381–392. doi:10.1176/appi.neuropsych.21.4.381 21/4/381 [pii]

115. Gouvea F, Lopes A, Greenberg B, Canteras M, Taub A, Mathis M et al (2010) Response to sham and active gamma ventral capsulotomy in otherwise intractable obsessive-compulsive disorder. Stereotact Funct Neurosurg 88(3):177–182. doi:10.1159/000313870 000313870 [pii]

116. Martin E, Jeanmonod D, Morel A, Zadicario E, Werner B (2009) High-intensity focused ultrasound for noninvasive functional neurosurgery. Ann Neurol 66(6):858–861. doi:10.1002/ana.21801

117. Rode J (1655) Compositiones medicae. Typis Pauli Frambotti

118. Penfield W (1958) Some mechanisms of consciousness discovered during electrical stimulation of the brain. Proc Natl Acad Sci USA 44(2):51–66

119. Penfield W, Welch K (1949) Instability of response to stimulation of the sensorimotor cortex of man. J Physiol 109(3–4):358–365, illust

120. Pool JL (1954) Psychosurgery in older people. J Am Geriatr Soc 2:456–465
121. Hariz MI, Blomstedt P, Zrinzo L (2010) Deep brain stimulation between 1947 and 1987: the untold story. Neurosurg Focus 29(2):E1
122. Delgado JM, Hamlin H, Chapman WP (1952) Technique of intracranial electrode implacement for recording and stimulation and its possible therapeutic value in psychotic patients. Confin Neurol 12(5–6):315–319
123. Delgado JMR, Graulich M (1972) Le conditionnement du cerveau et la liberté de l'esprit. Ch. Dessart
124. Baumeister AA (2000) The Tulane electrical brain stimulation program a historical case study in medical ethics. J Hist Neurosci 9(3):262–278. doi:10.1076/jhin.9.3.262.1787
125. Heath RG (1963) Electrical self-stimulation of the brain in man. Am J Psychiatry 120:571–577
126. Heath RG (1977) Modulation of emotion with a brain pacemaker. Treatment for intractable psychiatric illness. J Nerv Ment Dis 165(5):300–317
127. Heath RG (1972) Pleasure and brain activity in man. Deep and surface electroencephalograms during orgasm. J Nerv Ment Dis 154(1):3–18
128. Sem-Jacobsen CW (1965) Depth electrographic stimulation and treatment of patients with Parkinson's disease including neurosurgical technique. Acta Neurol Scand Suppl 13(1):365–377
129. Sem-Jacobsen CW (1966) Depth-electrographic observations related to Parkinson's disease. Recording and electrical stimulation in the area around the third ventricle. J Neurosurg 24(1):Suppl:388–402
130. Sem-Jacobsen CW (1968) Depth electrographic stimulation of the human brain and behavior: from fourteen years of studies and treatment of Parkinson's disease and mental disorders with implanted electrodes, 1 Jan 1965 edition, Springfield, Ill
131. Sheer D (1961) Electrical stimulation of the brain. An Interdisciplinary survey of neurobehavioral integrative system, Austin, Texas
132. Benabid AL, Pollak P, Louveau A, Henry S, de Rougemont J (1987) Combined (thalamotomy and stimulation) stereotactic surgery of the VIM thalamic nucleus for bilateral Parkinson disease. Appl Neurophysiol 50(1–6):344–346
133. Benabid AL, Pollak P, Gervason C, Hoffmann D, Gao DM, Hommel M et al (1991) Long-term suppression of tremor by chronic stimulation of the ventral intermediate thalamic nucleus. Lancet 337(8738):403–406 0140-6736(91)91175-T[pii]
134. Benabid AL, Pollak P, Seigneuret E, Hoffmann D, Gay E, Perret J (1993) Chronic VIM thalamic stimulation in Parkinson's disease, essential tremor and extra-pyramidal dyskinesias. Acta Neurochir Suppl (Wien) 58:39–44
135. Coubes P, Roubertie A, Vayssiere N, Hemm S, Echenne B (2000) Treatment of DYT1-generalised dystonia by stimulation of the internal globus pallidus. Lancet 355(9222):2220–2221. doi:10.1016/S0140-6736(00)02410-7 S0140-6736(00)02410-7 [pii]
136. Krack P, Batir A, Van Blercom N, Chabardes S, Fraix V, Ardouin C et al (2003) Five-year follow-up of bilateral stimulation of the subthalamic nucleus in advanced Parkinson's disease. N Engl J Med 349(20):1925–1934. doi:10.1056/NEJMoa035275 49/20/1925 [pii]
137. Deuschl G, Schade-Brittinger C, Krack P, Volkmann J, Schafer H, Botzel K et al (2006) A randomized trial of deep-brain stimulation for Parkinson's disease. N Engl J Med 355(9):896–908. doi:10.1056/NEJMoa060281 355/9/896 [pii]
138. Funkiewiez A, Ardouin C, Caputo E, Krack P, Fraix V, Klinger H et al (2004) Long term effects of bilateral subthalamic nucleus stimulation on cognitive function, mood, and behaviour in Parkinson's disease. J Neurol Neurosurg Psychiatry 75(6):834–839
139. Herzog J, Reiff J, Krack P, Witt K, Schrader B, Muller D et al (2003) Manic episode with psychotic symptoms induced by subthalamic nucleus stimulation in a patient with Parkinson's disease. Mov Disord 18(11):1382–1384. doi:10.1002/mds.10530
140. Romito LM, Raja M, Daniele A, Contarino MF, Bentivoglio AR, Barbier A et al (2002) Transient mania with hypersexuality after surgery for high frequency stimulation of the

subthalamic nucleus in Parkinson's disease. Mov Disord 17(6):1371–1374. doi:10.1002/mds.10265

141. Bejjani BP, Damier P, Arnulf I, Thivard L, Bonnet AM, Dormont D et al (1999) Transient acute depression induced by high-frequency deep-brain stimulation. N Engl J Med 340(19):1476–1480. doi:10.1056/NEJM199905133401905

142. Limousin P, Krack P, Pollak P, Benazzouz A, Ardouin C, Hoffmann D et al (1998) Electrical stimulation of the subthalamic nucleus in advanced Parkinson's disease. N Engl J Med 339(16):1105–1111. doi:10.1056/NEJM199810153391603

143. Houeto JL, Mesnage V, Mallet L, Pillon B, Gargiulo M, du Moncel ST et al (2002) Behavioural disorders, Parkinson's disease and subthalamic stimulation. J Neurol Neurosurg Psychiatry 72(6):701–707

144. Burkhard PR, Vingerhoets FJ, Berney A, Bogousslavsky J, Villemure JG, Ghika J (2004) Suicide after successful deep brain stimulation for movement disorders. Neurology 63(11):2170–2172 63/11/2170[pii]

145. Bejjani BP, Houeto JL, Hariz M, Yelnik J, Mesnage V, Bonnet AM et al (2002) Aggressive behavior induced by intraoperative stimulation in the triangle of Sano. Neurology 59(9):1425–1427

146. Jaafari N, Gire P, Houeto JL (2009) Deep brain stimulation, Parkinson's disease and neuropsychiatric complications. Presse Med 38(9):1335–1342. doi:10.1016/j.lpm.2008.11.019 S0755-4982(09)00048-7 [pii]

147. Houeto JL, Mallet L, Mesnage V, Tezenas du Montcel S, Behar C, Gargiulo M et al (2006) Subthalamic stimulation in Parkinson disease: behavior and social adaptation. Arch Neurol 63(8):1090–1095. doi:10.1001/archneur.63.8.1090 63/8/1090 [pii]

148. Aarsland D, Larsen JP, Lim NG, Janvin C, Karlsen K, Tandberg E et al (1999) Range of neuropsychiatric disturbances in patients with Parkinson's disease. J Neurol Neurosurg Psychiatry 67(4):492–496

149. Mallet L, Mesnage V, Houeto JL, Pelissolo A, Yelnik J, Behar C et al (2002) Compulsions, Parkinson's disease, and stimulation. Lancet 360(9342):1302–1304. doi:10.1016/S0140-6736(02)11339-0 S0140-6736(02)11339-0 [pii]

150. Fontaine D, Mattei V, Borg M, von Langsdorff D, Magnie MN, Chanalet S et al (2004) Effect of subthalamic nucleus stimulation on obsessive-compulsive disorder in a patient with Parkinson disease. Case report. J Neurosurg 100(6):1084–1086. doi:10.3171/jns.2004.100.6.1084

151. Nuttin B, Cosyns P, Demeulemeester H, Gybels J, Meyerson B (1999) Electrical stimulation in anterior limbs of internal capsules in patients with obsessive-compulsive disorder. Lancet 354(9189):1526. doi:10.1016/S0140-6736(99)02376-4 S0140-6736(99)02376-4 [pii]

152. Group O-DC (2002) Deep brain stimulation for psychiatric disorders. Neurosurgery 51(2):519

153. santé CCNdEplsdlvedl (2002) Avis sur la neurochirurgie fonctionnelle d'affections psychiatriques sévères. La Documentation française 153

154. France Comité consultatif national d'éthique pour les sciences de la vie et de la santé (2005) Avis sur la neurochirurgie fonctionnelle d'affections psychiatriques sévères. Ethique et recherche biomédicale Rapport 2002. la Documentation française, Paris

155. Carron R, Chabardes S, Hammond C (2012) Mechanisms of action of high-frequency deep brain stimulation. A review of the literature and current concepts. Neurochirurgie. doi:10.1016/j.neuchi.2012.02.006 S0028-3770(12)00013-6 [pii]

156. Garcia L, D'Alessandro G, Bioulac B, Hammond C (2005) High-frequency stimulation in Parkinson's disease: more or less? Trends Neurosci 28(4):209–216. doi:10.1016/j.tins.2005.02.005

157. Hemm S, Mennessier G, Vayssiere N, Cif L, El Fertit H, Coubes P (2005) Deep brain stimulation in movement disorders: stereotactic coregistration of two-dimensional electrical field modeling and magnetic resonance imaging. J Neurosurg 103(6):949–955. doi:10.3171/jns.2005.103.6.0949

158. Benazzouz A, Hallett M (2000) Mechanism of action of deep brain stimulation. Neurology 55(12 Suppl 6):S13–S16
159. Dostrovsky JO, Lozano AM (2002) Mechanisms of deep brain stimulation. Mov Disord 17(Suppl 3):S63–S68
160. Benabid AL, Benazzous A, Pollak P (2002) Mechanisms of deep brain stimulation. Mov Disord 17(Suppl 3):S73–S74
161. Nuttin BJ, Gabriels LA, Cosyns PR, Meyerson BA, Andreewitch S, Sunaert SG et al (2003) Long-term electrical capsular stimulation in patients with obsessive-compulsive disorder. Neurosurgery 52(6):1263–1272 (discussion 72–74)
162. Coenen VA, Honey CR, Hurwitz T, Rahman AA, McMaster J, Burgel U et al (2009) Medial forebrain bundle stimulation as a pathophysiological mechanism for hypomania in subthalamic nucleus deep brain stimulation for Parkinson's disease. Neurosurgery 64(6):1106–1114 (discussion 14–15). doi:10.1227/01.NEU.0000345631.54446.06
163. Hammond C, Ammari R, Bioulac B, Garcia L (2008) Latest view on the mechanism of action of deep brain stimulation. Mov Disord 23(15):2111–2121. doi:10.1002/mds.22120
164. Gradinaru V, Mogri M, Thompson KR, Henderson JM, Deisseroth K (2009) Optical deconstruction of parkinsonian neural circuitry. Science 324(5925):354–359. doi:10.1126/science.1167093 1167093 [pii]
165. Zhang F, Wang LP, Brauner M, Liewald JF, Kay K, Watzke N et al (2007) Multimodal fast optical interrogation of neural circuitry. Nature 446(7136):633–639. doi:10.1038/nature05744 nature05744 [pii]
166. Toda H, Hamani C, Fawcett AP, Hutchison WD, Lozano AM (2008) The regulation of adult rodent hippocampal neurogenesis by deep brain stimulation. J Neurosurg 108(1):132–138. doi:10.3171/JNS/2008/108/01/0132
167. Hamani C, Stone SS, Garten A, Lozano AM, Winocur G (2011) Memory rescue and enhanced neurogenesis following electrical stimulation of the anterior thalamus in rats treated with corticosterone. Exp Neurol 232(1):100–104. doi:10.1016/j.expneurol.2011.08.023
168. Stone SS, Teixeira CM, Devito LM, Zaslavsky K, Josselyn SA, Lozano AM et al (2011) Stimulation of entorhinal cortex promotes adult neurogenesis and facilitates spatial memory. J Neurosci 31(38):13469–13484. doi:10.1523/JNEUROSCI.3100-11.2011
169. Encinas JM, Hamani C, Lozano AM, Enikolopov G (2011) Neurogenic hippocampal targets of deep brain stimulation. J Comp Neurol 519(1):6–20. doi:10.1002/cne.22503
170. Ridha BH, Barnes J, van de Pol LA, Schott JM, Boyes RG, Siddique MM et al (2007) Application of automated medial temporal lobe atrophy scale to Alzheimer disease. Arch Neurol 64(6):849–854. doi:10.1001/archneur.64.6.849
171. Jack CR Jr, Shiung MM, Gunter JL, O'Brien PC, Weigand SD, Knopman DS et al (2004) Comparison of different MRI brain atrophy rate measures with clinical disease progression in AD. Neurology 62(4):591–600
172. Wang L, Swank JS, Glick IE, Gado MH, Miller MI, Morris JC et al (2003) Changes in hippocampal volume and shape across time distinguish dementia of the Alzheimer type from healthy aging. Neuroimage 20(2):667–682. doi:10.1016/S1053-8119(03)00361-6
173. Lozano A (2012) Functional neurosurgery—an illustrious past, an exciting future. In: XXth Congress of the European Society for stereotactic and functional neurosurgery, Cascais, Portugal, 27 Sept 2012
174. Mayberg HS, Silva JA, Brannan SK, Tekell JL, Mahurin RK, McGinnis S et al (2002) The functional neuroanatomy of the placebo effect. Am J Psychiatry 159(5):728–737
175. Carpenter WT Jr (2009) Placebo effect in depression. Am J Psychiatry 166(8):935. doi:10.1176/appi.ajp.2009.09030385 166/8/935 [pii]
176. Mx Cohen (2012) Scientific recording in deep brain stimulation. In: Denys D, Feenstra M, Schuurman R (eds) Deep brain stimulation: a new frontier in psychiatry. Springer, New York, pp 183–191
177. Fraix V, Houeto JL, Lagrange C, Le Pen C, Krystkowiak P, Guehl D et al (2006) Clinical and economic results of bilateral subthalamic nucleus stimulation in Parkinson's disease.

J Neurol Neurosurg Psychiatry 77(4):443–449. doi:10.1136/jnnp.2005.077677 77/4/443 [pii]

178. Kellner CH (2012) Brain stimulation in psychiatry: ECT, DBS, TMS and other modalities. Cambridge University Press, Cambridge

179. Kleiner-Fisman G, Herzog J, Fisman DN, Tamma F, Lyons KE, Pahwa R et al (2006) Subthalamic nucleus deep brain stimulation: summary and meta-analysis of outcomes. Mov Disord 21(Suppl 14):S290–S304. doi:10.1002/mds.20962

180. Bronstein JM, Tagliati M, Alterman RL, Lozano AM, Volkmann J, Stefani A et al (2011) Deep brain stimulation for Parkinson disease: an expert consensus and review of key issues. Arch Neurol 68(2):165. doi:10.1001/archneurol.2010.260 archneurol.2010.260 [pii]

181. Visser-Vandewalle V, van der Linden C, Temel Y, Celik H, Ackermans L, Spincemaille G et al (2005) Long-term effects of bilateral subthalamic nucleus stimulation in advanced Parkinson disease: a four year follow-up study. Parkinsonism Relat Disord 11(3):157–165. doi:10.1016/j.parkreldis.2004.10.011 S1353-8020(04)00199-3 [pii]

182. Fluchere F (2010) Suivi au long cours d'une cohorte de patients parkinsoniens traites par stimulation cerebrale profonde des noyaux sous thalamiques, et operes sous anesthesie generale. Université de la Méditéranée, Marseille

183. Vandewalle V, van der Linden C, Groenewegen HJ, Caemaert J (1999) Stereotactic treatment of Gilles de la Tourette syndrome by high frequency stimulation of thalamus. Lancet 353(9154):724 S0140673698059649[pii]

184. Lipsman N, Neimat JS, Lozano AM (2007) Deep brain stimulation for treatment-refractory obsessive-compulsive disorder: the search for a valid target. Neurosurgery 61(1):1–11 (discussion 3). doi:10.1227/01.neu.0000279719.75403.f7 00006123-200707000-00001 [pii]

185. Greenberg BD, Gabriels LA, Malone DA Jr, Rezai AR, Friehs GM, Okun MS et al (2010) Deep brain stimulation of the ventral internal capsule/ventral striatum for obsessive-compulsive disorder: worldwide experience. Mol Psychiatry 15(1):64–79. doi:10.1038/mp.2008.55 mp200855 [pii]

186. Abelson JL, Curtis GC, Sagher O, Albucher RC, Harrigan M, Taylor SF et al (2005) Deep brain stimulation for refractory obsessive-compulsive disorder. Biol Psychiatry 57(5):510–516. doi:10.1016/j.biopsych.2004.11.042 S0006-3223(04)01285-5 [pii]

187. Anderson D, Ahmed A (2003) Treatment of patients with intractable obsessive-compulsive disorder with anterior capsular stimulation. Case report. J Neurosurg 98(5):1104–1108. doi:10.3171/jns.2003.98.5.1104

188. Malone DA Jr, Dougherty DD, Rezai AR, Carpenter LL, Friehs GM, Eskandar EN et al (2009) Deep brain stimulation of the ventral capsule/ventral striatum for treatment-resistant depression. Biol Psychiatry 65(4):267–275. doi:10.1016/j.biopsych.2008.08.029 S0006-3223(08)01083-4 [pii]

189. Breiter HC, Rauch SL, Kwong KK, Baker JR, Weisskoff RM, Kennedy DN et al (1996) Functional magnetic resonance imaging of symptom provocation in obsessive-compulsive disorder. Arch Gen Psychiatry 53(7):595–606

190. Saxena S, Brody AL, Schwartz JM, Baxter LR (1998) Neuroimaging and frontal-subcortical circuitry in obsessive-compulsive disorder. Br J Psychiatry Suppl 35:26–37

191. Baxter LR Jr, Schwartz JM, Mazziotta JC, Phelps ME, Pahl JJ, Guze BH et al (1988) Cerebral glucose metabolic rates in nondepressed patients with obsessive-compulsive disorder. Am J Psychiatry 145(12):1560–1563

192. Abosch A, Cosgrove GR (2008) Biological basis for the surgical treatment of depression. Neurosurg Focus 25(1):E2. doi:10.3171/FOC/2008/25/7/E2

193. Aouizerate B, Cuny E, Martin-Guehl C, Guehl D, Amieva H, Benazzouz A et al (2004) Deep brain stimulation of the ventral caudate nucleus in the treatment of obsessive-compulsive disorder and major depression. Case report. J Neurosurg 101(4):682–686. doi:10.3171/jns.2004.101.4.0682

194. Halmi KA, Tozzi F, Thornton LM, Crow S, Fichter MM, Kaplan AS et al (2005) The relation among perfectionism, obsessive-compulsive personality disorder and obsessive-

compulsive disorder in individuals with eating disorders. Int J Eat Disord 38(4):371–374. doi:10.1002/eat.20190

195. Sherman BJ, Savage CR, Eddy KT, Blais MA, Deckersbach T, Jackson SC et al (2006) Strategic memory in adults with anorexia nervosa: are there similarities to obsessive compulsive spectrum disorders? Int J Eat Disord 39(6):468–476. doi:10.1002/eat.20300

196. Barbier J, Gabriels L, van Laere K, Nuttin B (2011) Successful anterior capsulotomy in comorbid anorexia nervosa and obsessive-compulsive disorder: case report. Neurosurgery 69(3):E745–E751 (discussion E51). doi:10.1227/NEU.0b013e31821964d2

197. Chang CH, Chen SY, Hsiao YL, Tsai ST, Tsai HC (2010) Hypomania with hypersexuality following bilateral anterior limb stimulation in obsessive-compulsive disorder. J Neurosurg 112(6):1299–1300. doi:10.3171/2009.10.JNS09918

198. Epstein J, Pan H, Kocsis JH, Yang Y, Butler T, Chusid J et al (2006) Lack of ventral striatal response to positive stimuli in depressed versus normal subjects. Am J Psychiatry 163(10):1784–1790. doi:10.1176/appi.ajp.163.10.1784 163/10/1784 [pii]

199. Tremblay LK, Naranjo CA, Graham SJ, Herrmann N, Mayberg HS, Hevenor S et al (2005) Functional neuroanatomical substrates of altered reward processing in major depressive disorder revealed by a dopaminergic probe. Arch Gen Psychiatry 62(11):1228–1236. doi:10.1001/archpsyc.62.11.1228 62/11/1228 [pii]

200. Schlaepfer TE, Cohen MX, Frick C, Kosel M, Brodesser D, Axmacher N et al (2008) Deep brain stimulation to reward circuitry alleviates anhedonia in refractory major depression. Neuropsychopharmacology 33(2):368–377. doi:10.1038/sj.npp.1301408 1301408 [pii]

201. Gorwood P (2008) Neurobiological mechanisms of anhedonia. Dialogues Clin Neurosci 10(3):291–299

202. Hauptman JS, DeSalles AA, Espinoza R, Sedrak M, Ishida W (2008) Potential surgical targets for deep brain stimulation in treatment-resistant depression. Neurosurg Focus 25(1):E3. doi:10.3171/FOC/2008/25/7/E3

203. Coenen VA, Schlaepfer TE, Maedler B, Panksepp J (2011) Cross-species affective functions of the medial forebrain bundle-implications for the treatment of affective pain and depression in humans. Neurosci Biobehav Rev 35(9):1971–1981. doi:10.1016/j.neubiorev.2010.12.009

204. Sturm V, Lenartz D, Koulousakis A, Treuer H, Herholz K, Klein JC et al (2003) The nucleus accumbens: a target for deep brain stimulation in obsessive-compulsive- and anxiety-disorders. J Chem Neuroanat 26(4):293–299 S0891061803001030[pii]

205. Bewernick BH, Hurlemann R, Matusch A, Kayser S, Grubert C, Hadrysiewicz B et al (2010) Nucleus accumbens deep brain stimulation decreases ratings of depression and anxiety in treatment-resistant depression. Biol Psychiatry 67(2):110–116. doi:10.1016/j.biopsych.2009.09.013 S0006-3223(09)01094-4 [pii]

206. Huff W, Lenartz D, Schormann M, Lee SH, Kuhn J, Koulousakis A et al (2010) Unilateral deep brain stimulation of the nucleus accumbens in patients with treatment-resistant obsessive-compulsive disorder: outcomes after one year. Clin Neurol Neurosurg 112(2):137–143. doi:10.1016/j.clineuro.2009.11.006 S0303-8467(09)00303-5 [pii]

207. Li N, Wang J, Wang XL, Chang CW, Ge SN, Gao L et al (2012) Nucleus accumbens surgery for addiction. World Neurosurg. doi:10.1016/j.wneu.2012.10.007

208. Voges J, Muller U, Bogerts B, Munte T, Heinze HJ (2012) DBS surgery for alcohol addiction. World Neurosurg. doi:10.1016/j.wneu.2012.07.011

209. Zhou H, Xu J, Jiang J (2011) Deep brain stimulation of nucleus accumbens on heroin-seeking behaviors: a case report. Biol Psychiatry 69(11):e41–e42. doi:10.1016/j.biopsych.2011.02.012 S0006-3223(11)00147-8 [pii]

210. Valencia-Alfonso CE, Luigjes J, Smolders R, Cohen MX, Levar N, Mazaheri A et al (2012) Effective deep brain stimulation in heroin addiction: a case report with complementary intracranial electroencephalogram. Biol Psychiatry 71(8):e35–e37. doi:10.1016/j.biopsych.2011.12.013

211. Sun B, Liu W (2012) Surgical treatments for drug addictons in humans. In: Denys D, Feenstra M, Schuurman R (eds) Deep Brain Stimulation: a new frontier in psychiatry. Springer, New York, pp 131–140

212. Ardouin C, Voon V, Worbe Y, Abouazar N, Czernecki V, Hosseini H et al (2006) Pathological gambling in Parkinson's disease improves on chronic subthalamic nucleus stimulation. Mov Disord 21(11):1941–1946. doi:10.1002/mds.21098

213. Temel Y, Blokland A, Steinbusch HW, Visser-Vandewalle V (2005) The functional role of the subthalamic nucleus in cognitive and limbic circuits. Prog Neurobiol 76(6):393–413. doi:10.1016/j.pneurobio.2005.09.005 S0301-0082(05)00104-8 [pii]

214. Nowinski WL, Belov D, Pollak P, Benabid AL (2005) Statistical analysis of 168 bilateral subthalamic nucleus implantations by means of the probabilistic functional atlas. Neurosurgery 57(4 Suppl):319–330 (discussion 30). doi:00006123-200510004-00014 [pii]

215. Parent A, Hazrati LN (1995) Functional anatomy of the basal ganglia. I. The cortico-basal ganglia-thalamo-cortical loop. Brain Res Brain Res Rev 20(1):91–127. doi:016501739400007C [pii]

216. Parent A, Hazrati LN (1995) Functional anatomy of the basal ganglia. II. The place of subthalamic nucleus and external pallidum in basal ganglia circuitry. Brain Res Brain Res Rev 20(1):128–154. doi:016501739400008D [pii]

217. Haynes WI, Mallet L (2012) What is the role of the subthalamic nucleus in OCD. Elements and insights from DBS. In: Denys D, Feenstra M, Schuurman R (eds) Deep brain stimulation: a new frontier in psychiatry. Springer, New York, pp 53–60

218. Chabardes S, Polosan M, Krack P, Bastin J, Krainik A, David O et al (2012) Deep brain stimulation for obsessive-compulsive disorder: subthalamic nucleus target. World Neurosurg. doi:10.1016/j.wneu.2012.03.010 S1878-8750(12)00413-5 [pii]

219. Mallet L, Polosan M, Jaafari N, Baup N, Welter ML, Fontaine D et al (2008) Subthalamic nucleus stimulation in severe obsessive-compulsive disorder. N Engl J Med 359(20):2121–2134. doi:10.1056/NEJMoa0708514 359/20/2121 [pii]

220. Jedynak CP (2005) Non à la nouvelle psychochirurgie des TOC. La Lettre du Neurologue 9:195–196

221. Berney A, Vingerhoets F, Perrin A, Guex P, Villemure JG, Burkhard PR et al (2002) Effect on mood of subthalamic DBS for Parkinson's disease: a consecutive series of 24 patients. Neurology 59(9):1427–1429

222. Doshi PK, Chhaya N, Bhatt MH (2002) Depression leading to attempted suicide after bilateral subthalamic nucleus stimulation for Parkinson's disease. Mov Disord 17(5):1084–1085. doi:10.1002/mds.10198

223. Thobois S, Mertens P, Guenot M, Hermier M, Mollion H, Bouvard M et al (2002) Subthalamic nucleus stimulation in Parkinson's disease: clinical evaluation of 18 patients. J Neurol 249(5):529–534. doi:10.1007/s004150200059

224. Heo JH, Lee KM, Paek SH, Kim MJ, Lee JY, Kim JY et al (2008) The effects of bilateral subthalamic nucleus deep brain stimulation (STN DBS) on cognition in Parkinson disease. J Neurol Sci 273(1–2):19–24. doi:10.1016/j.jns.2008.06.010 S0022-510X(08)00270-0 [pii]

225. Kaiser I, Kryspin-Exner I, Brucke T, Volc D, Alesch F (2008) Long-term effects of STN DBS on mood: psychosocial profiles remain stable in a 3-year follow-up. BMC Neurol 8:43. doi:10.1186/1471-2377-8-43 1471-2377-8-43 [pii]

226. Witt K, Daniels C, Reiff J, Krack P, Volkmann J, Pinsker MO et al (2008) Neuropsychological and psychiatric changes after deep brain stimulation for Parkinson's disease: a randomised, multicentre study. Lancet Neurol 7(7):605–614. doi:10.1016/S1474-4422(08)70114-5 S1474-4422(08)70114-5 [pii]

227. Ardouin C, Pillon B, Peiffer E, Bejjani P, Limousin P, Damier P et al (1999) Bilateral subthalamic or pallidal stimulation for Parkinson's disease affects neither memory nor executive functions: a consecutive series of 62 patients. Ann Neurol 46(2):217–223

228. Volkmann J, Allert N, Voges J, Weiss PH, Freund HJ, Sturm V (2001) Safety and efficacy of pallidal or subthalamic nucleus stimulation in advanced PD. Neurology 56(4):548–551

229. Daniele A, Albanese A, Contarino MF, Zinzi P, Barbier A, Gasparini F et al (2003) Cognitive and behavioural effects of chronic stimulation of the subthalamic nucleus in patients with Parkinson's disease. J Neurol Neurosurg Psychiatry 74(2):175–182
230. Castelli L, Perozzo P, Zibetti M, Crivelli B, Morabito U, Lanotte M et al (2006) Chronic deep brain stimulation of the subthalamic nucleus for Parkinson's disease: effects on cognition, mood, anxiety and personality traits. Eur Neurol 55(3):136–144. doi:10.1159/000093213 93213 [pii]
231. Wang X, Chang C, Geng N, Li N, Wang J, Ma J et al (2009) Long-term effects of bilateral deep brain stimulation of the subthalamic nucleus on depression in patients with Parkinson's disease. Parkinsonism Relat Disord 15(8):587–591. doi:10.1016/j.parkreldis.2009.02.006 S1353-8020(09)00056-X [pii]
232. Houeto JL, Welter ML, Bejjani PB, Tezenas du Montcel S, Bonnet AM, Mesnage V et al (2003) Subthalamic stimulation in Parkinson disease: intraoperative predictive factors. Arch Neurol 60(5):690–694. doi:10.1001/archneur.60.5.690 60/5/690 [pii]
233. Pillon B, Ardouin C, Damier P, Krack P, Houeto JL, Klinger H et al (2000) Neuropsychological changes between "off" and "on" STN or GPi stimulation in Parkinson's disease. Neurology 55(3):411–418
234. Saint-Cyr JA, Trepanier LL, Kumar R, Lozano AM, Lang AE (2000) Neuropsychological consequences of chronic bilateral stimulation of the subthalamic nucleus in Parkinson's disease. Brain 123(10):2091–2108
235. Hershey T, Revilla FJ, Wernle A, Gibson PS, Dowling JL, Perlmutter JS (2004) Stimulation of STN impairs aspects of cognitive control in PD. Neurology 62(7):1110–1114
236. Mayberg HS (2003) Modulating dysfunctional limbic-cortical circuits in depression: towards development of brain-based algorithms for diagnosis and optimised treatment. Br Med Bull 65:193–207
237. Seminowicz DA, Mayberg HS, McIntosh AR, Goldapple K, Kennedy S, Segal Z et al (2004) Limbic-frontal circuitry in major depression: a path modeling metanalysis. Neuroimage 22(1):409–418. doi:10.1016/j.neuroimage.2004.01.015 S1053811904000497 [pii]
238. Nobler MS, Oquendo MA, Kegeles LS, Malone KM, Campbell CC, Sackeim HA et al (2001) Decreased regional brain metabolism after ect. Am J Psychiatry 158(2):305–308
239. Mottaghy FM, Keller CE, Gangitano M, Ly J, Thall M, Parker JA et al (2002) Correlation of cerebral blood flow and treatment effects of repetitive transcranial magnetic stimulation in depressed patients. Psychiatry Res 115(1–2):1–14 S092549270200032X [pii]
240. Mayberg HS, Lozano AM, Voon V, McNeely HE, Seminowicz D, Hamani C et al (2005) Deep brain stimulation for treatment-resistant depression. Neuron 45(5):651–660. doi:10.1016/j.neuron.2005.02.014 S0896-6273(05)00156-X [pii]
241. Inagaki M, Yoshikawa E, Kobayakawa M, Matsuoka Y, Sugawara Y, Nakano T et al (2007) Regional cerebral glucose metabolism in patients with secondary depressive episodes after fatal pancreatic cancer diagnosis. J Affect Disord 99(1–3):231–236. doi:10.1016/j.jad.2006.08.019 S0165-0327(06)00349-1 [pii]
242. Kumano H, Ida I, Oshima A, Takahashi K, Yuuki N, Amanuma M et al (2007) Brain metabolic changes associated with predispotion to onset of major depressive disorder and adjustment disorder in cancer patients–a preliminary PET study. J Psychiatr Res 41(7):591–599. doi:10.1016/j.jpsychires.2006.03.006 S0022-3956(06)00061-6 [pii]
243. Kopell BH, Greenberg BD (2008) Anatomy and physiology of the basal ganglia: implications for DBS in psychiatry. Neurosci Biobehav Rev 32(3):408–422. doi:10.1016/j.neubiorev.2007.07.004 S0149-7634(07)00076-0 [pii]
244. Johansen-Berg H, Gutman DA, Behrens TE, Matthews PM, Rushworth MF, Katz E et al (2008) Anatomical connectivity of the subgenual cingulate region targeted with deep brain stimulation for treatment-resistant depression. Cereb Cortex 18(6):1374–1383. doi:10.1093/cercor/bhm167 bhm167 [pii]

245. Sedrak M, Gorgulho A, De Salles AF, Frew A, Behnke E, Ishida W et al (2008) The role of modern imaging modalities on deep brain stimulation targeting for mental illness. Acta Neurochir Suppl 101:3–7
246. Hamani C, Mayberg H, Snyder B, Giacobbe P, Kennedy S, Lozano AM (2009) Deep brain stimulation of the subcallosal cingulate gyrus for depression: anatomical location of active contacts in clinical responders and a suggested guideline for targeting. J Neurosurg 111(6):1209–1215. doi:10.3171/2008.10.JNS08763
247. Lozano AM, Mayberg HS, Giacobbe P, Hamani C, Craddock RC, Kennedy SH (2008) Subcallosal cingulate gyrus deep brain stimulation for treatment-resistant depression. Biol Psychiatry 64(6):461–467. doi:10.1016/j.biopsych.2008.05.034 S0006-3223(08)00703-8 [pii]
248. McNeely HE, Mayberg HS, Lozano AM, Kennedy SH (2008) Neuropsychological impact of Cg25 deep brain stimulation for treatment-resistant depression: preliminary results over 12 months. J Nerv Ment Dis 196(5):405–410. doi:10.1097/NMD.0b013e3181710927 00005053-200805000-00007 [pii]
249. Coenen VA, Bewernick B, Kayser S, Maedler B, Schlaepfer TE (2012) Deep brain stimulation of the human medial forebrain bundle (slmfb-dbs) for refractory depression— results from the foresee study. In: XXth Congress of the European Society for stereotactic and functional neurosurgery, Cascais, Portugal, 27 Sept 2012
250. Jimenez F, Velasco F, Salin-Pascual R, Hernandez JA, Velasco M, Criales JL et al (2005) A patient with a resistant major depression disorder treated with deep brain stimulation in the inferior thalamic peduncle. Neurosurgery 57(3):585–593 (discussion 93). doi:00006123-200509000-00027 [pii]
251. Jimenez-Ponce F, Velasco-Campos F, Castro-Farfan G, Nicolini H, Velasco AL, Salin-Pascual R et al (2009) Preliminary study in patients with obsessive-compulsive disorder treated with electrical stimulation in the inferior thalamic peduncle. Neurosurgery 65(6 Suppl):203–209 (discussion 9). doi:10.1227/01.NEU.0000345938.39199.90 00006123-200912001-00026 [pii]
252. Hong S, Hikosaka O (2008) The globus pallidus sends reward-related signals to the lateral habenula. Neuron 60(4):720–729. doi:10.1016/j.neuron.2008.09.035 S0896-6273(08)00837-4 [pii]
253. Matsumoto M, Hikosaka O (2009) Representation of negative motivational value in the primate lateral habenula. Nat Neurosci 12(1):77–84. doi:10.1038/nn.2233 nn.2233 [pii]
254. Geisler S, Trimble M (2008) The lateral habenula: no longer neglected. CNS Spectr 13(6):484–489
255. Hikosaka O, Sesack SR, Lecourtier L, Shepard PD (2008) Habenula: crossroad between the basal ganglia and the limbic system. J Neurosci 28(46):11825–11829. doi:10.1523/JNEUROSCI.3463-08.2008 28/46/11825 [pii]
256. Morra JT (2007) The neural substrate of disappointment revealed? J Neurosci 27(40):10647–10648. doi:10.1523/JNEUROSCI.3026-07.2007 27/40/10647 [pii]
257. Winter C, Vollmayr B, Djodari-Irani A, Klein J, Sartorius A (2011) Pharmacological inhibition of the lateral habenula improves depressive-like behavior in an animal model of treatment resistant depression. Behav Brain Res 216(1):463–465. doi:10.1016/j.bbr.2010.07.034 S0166-4328(10)00535-8 [pii]
258. Sartorius A, Henn FA (2007) Deep brain stimulation of the lateral habenula in treatment resistant major depression. Med Hypotheses 69(6):1305–1308. doi:10.1016/j.mehy.2007.03.021 S0306-9877(07)00247-2 [pii]
259. Sartorius A, Kiening KL, Kirsch P, von Gall CC, Haberkorn U, Unterberg AW et al (2010) Remission of major depression under deep brain stimulation of the lateral habenula in a therapy-refractory patient. Biol Psychiatry 67(2):e9–e11. doi:10.1016/j.biopsych.2009.08.027 S0006-3223(09)01047-6 [pii]
260. de Koning PP, Figee M, van den Munckhof P, Schuurman PR, Denys D (2011) Current status of deep brain stimulation for obsessive-compulsive disorder: a clinical review of different targets. Curr Psychiatry Rep 13(4):274–282. doi:10.1007/s11920-011-0200-8

261. Sarnecki T, Temel Y (2011) Deep brain stimulation for treatment-resistant depression: a review. Open Neurosurg J 4:1–6

262. Pansaon Piedad JC, Rickards HE, Cavanna AE (2012) What patients with gilles de la tourette syndrome should be treated with deep brain stimulation and what is the best target? Neurosurgery 71(1):173–192. doi:10.1227/NEU.0b013e3182535a00

263. Rogers MH, Anderson PB (2009) Deep brain stimulation: applications, complications and side effects. Nova Biomedical Books, New York

264. Maciunas RJ, Maddux BN, Riley DE, Whitney CM, Schoenberg MR, Ogrocki PJ et al (2007) Prospective randomized double-blind trial of bilateral thalamic deep brain stimulation in adults with Tourette syndrome. J Neurosurg 107(5):1004–1014. doi:10. 3171/JNS-07/11/1004

265. Welter ML, Mallet L, Houeto JL, Karachi C, Czernecki V, Cornu P et al (2008) Internal pallidal and thalamic stimulation in patients with Tourette syndrome. Arch Neurol 65(7):952–957. doi:10.1001/archneur.65.7.952 65/7/952 [pii]

266. Hoflich GK, Kasper S, Hufnagel A et al (1993) Application of transcranial magnetic stimulation in treatment of drug-resistant major depression: a report of two cases. Hum Psychopharmacol Bull 8:361–365

267. Pascual-Leone A, Rubio B, Pallardo F, Catala MD (1996) Rapid-rate transcranial magnetic stimulation of left dorsolateral prefrontal cortex in drug-resistant depression. Lancet 348(9022):233–237. S0140673696012196 [pii]

268. Martin JL, Barbanoj MJ, Schlaepfer TE, Thompson E, Perez V, Kulisevsky J (2003) Repetitive transcranial magnetic stimulation for the treatment of depression. Systematic review and meta-analysis. Br J Psychiatry 182:480–491

269. Benadhira R, Saba G, Samaan A, Dumortier G, Lipski H, Gastal D et al (2005) Transcranial magnetic stimulation for refractory depression. Am J Psychiatry 162(1):193. doi:10.1176/ appi.ajp.162.1.193 162/1/193 [pii]

270. Januel D, Dumortier G, Verdon CM, Stamatiadis L, Saba G, Cabaret W et al (2006) A double-blind sham controlled study of right prefrontal repetitive transcranial magnetic stimulation (rTMS): therapeutic and cognitive effect in medication free unipolar depression during 4 weeks. Prog Neuropsychopharmacol Biol Psychiatry 30(1):126–130. doi:10.1016/j. pnpbp.2005.08.016 S0278-5846(05)00279-4 [pii]

271. Barker AT, Jalinous R, Freeston IL (1985) Non-invasive magnetic stimulation of human motor cortex. Lancet 1(8437):1106–1107. S0140-6736(85)92413-4 [pii]

272. Rossi S, De Capua A, Ulivelli M, Bartalini S, Falzarano V, Filippone G et al (2007) Effects of repetitive transcranial magnetic stimulation on chronic tinnitus: a randomised, crossover, double blind, placebo controlled study. J Neurol Neurosurg Psychiatry 78(8):857–863. doi:10.1136/jnnp.2006.105007 jnnp.2006.105007 [pii]

273. Rosenberg O, Roth Y, Kotler M, Zangen A, Dannon P (2011) Deep transcranial magnetic stimulation for the treatment of auditory hallucinations: a preliminary open-label study. Ann Gen Psychiatry 10(1):3. doi:10.1186/1744-859X-10-3 1744-859X-10-3 [pii]

274. Husted DS, Shapira NA (2004) A review of the treatment for refractory obsessive-compulsive disorder: from medicine to deep brain stimulation. CNS Spectr 9(11):833–847

275. Jaafari N, Rachid F, Rotge JY, Polosan M, El-Hage W, Belin D et al (2012) Safety and efficacy of repetitive transcranial magnetic stimulation in the treatment of obsessive-compulsive disorder: a review. World J Biol Psychiatry 13(3):164–177. doi:10.3109/ 15622975.2011.575177

276. Saillet S, Langlois M, Feddersen B, Minotti L, Vercueil L, Chabardes S et al (2009) Manipulating the epileptic brain using stimulation: a review of experimental and clinical studies. Epileptic Disord 11(2):100–112. doi:10.1684/epd.2009.0255 epd.2009.0255 [pii]

277. Williams JA, Imamura M, Fregni F (2009) Updates on the use of non-invasive brain stimulation in physical and rehabilitation medicine. J Rehabil Med 41(5):305–311. doi:10. 2340/16501977-0356

278. Passard A, Attal N, Benadhira R, Brasseur L, Saba G, Sichere P et al (2007) Effects of unilateral repetitive transcranial magnetic stimulation of the motor cortex on chronic

widespread pain in fibromyalgia. Brain 130(Pt 10):2661–2670. doi:10.1093/brain/awm189 awm189 [pii]

279. (ANAES) ANdAedÉeS (ed) (1998) Indications et Modalités de l'Electroconvulsothérapie— Recommandations Professionnelles. Service Communication et Diffusion, Paris

280. Grunhaus L, Schreiber S, Dolberg OT, Polak D, Dannon PN (2003) A randomized controlled comparison of electroconvulsive therapy and repetitive transcranial magnetic stimulation in severe and resistant nonpsychotic major depression. Biol Psychiatry 53(4):324–331. S0006322302014993 [pii]

281. Dannon PN, Grunhaus L (2003) Repetitive transcranial magnetic stimulation is effective following repeated courses in the treatment of major depressive disorder–a case report. Hum Psychopharmacol 18(4):313–315. doi:10.1002/hup.478

282. Janicak PG, Dowd SM, Martis B, Alam D, Beedle D, Krasuski J et al (2002) Repetitive transcranial magnetic stimulation versus electroconvulsive therapy for major depression: preliminary results of a randomized trial. Biol Psychiatry 51(8):659–667. S0006322301013543 [pii]

283. Pridmore S, Bruno R, Turnier-Shea Y, Reid P, Rybak M (2000) Comparison of unlimited numbers of rapid transcranial magnetic stimulation (rTMS) and ECT treatment sessions in major depressive episode. Int J Neuropsychopharmacol 3(2):129–134. doi:10.1017/ S1461145700001784 S1461145700001784 [pii]

284. Arsonval A (1896) Dispositifs pour la mesure des courants alternatifs de toutes fréquences. C R Soc Biol (Paris) 2:450–451

285. Magnuson CE, Stevens HC (1914) Visual sensations created by a magnetic field. Philosoph Mag 28:188–207

286. Baxter LR Jr, Schwartz JM, Phelps ME, Mazziotta JC, Guze BH, Selin CE et al (1989) Reduction of prefrontal cortex glucose metabolism common to three types of depression. Arch Gen Psychiatry 46(3):243–250

287. Kito S, Fujita K, Koga Y (2008) Changes in regional cerebral blood flow after repetitive transcranial magnetic stimulation of the left dorsolateral prefrontal cortex in treatment-resistant depression. J Neuropsychiatry Clin Neurosci 20(1):74–80. doi:10.1176/appi. neuropsych.20.1.74 20/1/74 [pii]

288. Richieri R, Adida M, Dumas R, Fakra E, Azorin JM, Pringuey D et al (2010) Affective disorders and repetitive transcranial magnetic stimulation: therapeutic innovations. Encephale 36(Suppl 6):S197–S201. doi:10.1016/S0013-7006(10)70057-9 S0013-7006(10)70057-9 [pii]

289. Brunelin J, Poulet E, Boeuve C, Zeroug-vial H, d'Amato T, Saoud M (2007) Efficacy of repetitive transcranial magnetic stimulation (rTMS) in major depression: a review. Encephale 33(2):126–134. MDOI-ENC-4-2007-33-2-0013-7006-101019-200730012 [pii]

290. Millet B (2009) Electrostimulation techniques in treatment for severe depression. Encephale 35(Suppl 7):S325–S329. doi:10.1016/S0013-7006(09)73496-7 S0013-7006(09)73496-7 [pii]

291. Holtzheimer PE 3rd, Russo J, Avery DH (2001) A meta-analysis of repetitive transcranial magnetic stimulation in the treatment of depression. Psychopharmacol Bull 35(4):149–169

292. Kozel FA, George MS (2002) Meta-analysis of left prefrontal repetitive transcranial magnetic stimulation (rTMS) to treat depression. J Psychiatr Pract 8(5):270–275. 00131746-200209000-00003 [pii]

293. Gross M, Nakamura L, Pascual-Leone A, Fregni F (2007) Has repetitive transcranial magnetic stimulation (rTMS) treatment for depression improved? A systematic review and meta-analysis comparing the recent vs. the earlier rTMS studies. Acta Psychiatr Scand 116(3):165–173. doi:10.1111/j.1600-0447.2007.01049.x ACP1049 [pii]

294. Lam RW, Chan P, Wilkins-Ho M, Yatham LN (2008) Repetitive transcranial magnetic stimulation for treatment-resistant depression: a systematic review and metaanalysis. Can J Psychiatry 53(9):621–631

295. Schutter DJ, Laman DM, van Honk J, Vergouwen AC, Koerselman GF (2009) Partial clinical response to 2 weeks of 2 Hz repetitive transcranial magnetic stimulation to the right

parietal cortex in depression. Int J Neuropsychopharmacol 12(5):643–650. doi:10.1017/S1461145708009553 S1461145708009553 [pii]

296. Velasco F, Arguelles C, Carrillo-Ruiz JD, Castro G, Velasco AL, Jimenez F et al (2008) Efficacy of motor cortex stimulation in the treatment of neuropathic pain: a randomized double-blind trial. J Neurosurg 108(4):698–706. doi:10.3171/JNS/2008/108/4/0698

297. Friedland DR, Gaggl W, Runge-Samuelson C, Ulmer JL, Kopell BH (2007) Feasibility of auditory cortical stimulation for the treatment of tinnitus. Otol Neurotol 28(8):1005–1012. doi:10.1097/MAO.0b013e318159ebf5 00129492-200712000-00004 [pii]

298. Priori A, Lefaucheur JP (2007) Chronic epidural motor cortical stimulation for movement disorders. Lancet Neurol 6(3):279–286. doi:10.1016/S1474-4422(07)70056-X S1474-4422(07)70056-X [pii]

299. Brown JA, Lutsep HL, Weinand M, Cramer SC (2006) Motor cortex stimulation for the enhancement of recovery from stroke: a prospective, multicenter safety study. Neurosurgery 58(3):464–473. doi:10.1227/01.NEU.0000197100.63931.04 00006123-200603000-00007 [pii]

300. Amiaz R, Levy D, Vainiger D, Grunhaus L, Zangen A (2009) Repeated high-frequency transcranial magnetic stimulation over the dorsolateral prefrontal cortex reduces cigarette craving and consumption. Addiction 104:653–660

301. Kopell BH (2011) Epidural cortical stimulation (EpCS) of the left dorsolateral prefrontal cortex for refractory major depressive disorder. Neurosurgey

302. Nahas Z, Anderson BS, Borckardt J, Arana AB, George MS, Reeves ST et al (2010) Bilateral epidural prefrontal cortical stimulation for treatment-resistant depression. Biol Psychiatry 67(2):101–109. doi:10.1016/j.biopsych.2009.08.021 S0006-3223(09)01020-8 [pii]

303. Kito S, Fujita K, Koga Y (2008) Regional cerebral blood flow changes after low-frequency transcranial magnetic stimulation of the right dorsolateral prefrontal cortex in treatment-resistant depression. Neuropsychobiology 58(1):29–36. doi:10.1159/000154477 000154477 [pii]

304. Canavero S, Bonicalzi V (2002) Therapeutic extradural cortical stimulation for central and neuropathic pain: a review. Clin J Pain 18(1):48–55

305. Lefaucheur JP (2004) Transcranial magnetic stimulation in the management of pain. Suppl Clin Neurophysiol 57:737–748

306. Lefaucheur JP, Drouot X, Menard-Lefaucheur I, Nguyen JP (2004) Neuropathic pain controlled for more than a year by monthly sessions of repetitive transcranial magnetic stimulation of the motor cortex. Neurophysiol Clin 34(2):91–95. doi:10.1016/j.neucli.2004.02.001 S098770530400005X [pii]

307. Migita K, Uozumi T, Arita K, Monden S (1995) Transcranial magnetic coil stimulation of motor cortex in patients with central pain. Neurosurgery 36(5):1037–1039 (discussion 9–40)

308. Dougherty DD, Thase ME, Howland RH, Evans KC, Harsch H, Kondziolka D (eds) (2008) Feasibility study of an implantable cortical stimulation system for patients with major depressive disorder. Society of Biological Psychiatry 63rd Annual Meeting, Washington, D.C

309. Kopell BH, Halverson J, Butson CR, Dickinson M, Bobholz J, Harsch H et al (2011) Epidural cortical stimulation of the left dorsolateral prefrontal cortex for refractory major depressive disorder. Neurosurgery 69(5):1015–1029 (discussion 29). doi:10.1227/NEU.0b013e318229cfcd

310. Spielmans GI (2012) Unimpressive efficacy and unclear safety assessment of epidural cortical stimulation for refractory major depressive disorder. Neurosurgery 70(1):E268–E269; author reply E9. doi:10.1227/NEU.0b013e31823a3206

311. Achem (1994)

312. Handforth (1998)

313. Elger G, Hoppe C, Falkai P, Rush AJ, Elger CE (2000) Vagus nerve stimulation is associated with mood improvements in epilepsy patients. Epilepsy Res 42(2–3):203–210. S0920-1211(00)00181-9 [pii]

314. Carpenter LL, Friehs GM, Price LH (2003) Cervical vagus nerve stimulation for treatment-resistant depression. Neurosurg Clin N Am 14(2):275–282
315. Harden CL, Pulver MC, Ravdin LD, Nikolov B, Halper JP, Labar DR (2000) A pilot study of mood in epilepsy patients treated with vagus nerve stimulation. Epilepsy Behav 1(2):93–99. doi:10.1006/ebeh.2000.0046 S1525-5050(00)90046-5 [pii]
316. Hoppe C, Helmstaedter C, Scherrmann J, Elger CE (2001) Self-reported mood changes following 6 months of vagus nerve stimulation in epilepsy patients. Epilepsy Behav 2(4):335–342. doi:10.1006/ebeh.2001.0194 S1525-5050(01)90194-5 [pii]
317. Nemeroff CB, Mayberg HS, Krahl SE, McNamara J, Frazer A, Henry TR et al (2006) VNS therapy in treatment-resistant depression: clinical evidence and putative neurobiological mechanisms. Neuropsychopharmacology 31(7):1345–1355. doi:10.1038/sj.npp.1301082 1301082 [pii]
318. Yatham LN (2004) Newer anticonvulsants in the treatment of bipolar disorder. J Clin Psychiatry 65(Suppl 10):28–35
319. Groves DA, Brown VJ (2005) Vagal nerve stimulation: a review of its applications and potential mechanisms that mediate its clinical effects. Neurosci Biobehav Rev 29(3):493–500. doi:10.1016/j.neubiorev.2005.01.004
320. Zobel A, Joe A, Freymann N, Clusmann H, Schramm J, Reinhardt M et al (2005) Changes in regional cerebral blood flow by therapeutic vagus nerve stimulation in depression: an exploratory approach. Psychiatry Res 139(3):165–179. doi:10.1016/j.pscychresns.2005.02.010 S0925-4927(05)00091-0 [pii]
321. Henry TR, Bakay RA, Votaw JR, Pennell PB, Epstein CM, Faber TL et al (1998) Brain blood flow alterations induced by therapeutic vagus nerve stimulation in partial epilepsy: I. Acute effects at high and low levels of stimulation. Epilepsia 39(9):983–990
322. Drevets WC, Price JL, Bardgett ME, Reich T, Todd RD, Raichle ME (2002) Glucose metabolism in the amygdala in depression: relationship to diagnostic subtype and plasma cortisol levels. Pharmacol Biochem Behav 71(3):431–447. S0091305701006876 [pii]
323. Mayberg HS, Brannan SK, Tekell JL, Silva JA, Mahurin RK, McGinnis S et al (2000) Regional metabolic effects of fluoxetine in major depression: serial changes and relationship to clinical response. Biol Psychiatry 48(8):830–843. S0006-3223(00)01036-2 [pii]
324. Kosel M, Brockmann H, Frick C, Zobel A, Schlaepfer TE (2011) Chronic vagus nerve stimulation for treatment-resistant depression increases regional cerebral blood flow in the dorsolateral prefrontal cortex. Psychiatry Res 191(3):153–159. doi:10.1016/j.pscychresns.2010.11.004 S0925-4927(10)00385-9 [pii]
325. Jobe PC, Dailey JW, Wernicke JF (1999) A noradrenergic and serotonergic hypothesis of the linkage between epilepsy and affective disorders. Crit Rev Neurobiol 13(4):317–356
326. Rauch SL (2003) Neuroimaging and neurocircuitry models pertaining to the neurosurgical treatment of psychiatric disorders. Neurosurg Clin N Am 14(2):213–223, vii–viii
327. Hammond EJ, Uthman BM, Wilder BJ, Ben-Menachem E, Hamberger A, Hedner T et al (1992) Neurochemical effects of vagus nerve stimulation in humans. Brain Res 583(1–2):300–303
328. Ben-Menachem E, Hamberger A, Hedner T, Hammond EJ, Uthman BM, Slater J et al (1995) Effects of vagus nerve stimulation on amino acids and other metabolites in the CSF of patients with partial seizures. Epilepsy Res 20(3):221–227. doi:0920121194000839 [pii]
329. Roux FX, Turak B, Landre E (2008) Vagus nerve stimulation for the treatment of refractory epilepsy. Neurochirurgie 54(3):332–339. doi:10.1016/j.neuchi.2008.02.048 S0028-3770(08)00092-1 [pii]
330. Rush AJ, George MS, Sackeim HA, Marangell LB, Husain MM, Giller C et al (2000) Vagus nerve stimulation (VNS) for treatment-resistant depressions: a multicenter study. Biol Psychiatry 47(4):276–286. S0006-3223(99)00304-2 [pii]
331. George MS, Sackeim HA, Rush AJ, Marangell LB, Nahas Z, Husain MM et al (2000) Vagus nerve stimulation: a new tool for brain research and therapy. Biol Psychiatry 47(4):287–295. S0006-3223(99)00308-X [pii]

332. Sackeim HA, Rush AJ, George MS, Marangell LB, Husain MM, Nahas Z et al (2001) Vagus nerve stimulation (VNS) for treatment-resistant depression: efficacy, side effects, and predictors of outcome. Neuropsychopharmacology 25(5):713–728. doi:10.1016/S0893-133X(01)00271-8 S0893133X01002718 [pii]
333. Shuchman M (2007) Approving the vagus-nerve stimulator for depression. N Engl J Med 356(16):1604–1607. doi:10.1056/NEJMp078035 356/16/1604 [pii]
334. Rush AJ, Marangell LB, Sackeim HA, George MS, Brannan SK, Davis SM et al (2005) Vagus nerve stimulation for treatment-resistant depression: a randomized, controlled acute phase trial. Biol Psychiatry 58(5):347–354. doi:10.1016/j.biopsych.2005.05.025 S0006-3223(05)00620-7 [pii]
335. Nahas Z, Marangell LB, Husain MM, Rush AJ, Sackeim HA, Lisanby SH et al (2005) Two-year outcome of vagus nerve stimulation (VNS) for treatment of major depressive episodes. J Clin Psychiatry 66(9):1097–1104
336. Schlaepfer TE, Frick C, Zobel A, Maier W, Heuser I, Bajbouj M et al (2008) Vagus nerve stimulation for depression: efficacy and safety in a European study. Psychol Med 38(5):651–661. doi:10.1017/S0033291707001924 S0033291707001924 [pii]
337. Cristancho P, Cristancho MA, Baltuch GH, Thase ME, O'Reardon JP (2011) Effectiveness and safety of vagus nerve stimulation for severe treatment-resistant major depression in clinical practice after FDA approval: outcomes at 1 year. J Clin Psychiatry. doi:10.4088/JCP.09m05888blu
338. Schatzberg AF, Kraemer HC (2000) Use of placebo control groups in evaluating efficacy of treatment of unipolar major depression. Biol Psychiatry 47(8):736–744. doi:S0006-3223(00)00846-5 [pii]
339. George MS, Rush AJ, Marangell LB, Sackeim HA, Brannan SK, Davis SM et al (2005) A one-year comparison of vagus nerve stimulation with treatment as usual for treatment-resistant depression. Biol Psychiatry 58(5):364–373. doi:10.1016/j.biopsych.2005.07.028 S0006-3223(05)00917-0 [pii]
340. Morris GL 3rd, Mueller WM (1999) Long-term treatment with vagus nerve stimulation in patients with refractory epilepsy. The Vagus Nerve Stimulation Study Group E01-E05. Neurology 53(8):1731–1735
341. Rychlicki F, Zamponi N, Trignani R, Ricciuti RA, Iacoangeli M, Scerrati M (2006) Vagus nerve stimulation: clinical experience in drug-resistant pediatric epileptic patients. Seizure 15(7):483–490. doi:10.1016/j.seizure.2006.06.001
342. Khurana DS, Reumann M, Hobdell EF, Neff S, Valencia I, Legido A et al (2007) Vagus nerve stimulation in children with refractory epilepsy: unusual complications and relationship to sleep-disordered breathing. Childs Nerv Syst 23(11):1309–1312. doi:10.1007/s00381-007-0404-8
343. Sackeim HA, Keilp JG, Rush AJ, George MS, Marangell LB, Dormer JS et al (2001) The effects of vagus nerve stimulation on cognitive performance in patients with treatment-resistant depression. Neuropsychiatry Neuropsychol Behav Neurol 14(1):53–62

Chapter 4
Disorders for Which Psychosurgery is Relevant Today

Abstract Obsessive-compulsive disorder with verification or washing rituals, for example, can be extremely debilitating and in 10 % of cases do not respond to psychotherapy or medication. Highly focused surgical procedures have been proposed, in particular lesions in the internal capsule and the cingulum to interrupt loops causing this disorder. These relatively effective interventions, capsulotomy, or cingulotomy, are however irreversible, and can make some definitive complications. With the advent of deep brain stimulation targets such as the internal capsule were taken and others, such as the subthalamic nucleus accumbens, came to be added. This stimulation through electrodes implanted in the brain has the advantage of being reversible and adaptable.

Obsessive-Compulsive Disorders

Abstract Obsessive-compulsive disorder with verification or washing rituals, for example, can be extremely debilitating and in 10 % of cases do not respond to psychotherapy or medication. Highly focused surgical procedures have been proposed, in particular lesions in the internal capsule and the cingulum to interrupt loops causing this disorder. These relatively effective interventions, capsulotomy or cingulotomy, are however irreversible and can make some definitive complications. With the advent of deep brain stimulation targets such as the internal capsule were taken and others, such as the subthalamic nucleus accumbens, came to be added. This stimulation through electrodes implanted in the brain, has the advantage of being reversible and adaptable.

Obsessive-compulsive disorder (OCD) concern about 1–2 % of the population of Western countries and 10 % of them would rebel at all psychotherapeutic or drug treatments [1]. This "doubting mania" is one of the most disabling anxiety disorders because of intrusive thoughts—obsessions—and repetitive and ritualistic behaviors—compulsions—which the patient is unable to overcome. These

M. Lévêque, *Psychosurgery*, DOI: 10.1007/978-3-319-01144-8_4,
© Springer International Publishing Switzerland 2014

obsessions, besieging mind, these "internal enemies"[1] as Cottraux names them can be of the order of the impulse, such as the fear of committing a wrongful act (the fear of knives for fear of using them to hurt) but can also take the form of unpleasant or even guilt causing obsessive ideations such as sacrilegious phrases addressing God or mental tasks that the subject imposes on himself. Compulsions are manifested by "conjuring rituals" or magical thinking that the patient recognizes as absurd, but which are necessary to reduce anxiety caused by their obsessions. It may be rituals involving dressing, washing, tidying up, verification… These anxiety and rituals sometimes become increasingly pervasive in the life of the patient, to the point that it gradually leads to marginalization or even social ostracism. OCD should be differentiated from "*obsessive personality*" traits which are expressed as a desire for perfection or control but for which affected individuals only complain very rarely.

Frequently Associated Psychiatric Disorders

Psychiatric comorbidity associated with OCD is important. It is estimated that nearly two-thirds of patients also suffer from depression. Other mood disorders may be observed in particular episodes of hypomania in one in ten patients. An estimated 15 % of patients presented or will present bipolar disorder with alternating episodes of depression and hypomania. The use of antidepressant drugs in these patients together with OCD and bipolar disorder can trigger manic turns and promote rapidly alternating depression and mania. Other anxiety disorders are found in almost two-thirds of patients with OCD among them panic disorders (12 %), phobias (40 %), nearly half of which turn out to be social phobias. The syndrome of Gilles de la Tourette[2] is found in 7 % of patients while schizophrenia affects one patient in ten instead of one in a hundred among the general population.

A Severe Impact on Quality of Life

It is estimated that more than half of patients with OCD believes that this disease affects their family or business relationships, and nearly a third consider that it severely impacts their work. The impact on their lives is a result of the considerable time devoted to repeating these rituals but also the anxious or depressive manifestations of the illness. Patients who are aware of the absurdity of their compulsions derive a sense of shame forcing them, generally, to conceal the nature

---

[1] Cottraux, J. (1998). Les ennemis intérieurs obsessions et compulsions. Paris, O. Jacob.

[2] Cf. Gilles de la Tourette syndrome, p. 296.

of their disease and its rituals. On average, they wait 7 years before consulting a psychiatrist.

Evaluating OCD and Its Severity

The different types of OCD, their severity, and their impact in the life of the patient led to the development of diagnostic scales in order to assess the effectiveness of treatments. The most used is the *Yale-Brown Obsessive-Compulsive Scale (Y-BOCS)*. The *Y-BOCS* scale (Table 4.1) is a synthetic global standard assessment tool which also exists in a version for juvenile OCD or for self-evaluation. Y-BOCS contains ten criteria, each rated on four points: five items relating to obsessions and five to compulsions. An overall score between 16 and 18 signifies sufficient intensity to warrant treatment while severe cases are characterized by a score above 30. Below 16 is considered subclinical OCD or OC syndrome (OCS), a mild form of OCD which is four times more common than OCD.

Table 4.1 Yale-brown obsessive-compulsive scale (Y-BOCS)

How much of your time is occupied by obsessive thoughts?
0   None
1   Less than 1 h per day
2   1–3 h per day
3   3–8 h per day
4   More than 8 h per day

How much do your obsessive thoughts interfere with functioning in your social, work, or other roles?
0   None
1   Slight interference, but no impairment
2   Definite interference, but manageable
3   Substantial interference
4   Extreme interference, incapacitating

How much distress do your obsessive thoughts cause you?
0   None
1   Mild, not too disturbing
2   Moderate, disturbing, but still manageable
3   Severe, very disturbing
4   Extreme, near constant and disabling distress

How much of an effort do you make to resist the obsessive thoughts?
0   Always make an effort to resist, or don't even need to resist
1   Try to resist most of the time
2   Make some effort to resist
3   Reluctantly yield to all obsessive thoughts
4   Completely and willingly yield to all obsessions

(continued)

Table 4.1 (continued)

How much control do you have over your obsessive thoughts?

0   Complete control

1   Much control, usually able to stop or divert obsessions with some effort and concentration

2   Moderate control, sometimes able to stop or divert obsessions

3   Little control, rarely successful in stopping or dismissing obsessions

4   No control, rarely able to even momentarily alter obsessive thinking

How much time do you spend performing compulsive behaviors?

0   None

1   Less than 1 h per day

2   1–3 h per day

3   3–8 h per day

4   More than 8 h per day

How much do your compulsive behaviors interfere with functioning in your social, work, or other roles?

0   None

1   Slight interference, but no impairment

2   Definite interference, but manageable

3   Substantial interference

4   Extreme interference, incapacitating

How anxious would you become if you were prevented from performing your compulsive behaviors?

0   No anxiety

1   Only slightly anxious

2   Some anxiety, but manageable

3   Prominent and disturbing anxiety

4   Extreme, incapacitating anxiety

How much of an effort do you make to resist the compulsions?

0   Always make an effort to resist, or don't even need to resist

1   Try to resist most of the time

2   Make some effort to resist

3   Reluctantly yield to all compulsions

4   Completely and willingly yield to all compulsions

How much control do you have over the compulsions?

0   Complete control

1   Much control, usually able to stop or divert compulsive behavior with some effort and concentration

2   Moderate control, sometimes able to stop or divert compulsive behavior

3   Little control, rarely successful in stopping or dismissing compulsive behavior

4   No control, rarely able to even momentarily alter compulsive behavior

Y-BOCS is often used alongside a *Global Assessment of Functioning* (GAF) scale (Table 4.2), which assesses the impact of the disease on the subject's life.

The severity of OCD will be determined from the scores on each of these scales but also from the degree of response to treatment.

Table 4.2 Global assessment of functioning (GAF) scale

100–91	Superior functioning in a wide range of activities, life's problems never seem to get out of hand, is sought out by others because of his or her many positive qualities. No symptoms
90–81	Absent or minimal symptoms (e.g., mild anxiety before an exam), good functioning in all areas, interested and involved in a wide range of activities, socially effective, generally satisfied with life, no more than everyday problems or concerns (e.g., an occasional argument with family members)
80–71	If symptoms are present, they are transient and expectable reactions to psychosocial stressors (e.g., difficulty concentrating after family argument); no more than slight impairment in social, occupational, or school functioning (e.g., temporarily falling behind in schoolwork)
70–61	Some mild symptoms (e.g., depressed mood and mild insomnia) OR some difficulty in social, occupational, or school functioning (e.g., occasional truancy, or theft within the household), but generally functioning pretty well, has some meaningful interpersonal relationships
60–51	Moderate symptoms (e.g., flat affect and circumstantial speech, occasional panic attacks) OR moderate difficulty in social, occupational, or school functioning (e.g., few friends, conflicts with peers or co-workers)
50–41	Serious symptoms (e.g., suicidal ideation, severe obsessional rituals, frequent shoplifting) OR any serious impairment in social, occupational, or school functioning (e.g., no friends, unable to keep a job)
40–31	Some impairment in reality testing or communication (e.g., speech is at times illogical, obscure, or irrelevant) OR major impairment in several areas, such as work or school, family relations, judgment, thinking, or mood (e.g., depressed man avoids friends, neglects family, and is unable to work; child frequently beats up younger children, is defiant at home, and is failing at school)
30–21	Behavior is considerably influenced by delusions or hallucinations OR serious impairment, in communication or judgment (e.g., sometimes incoherent, acts grossly inappropriately, suicidal preoccupation) OR inability to function in almost all areas (e.g., stays in bed all day, no job, home, or friends)
20–11	Some danger of hurting self or others (e.g., suicide attempts without clear expectation of death; frequently violent; manic excitement) OR occasionally fails to maintain minimal personal hygiene (e.g., smears feces) OR gross impairment in communication (e.g., largely incoherent or mute)
10–1	Persistent danger of severely hurting self or others (e.g., recurrent violence) OR persistent inability to maintain minimal personal hygiene OR serious suicidal act with clear expectation of death
0	Inadequate information

Physiopathology

Advances in functional imaging have elucidated some aspects of the pathophysiology of OCD. However, it still remains largely misunderstood. Imaging revealed hypermetabolism and localized increase in blood flow to regions of the orbitofrontal cortex,[3] anterior cingulate[4] and caudate nucleus[5] and a concurrent decrease in the activity of the dorsomedial prefrontal cortex [2, 3]. MRI has also shown that the volume of the structures differs from the volume in control subjects [4–8]. This activity is exacerbated during states of obsession and compulsion [9, 10]. Conversely, the recovery of these patients—obtained by any method—causes a decrease in activity in these regions [11–13]. It has also been shown that modification in the activity of these structures at the beginning of treatment was predictive of a favorable clinical response [2, 3, 14, 15]. These data confirm the involvement of the motor, cognitive, and emotional cortico-striato-thalamo-cortical (CSTC) loops[6] [16]. The activating effect the loop has on the cortex is, as we have seen, dependent on whether the stimulating *direct route*, or the inhibiting *indirect route* is predominant. If we take the example of degenerative neurological disorders manifested by excessive movement,[7] such as Huntington's disease or hemiballismus, lack of inhibition due to an alteration in the indirect pathway is at the origin of these abnormal movements. According to this model, intrusive thoughts and behaviors characteristic of OCD or Gilles de la Tourette syndrome, result from an overactive ventromedial striatum (caudate nucleus) involved in the *direct pathway* and insufficiently offset by the indirect, *inhibitory pathway*.[8] This phenomenon induces in the subject involuntary thinking and the persistent feeling of being at fault or that *something is not right* leading to obsessive thoughts [19]. Anatomically, the direct route involves the ventromedial part of the caudate nucleus at the level of the striatum, while the indirect route involves the dorsolateral part of the same nucleus [20, 21]. Additionally, abnormalities of the anterior cingulate cortex, which is involved in the famous memory circuit (Papez circuit), point to possible links between memory processes and OCD. Some authors have suggested that abnormalities in this circuit could be the cause of incessant receptions involving washing or checking [22, 23]. Finally, a third circuit, intimately connected to the previous two via the thalamus and the orbitofrontal cortex, connects the amygdala[9] and its "extension," the bed nucleus of the stria terminalis, responsible for anxious manifestations encountered in OCD [24].

---

[3] Cf. p. 93.

[4] Cf. p. 95.

[5] Cf. p. 128.

[6] Cf. p. 139.

[7] Conversely, taking Parkinson's disease as an example, the lack of dopamine leads to an imbalance between the direct pathway, which initiates the movement, and the indirect pathway which slows it. This imbalance benefits the indirect pathway, provoking muscular rigidity and the disease's characteristic akinesia.

[8] Some tumoral or haemorrhagic lesions of the striatum have been recorded as the potential cause of an obsessive-compulsive disorder, in [17, 18].

[9] Cf. p. 98.

Therapeutic Management

The management of patients with severe OCD, that is to say those whose Y-BOCS score is greater than 16, relies on medication and psychotherapeutic approaches [25]. In cases of treatment failure and extremely debilitating forms of the disease, surgical options may be considered.

Cognitive-Behavioral Therapies (CBT)

Cognitive therapies help patients identify intrusive thoughts and irrational beliefs within their interior monologues in order for them to change their thinking strategies. Behavioral therapies, often coupled with the previous ones, are essentially based on a technique called exposure and response prevention (ERP), which involves exposing patients to stimuli they fear while encouraging them to defer then eliminate their ritualistic response. In general, these therapies are continued for at least 1 year at a rate of one to two sessions per week and are considered effective in 50–70 % of cases. CBT is usually associated with a drug-based treatment.

Pharmacological Treatments

Drug-based treatments primarily involve antidepressants. Among them, serotonin reuptake inhibitors (SRI) have demonstrated their effectiveness, irrespective of their antidepressant effects. Therefore they are used as first-line monotherapy in this disease [26]. In this family of antidepressants, clomipramine *Anafranil®* with its serotonergic[10] and noradrenergic properties[11] has proven most effective. Nevertheless, its antagonistic effect on histaminic, muscarinic, adrenergic alpha-1, and serotonergic 5-HT2 receptors causes frequent side effects (dry mouth, urinary retention, constipation, dizziness, sexual dysfunction, cardiac rhythm problems) and limits its use. The chronic nature of this pathology and the long-term treatment it requires make these side effects even more difficult to accept. For this last reason, preference is now given to specific serotonin reuptake inhibitors (SSRIs) like fluoxetine (*Prozac®*), paroxetine (*Deroxat®*), or citalopram (*Seropram®*) which are significantly less effective but burdened with fewer side effects. The initial duration of this treatment is generally 12–24 months and it is acceptable for the effect on the obsessive symptoms to be delayed by approximately 8–12 weeks. By comparison, the delay normally required for depressive symptoms to be lessened is half. Clinical improvement occurs in 50–60 % of patients, but the rate of recurrence is around 90 % if treatment is interrupted abruptly. Factors suggesting a

---

[10] Cf. p. 149.

[11] Ibid.

Table 4.3 Example of classification for different stages of OCD based on response to treatment

I	SRI or CBT
II	SRI and CBT
III	2 SRI and CBT
IV	3 SRI and CBT
V	3 SRI (including clomipramine) and CBT
VI	3 SRI (including increase of clomipramine) and CBT
VII	3 SRI (including increase of clomipramine), CBT and other medications (BZD, neuroleptics)
VIII	3 SRI (including clomipramine IV) CBT and psychoeducation
IX	3 SRI (including clomipramine) CBT, psychoeducation and others categories of antidepressants
X	Neurosurgery

poor potential response to inhibitors of serotonin reuptake include onset of the disorder at a young age, family history, lack of employment, severity, complexity of the OCD, or washing rituals. Anxiolytics, including clonazepam, may be a beneficial complementary therapy when combined with previous treatments. They are reserved for patients with severe and short-term anxiety. So-called atypical antipsychotic agents such as risperidone or olanzapine, prescribed in combination with an SRI, were successful in patients with a treatment-resistant disorder. Nevertheless, the effectiveness of this association needs to be confirmed given that studies were only performed on small series of patients. The severity of the OCD is thus determined from scores on the Y-BOCS and GAF scales as well as response to the treatments mentioned above. Depending on the classifications of response to treatment, up to ten stages of severity can be identified (Table 4.3).

Surgical Treatments

When the OCD becomes an excessive handicap in the patient's life and all pharmacological treatments have failed, some authors deem it a "malignant" OCD [27]. Faced with a severe form, confirmed by clinical (Y-BOCS) and social functioning (GAF) scores, refractory to all available treatments, the practitioner must consider the possibilities of a neurosurgical treatment. Two types of interventions are possible: lesional surgery or deep brain stimulation (Fig. 4.1). In France, in 2002, the National Ethics Advisory Committee issued an opinion unfavorable to lesional psychosurgical interventions—without banning it outright—in favor of reversible deep brain stimulation [28].

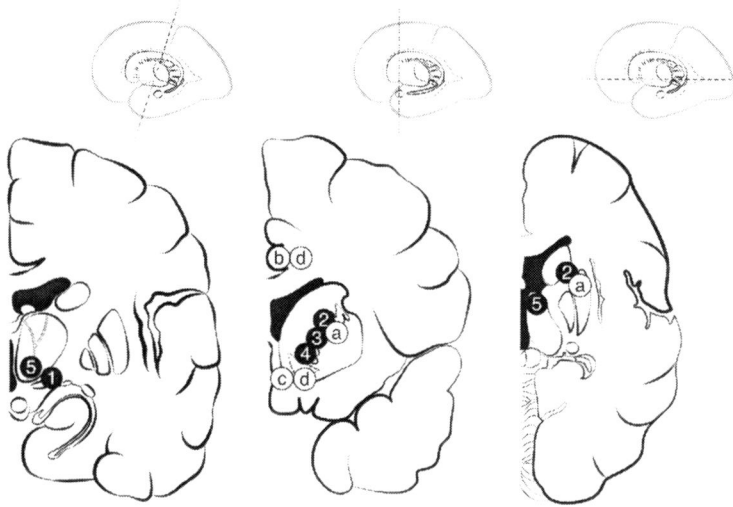

Fig. 4.1 Lesional or deep brain stimulation (*DBS*) targets in *OCD* treatment. (*a*) Thermocapsulotomy or gamma knife anterior capsulotomy [29–31], (*b*) cingulotomy [32, 33], (*c*) subcaudate tractotomy [34], (*d*) limbic leucotomy [35], (1) *DBS* of the subthalamic nucleus [36, 37], (2) *DBS* of the anterior limb of the internal capsule [38, 39], (3) *DBS* of the ventral striatum (*VC/VS*) [40], (4) *DBS* of the nucleus accumbens [41–43], (5) *DBS* of the inferior thalamic peduncle [44]

Lesional Surgery

Four types of interventions have been carried out in recent years. All four interrupt the connections between the orbitofrontal cortex and the rest of the limbic system and the thalamus. The technical details and modalities of each of these gestures were described earlier.

Bilateral Anterior Capsulotomy

The anterior limb of the internal capsule contains the thalamo-cortical connections of the cortico-striato-thalamo-cortical (CSTC) loop.[12] Hyperactivity in these connections, schematically speaking, results in the continuous return of the same concerns. Two procedures, performed under local anesthesia, are currently used to lesion the anterior capsule: thermocoagulation and radiosurgery.[13] Both methods achieve similar results [31], with 50–60 % of patients considered *responders* [29–31, 45, 46], with Y-BOCS scores decreased by at least 35 %. Side effects for this type of treatment, in addition to headaches or transient confusion, include a weight

---

[12] Cf. p. 139.

[13] Stereotaxic capsulotomy performed with thermocoagulation, cf. p. 167 or with radiosurgery, cf. p. 187.

gain of about 6 kg in the first year [31, 47]. Furthermore, one-third of patients complained of fatigue and urinary incontinence during the first month [48]. Regarding cognitive functions, results differ from one series of patients to another. Thus, a team led by Rück [31], in Stockholm has identified, among 25 patients treated, 10 patients with apathy while a Brazilian team has observed improved cognitive functions subsequent to mitigation of the obsessive-compulsive symptoms [49]. It is therefore difficult to draw any conclusions, especially given that no rigorous neuropsychological assessments were carried out in either study. It would appear, however, that there are fewer neuropsychological side effects associated with radiosurgery, than with thermocoagulation provided that the maximum dose of radiation delivered remains under 160 Gy [50].

Bilateral Anterior Cingulotomy

Currently, the cingulotomy appears to be the most commonly used lesional technique in the treatment of OCD, particularly in the United States. Although functional imaging studies do show an overactive anterior cingulate in patients suffering from OCD, the first interventions to target the anterior cingulate with lesioning were conducted by Ballantine, long before imaging data was available [51]. His team in Boston considered that obsessive-compulsive disorders were primarily an anxiety disorder and saw this part of the limbic system as a prime target. Within this system, the anterior cingulate had previously been targeted by Foltz and White [52] in the treatment of intractable pain with an efficacy proportional to the anxiety component of the pain. Unlike capsulotomy, this procedure is performed almost[14] exclusively by thermocoagulation[15] and its effects are delayed by 6 months to a year. A recent publication by Dougherty, concerning 44 patients reported that a third of these were responders more than 3 years after the procedure [33]. Other teams have presented superior results, nearly 50 % responders, but with a shorter follow-up period and fewer patients [3, 48, 53–58]. Among the complications reported were epileptic seizures in 1–9 % of patients, usually ones who had experienced seizures in the past [48, 59]. For the most part these could be controlled by an anti-epileptic treatment. Transient fever, transient urinary disorders, and postoperative headaches are also potential complications. Very few studies have focused on neuropsychological complications of this type of

---

[14] Cingulotomies were performed by cryotherapy (−70 °C) but the controversial practice was used in opium addiction treatment (cf. p. 178 and 363).

[15] This is probably due to historical reasons: the capsulotomy was first developed in Europe, especially in Sweden, the birthplace of Gamma Knife® radiosurgery, whereas the cingulotomy was developed by the Boston team, which at that time had little or no experience in radiosurgery. To date, only a South-Korean team treated OCD patients by cingulotomy with radiosurgery (CyberKnife®) (M. C. Kim, and T. K. Lee. 2008. Stereotactic lesioning for mental illness. Acta Neurochir Suppl 101:39–43).

intervention. Given that the cingulate gyrus is part of the Papez circuit,[16] the "memory circuit" (Fig. 2.24, p. 85), bilateral lesions of the gyrus have the potential to cause memory impairment. The few publications on the subject differ: some teams mention a moderate and transient impairment of memory in 3–20 % of patients [57, 59] while a Korean study observed no damage but, on the contrary, improved executive functions related to the alleviation of symptoms of OCD [56].

Subcaudate Tractotomy and Limbic Leucotomy

Developed by the English neurosurgeon G. Knight in 1964, this intervention is equivalent to the cortical undercutting,[17] developed by the American W. Scoville 20 years earlier except that it is performed by stereotactic thermocoagulation. The intervention aims to interrupt the bundles passing under the head of the caudate nucleus and connecting the orbitofrontal cortex[18] to the thalamus and the amygdala. This lesion located under the head of the caudate nucleus leads to improvement in a third to half of cases [34, 60, 61]. Neuropsychological tests do not show long-term cognitive disorders or personality changes associated with this procedure [62]. In instances of failure of the cingulotomy, a complementary, minimal tractotomy can be performed. This combination is called a limbic leucotomy. This procedure developed by Kelly provides an equivalent improvement [63]. These two types of interventions, which are practically never used today,[19] can lead to epileptic seizures, transient confusion, and minor personality changes [64].

Deep Brain Stimulation

Use of the above neurosurgical techniques has tended to diminish in favor of deep brain stimulation, which has the advantage of being reversible and adaptable. Patients must meet certain criteria to be eligible for this type of intervention. In France, they are performed exclusively within the context of research protocols often involving several university hospitals. The evaluation of the patient and the decision to operate must be made by a team of experts working independently from the neurosurgeons who will carry out the procedure. Once the patient has given informed consent to the procedure, he must commit to preoperative neuropsychological testing and participation in the postoperative monitoring and

---

[16] The Papez circuit cf. p. 133.

[17] Cortical undercutting cf. p. 47.

[18] Cf. p. 93.

[19] The last mention of this intervention in literature was in 2006. Two OCD patients were operated using neuronavigation. (P. A. Woerdeman, P. W. Willems, H. J. Noordmans, J. W. Berkelbach van der Sprenkel, and P. C. van Rijen. 2006. Frameless stereotactic subcaudate tractotomy for intractable obsessive-compulsive disorder. Acta Neurochir (Wien) 148:633–637).

rehabilitation program [65]. It is estimated that about 100 patients have received such treatment to date [66].

Inclusion and Exclusion Criteria

The inclusion criteria for this type of surgery can differ significantly from one country to the next and according to the study protocols [32, 40, 67, 68]. The criteria in use in France stipulate that to be candidates for this procedure patients must be over 21 and suffer from an OCD with a Y-BOCS score above 25 and a strong psychosocial impact. The disease must evolve for at least 5 years, and during this period the patient must have undergone two unsuccessful cognitive-behavioral therapies (CBT) conducted in an appropriate setting and by different therapists. At least 40 h of a mix, wherever possible, of group and individual therapy. Moreover, the failure of the drug-based treatment must be formally established. To do this, at least three selective serotonin reuptake inhibitors (SSRIs), including clomipramine, must have been tested for a minimum of 12 weeks at the maximum tolerable dose. Other molecules, such as chlorpromazine (Thorazine®) risperidone (*Risperdal®*), lithium, clonazepam, buspirone, and pindolol, used in combination with clomipramine must also have been unsuccessful. The above shows that deep brain stimulation is considered exclusively for patients without any other treatment options [36, 65, 69]. Before deep brain stimulation is indicated, the team must ensure the absence of any cognitive deterioration, personality disorder, or other psychiatric disorder such as schizophrenia, addictive behavior, or bipolar disease. Given that the procedure necessitates magnetic resonance imaging (MRI) of the brain, the subject must not have any contraindication to MRIs. Likewise there must be no contraindications to the surgical act itself, such as altered coagulation or any brain abnormality, which may potentially deflect the trajectory of the electrodes during their descent [36].

Anatomical Targets

The choice of anatomical targets owes as much to serendipity as to results obtained with lesional surgery. As the journalist J.-Y. Nau wrote about the choice of the subthalamic nucleus, "*should we invoke here simple luck or rather emphasize the acuity of the observer?*" [70]. For, it is following clinical improvement of three patients with OCD [71, 72] who were being treated by deep brain stimulation for Parkinson's disease that the French teams of Polosan, and Mallet decided to study this target [36]. However, the decision of the Belgian team led by Nuttin to implant electrodes in the anterior limb of the internal capsule stems primarily from the satisfactory results obtained by capsulotomys[20] in patients with OCD [38].

---

[20] The capsulotomy for OCD cf. p. 284.

The choice of the nucleus accumbens is also a result of clinical observations in patients whose electrodes targeted the ALIC, but in whom the *effective* terminals were located closer to the nucleus accumbens the high intensity of stimulation suggested that this structure was also being stimulated (Fig. 4.1) [41].

The Anterior Limb of the Internal Capsule and "VC/VS"

Of the four patients initially operated in the ALIC by Nuttin's team, three showed a significant reduction in their symptoms including one over 90 % [38, 73–75]. Extensive research combining past authors and American teams showed that for 26 patients, 50 % were responders[21] at 3 months, 46 % at 6 months (N = 24), 48 % at 1 year (N = 21), 65 % at 2 years (N = 17), and 58 % at 3 years (N = 12) (Table 4.4). In this study, which was conducted over 8 years, the target area was gradually shifted to a more inferior and posterior position [40]. The researchers observed that better responses were obtained at a lower intensity of stimulation with this positioning of electrodes. The new location was at the junction between the ventral part of the internal capsule (VC) and the ventral striatum (VS), hence the name of this target: *VC/VS*. In their article, Greenberg and his colleagues also reported a decrease in depressive symptoms and a marked improvement in the overall functioning of these patients according to the *GAF* scale.[22] Two infections and hematoma were deplored after surgery as well as an epileptic seizure in one patient. During stimulation, the authors noticed occasional hypomanic states of excitement, irritability, or mood changes including suicidal ideation. These mood changes, for the most part, could be corrected by adjusting the stimulation parameters. Neuropsychological tests did not reveal any cognitive impairment following these interventions. The same year, a New York team led by Goodman reported that four out of six patients implanted with electrodes in this same VC/VS target were responders after 1 year of stimulation [76]. The authors also reported mood disorders, notably hypomania, during stimulation. But it was quickly corrected after adjustments were made to the stimulation parameters.

The Nucleus Accumbens

The VC/VS region is in the vicinity of the nucleus accumbens itself belonging to the ventral striatum. Between 2003 and 2008, a German team led by Sturm and Huff in Cologne implanted ten patients with a unilateral electrode in the right nucleus accumbens [41, 77]. After a year of stimulation, one patient was responding while the Y-BOCS score of five others had been reduced by a quarter. Side effects were similar both in kind and incidence to those described for a VC/VS target. In 2010, a Dutch team tried to improve on these results by

---

[21] Responders are patients in which the Y-BOCS score decreased by at least 35 % after treatment.

[22] Cf. definition: p. 273—Table 4.2.

implanting 16 patients bilaterally[23] [42]. During a first, "open" phase lasting 8 months, nine of these patients were responders with a mean decrease of 72 % in their Y-BOCS scores. During the subsequent double-blinded phase, which only involved 14 of the patients—7 patients being stimulated and 7 not being stimulated (all were unaware of their status)—the psychiatrist Denys and his colleagues observed a mean decrease of 25 % in the Y-BOCS score of those receiving stimulation versus the control group. A regression of the symptoms of depression was also reported with a decrease of more than 50 % according to the HAD scale.[24] This latter finding explains why this target has also been used in the treatment of severe depression.[25] No surgical complications were reported while eight patients presented, especially in the beginning, hypomanic states—confirming the role of this structure in the regulation of mood. These states were resolved by adjusting the stimulation parameters. The results of other smaller studies validate these findings [41, 43, 78].

The Subthalamic Nucleus[26]

Starting in 2005 as part of a national protocol, several French teams began targeting the associative and limbic parts of the subthalamic nucleus. The results of their work, collected in a 2008 article in the *New England Journal of Medicine* [36], were encouraging: three-quarters of the 16 patients had Y-BOCS scores decreased by more than a quarter. The average Y-BOCS score was 28 after 3 months of stimulation versus 19 for the control group (patients who had received a placebo "stimulation").[27] In addition, six out of the ten patients were able to regain a satisfying family and social life as evidenced by the mean GAF score which increased from 43 to 56. The main criticism of this rigorous, randomized, and double-blinded study (Fig. 4.2) was its short follow-up observation period of only 3 months. An as yet unpublished 3 years follow-up study does, however, seem to confirm these initial positive results [79]. Adverse effects were also deplored including the occurrence of two infections and one cerebral hematoma leading to paralysis in a finger. Movement and psychological disorders were observed in seven patients, but declined after adjustment of the stimulation parameters. Neuropsychological tests performed for all patients before and after surgery revealed no abnormalities.

---

[23] Immediately following an increase in the stimulation voltage, excessive self-confidence as well as irritability and impulsiveness was observed in both patients. Everything returned to normal after the stimulation was decreased. In J. Luigjes, M. Mantione, W. Van Den Brink et al. (2011) Deep brain stimulation increases impulsivity in two patients with obsessive-compulsive disorder. Int Clin Psychopharmacol 26: 338–340).

[24] Hetero-evaluation scale for the severity of depression cf. p. 314 Table 4.8.

[25] Cf. p. 213.

[26] Cf. p. 218.

[27] The patient who is not being stimulated is unaware of whether or not she is being stimulated.

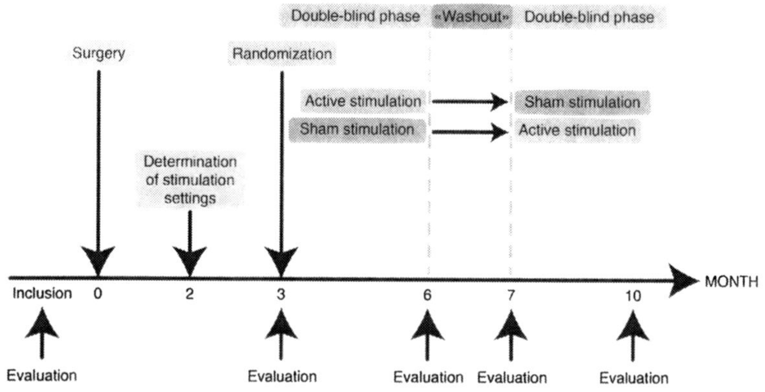

Fig. 4.2 Example of a "design" for a French study of subthalamic *DBS* in *OCD*

The Inferior Thalamic Peduncle

Targeting of the inferior thalamic peduncle, a much rarer practice, aims to modulate the activity of the bundles connecting the thalamus to the orbitofrontal cortex. A Mexican study by F. Jiménez-Ponce conducted from 2003 to 2007 on five patients showed a response to stimulation in each of them with an average decrease in the Y-BOCS score from 35 to 18 after 1 year, while the average overall performance increased by 20–70 %. The authors reported no complications [44].

Conclusion

The clinical efficacy of psychosurgery in the treatment of severe OCD is now established. After the listing of surgical techniques and targets, the question arises whether it is the best move and what structure should be targeted. A recent review

Table 4.4 Result of deep brain stimulation in the treatment of OCD

Study	Pts	Target	Follow-up	Response (%)
Belgium, 1999 [38]	4	Anterior limb of the internal capsule	–	75
Belgium, 2003 [39]	6	Anterior limb of the internal capsule	3–31	50
Germany, 2003 [41]	5	Nucleus accumbens	24–30	60
Abelson, 2005 [80]	4	Anterior limb of the internal capsule	4–23	50
United States, 2006 [81]	10	VC/VS	36	40
France, 2008 [36]	16	Subthalamic nuclei	3	75[a]
Mexico, 2009 [44]	5	Inferior thalamic peduncle	21	100
Germany, 2010 [77]	10	Nucleus accumbens (unilateral)	12	10
Netherlands, 2010 [42]	16	Nucleus accumbens	21	56
United States, 2010 [76]	6	VC/VS	12	33
France, 2012 [37]	4	Subthalamic nuclei	6	100

[a] Response is defined as a decrease of at least 25 % in the Y-BOCS score

of the literature prepared by the Queen Square team in London summarizing 18 publications compared the efficacy of capsulotomies in 85 patients with stimulation of the internal capsule or the nucleus accumbens in 64 patients [82]. In terms of efficacy, the comparison seemed to favor the capsulotomy with 68 % response versus 46 % with long-term stimulation.[28] However, a small number of patients who underwent a capsulotomy, were more prone to apathy and disinhibition. Meanwhile, weight gain seems exclusive to capsulotomies. Potentially greater efficacy with the lesional technique versus greater innocuous of deep brain stimulation, the debate remains ongoing and can only be resolved by further studies.

Gilles de la Tourette Syndrome

Abstract Gilles de la Tourette syndrome is an extreme form of tics whose manifestations are simple or complex, motor or vocal. Typically, the disease occurs between 5 and 7 years to worsen in adolescence and decline generally in adulthood. This rare neuropsychiatric disorder can be debilitating and sometimes responds poorly to drug treatment. Sixty neurosurgical lesions have been performed so far, and the best results seem to result from the thalamic target. At the end of the 1990s, because of its advantages—flexibility and reversibility—deep brain stimulation began to replace ablative surgery. Today, thalamic and/or pallidal targets seem promising.

Gilles de la Tourette syndrome is a neuropsychiatric disorder generally well recognized by the general public due to the profanity or vulgarity that some patients may express in an irrepressible manner. Described in 1885 by a pupil of Charcot, the neurologist Georges Albert Édouard Brutus Gilles de la Tourette, the *tics disease* as he called it, is a rare disease affecting between 0.1 and 1 % of the population [83]. Usually diagnosed during the first and second childhood or adolescence, this syndrome is associated with motor and vocal tics whose manifestations and severity may fluctuate over weeks or years. These tics remain controllable by will power for short moment, but subjects describe these moments of control as "apnea" inevitably followed by a resurgence of symptoms or *bounce* [84].

---

[28] A patient is "responding" when his Y-BOCS score decreases by at least a third. An "excellent" result is when this score is halved and remission to a score under 8. In the capsulotomy group an excellent result was observed in 26 % versus 11 % in the stimulation group as well as remission in 9 % versus 2 %.

Clinical Aspects

The syndrome of Gilles de la Tourette is considered primarily movement disorder due to its simple or complex motor and oral tics. Motor tics are manifested by short, stereotypical, involuntary, or semi-voluntary movements such as blinking or clearing of the throat for simple forms or more complex sequences of gestures often normal in appearance but made in an inappropriate context: When the patient makes an obscene gesture, it is called copropraxia. When he cannot help imitating the movements of the speaker, it is called echopraxia. Verbal tics can be simple cries or mumbling, or more complex sequences such as sentences or foul language. These tics can adapt to context as in the case of the practitioner with the German sounding name who is called a *dirty German* by his patient [85]. This more elaborate manifestation, although well known to the general public, is encountered in only 10 % of patients. Generally these symptoms will manifest with even more force and frequency when the patient is experiencing fatigue, boredom, or stress [86]. Conversely, most patients notice a reduction in their symptoms during physical or mental effort. Different scales have been proposed to assess the severity and impact of these tics, the two most used in clinical research is the *Yale Global Tic Severity Scales* (YGTSS) [87] and the *Rush Videotape Rating Scale* (RVRS) [88]. Motor tics are usually the first to appear in childhood with an incidence three to four times higher among boys than girls [89]. In 96 % of cases, the first symptoms appear before the age of 11 [90], the symptoms broaden and worsen toward prepuberty and usually fade in early adulthood. It is estimated that by 18, half of patients no longer present symptoms [87, 91]. When the first signs occur in adulthood, an infection, head trauma, drug use, or neuroleptics are probably the source of this so-called *secondary* form of the disease [92, 93].

Associated Disorders

The mental component of this neurological movement disorder comes from "*the ambiguity in the value placed on coprolalia and copropraxia that approximate behavioral disorders*",[29] and numerous psychiatric comorbidities that, in nearly 90 % of patients, are associated: *Attention Deficit Hyperactivity Disorder* (ADHD) obsessive-compulsive behavior, depression, anxiety disorders, personality disorders, and self-mutilation [94]. Moreover, this condition can cause great suffering through mockery, stigma, and the grave effects on family life or careers. The frequency of hyperactivity and attention deficit disorder in patients with Gilles de

---

[29] See on the subject the excellent thesis by B. Moutaud: "C'est un problème neurologique ou psychiatrique?" Ethnologie de la stimulation cérébrale profonde appliquée au disorder obsessionnel compulsif. Paris: Ecole Doctorale "Education, langage, sociétés," Université Paris Descartes; 2009—Available online.

la Tourette syndrome fluctuates from 21 to 90 % depending on the report. The frequency of obsessive-compulsive behaviors is less variable and affects one in two subjects with themes of sexual, religious, violent, or symmetry obsessions and compulsions manifested by rituals of counting, organizing, and self-mutilation [95, 96]. An autoaggression that causes patients to inflict burns, scars, or bites on themselves [97].

Physiopathology

Studies of identical twins have shown that in 89–94 % of cases both were affected which suggests a genetic link even if, for the moment, no gene has been formally isolated [98]. Some factors such as low birth weight during the first trimester of pregnancy or a stressful life could promote the expression of the disease [99]. The biochemical, neurophysiological, and imaging tend to show that this syndrome is due to a developmental abnormality of synaptic transmission, leading to a disinhibition of the cortico-striato-thalamo-cortical loop (CSTC) [92, 100]. These CSTC loops modulate the activity of the frontal cortex by facilitating or repressing motors or behavioral programs as needed. Autopsies have shown that dopaminergic transmission may be involved, which may explain the effectiveness of antipsychotics in the treatment of the disease. The dopaminergic hyperactivity is due to an increase in the sensitivity of dopamine receptors at a presynaptic abnormality or to increase dopamine,[30] resulting in an inhibition of the indirect pathway in the CSTC loop, which leads to thalamo-cortical hyperactivity and motor or verbal tics as a consequence of this lack of inhibition [91, 101, 102]. Within the thalamus,[31] two nuclei groups seem affected by this hyperactivity: first, the medial and ventral nuclei, more involved in motor control, and second, the intralaminar nuclei—the most voluminous of these being the centromedian and parafascicular nuclei (CM-Pf) linked also to cognitive and emotional functions. Research using functional MRI confirms the involvement of these CSTC loop structures: when patients tried to contain their tics there was a decrease in the activity of the putamen, the globus pallidus, and the thalamus, accompanied by an increase in the activity of the head of the caudate nucleus and frontal, temporal, and cingulate cortices [103]. The overlaps between the motor and behavioral manifestations of the syndrome of Gilles de la Tourette make an interesting model for understanding neurobehavioral phenomena, such as Lesch-Nyhan[32] syndrome which is characterized by abnormal movements like dystonia and aggressive behavior disorders like self-mutilation [92, 104, 105].

---

[30] Cf. p. 146.

[31] Cf. p. 123.

[32] Cf. p. 354.

Pharmacological Treatments

Whether pharmacological or psychotherapeutic, with cognitive-behavioral therapies (CBT), the treatment of Gilles de la Tourette syndrome does not seek to suppress tics but rather give some degree of control over symptoms in order to mitigate the embarrassment and discomfort they generate [92]. Very few double-blinded and placebo controlled studies have been undertaken to evaluate the effectiveness of neuroleptics or new antipsychotics, which at present, along with CBT, remain the standard treatment [92, 106, 107]. These blockers of dopamine receptors allow a significant improvement in tics but often at the price of side effects, such as depression, apathy, weight gain or—in the longer term—tardive dyskinesia. Cannabis as well as some anxiolytics like clonazepam or nicotine patches may be beneficial, but no randomized trials have been performed to confirm their effect [108]. The management of the disease includes treatment of associated psychiatric comorbidities using amphetamine derivatives when there is an ADHD component and antidepressants, including selective serotonin reuptake inhibitors (SSRIs), when obsessive-compulsive behaviors are present.

Surgical Treatments

A smaller segment of the patient population keeps symptoms, sometimes excessively disabling ones, of the disease into adulthood. When pharmacologic treatments are ineffective or encumbered by severe side effects, the question of surgical treatment arises. Since 1962, 65 patients have been treated by lesional surgeries [109]. These have now almost entirely disappeared in favor of deep brain stimulation, which has the advantage of being reversible and adaptable. Since 1999, nearly a 100 patients have undergone this procedure [89, 109–114] (Fig. 4.3).

Ablative Techniques

Since the early 1960s, many anatomical structures have been targeted using lesional techniques. The "traditional" psychosurgery interventions have of course been tried for this disorder often equated with an obsessive-compulsive disorder. This includes the oldest technique, the prefrontal leucotomy[33] but also the cingulotomy[34] or limbic leucotomy.[35] More specific interventions have been proposed: thalamotomy (median and intralaminar nuclei of the thalamus) or targets such as the zona incerta, the red nucleus or the dentate nucleus of the cerebellum.

---

[33] Cf. The first intervention p. 34.

[34] Cf. p. 173.

[35] Ibid.

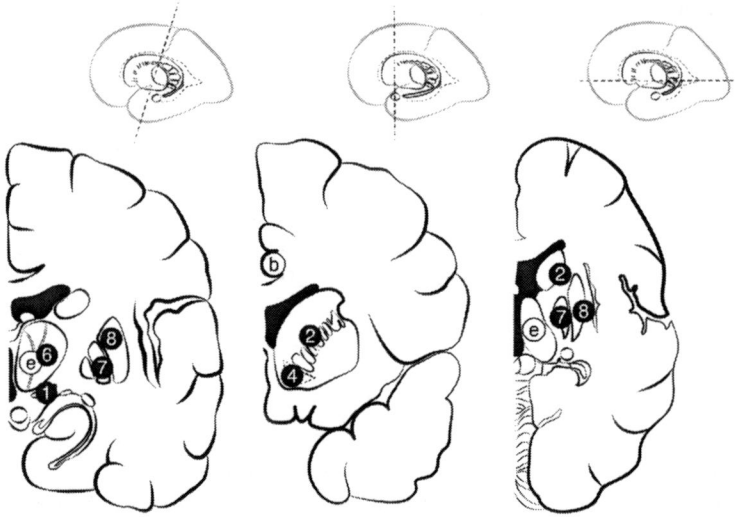

Fig. 4.3 Lesional or deep brain stimulation (*DBS*) targets in Gilles de la Tourette syndrome. (*b*) Cingulotomy [115], (*e*) medial thalamotomy [116, 117], (1) *DBS* of the subthalamic nucleus [118], (2) *DBS* of the anterior limb of the internal capsule [119, (4) *DBS* of the nucleus accumbens [120], (6) *DBS* of the centromedian and parafascicular thalamic nuclei [121, 122], (7) *DBS* of the internal globus pallidus [110, 123], (8) *DBS* of the external globus pallidus [124]

The many techniques used, the small numbers of patients, non-standardized selection of patients, and the absence of reliable estimates[36] make comparisons between each of these interventions difficult [91]. Psychiatric comorbidities, particularly frequent in severe forms of Gilles de la Tourette syndrome, are confounding factors further complicating the analysis. However, it would seem that the population of patients (39 of 65) in which the thalamic target was chosen achieved the best results with 45–100 % reduction of tics after a minimum follow-up, when one is mentioned, of 12–24 months [122, 125–131]. Lesional surgery, though not without success when applied to the thalamic target, does however raise ethical concerns over the multiplicity of targets "tested" and the young age, 11- and 12-years old [132], of the youngest surgery patients. Moreover, the majority of publications relating to these interventions did not mention the side effects of surgery. Of 22 patients for whom this information is available, 20 had complications such as dystonia (7 patients), hemiplegia (4), dysarthria (4), cognitive impairment (2), or a severe, unspecified neurological deficit (3) [109]. These complications encouraged the development, beginning in 1999, of reversible deep brain stimulation techniques [122].

---

[36] In a majority of cases, the results were evaluated by the same team which had determined the appropriateness of the surgical treatment (The debatable results of clinical studies: p. 184).

Deep Brain Stimulation

To date, six anatomical targets have been explored by the deep brain stimulation technique in the treatment of Gilles de la Tourette syndrome: the median part of the thalamus and its peri-fascicular nucleus, the nucleus accumbens, the subthalamic nucleus, the internal and external globus pallidus, and the anterior limb of the internal capsule (Table 4.5). Of the anatomical structures targeted for 30 years by lesional surgery, only the thalamic target is still used today. This is due to the satisfactory clinical results obtained and greater pathophysiological understanding which suggests a lack of inhibition in the thalamus. Thus a thalamic target, more precisely the anterior intralaminar nucleus of the thalamus, was chosen by the Dutch team of V. Vandewalle in 1999 [122]. The patient, a 42-year-old man saw his tics reduced by 90 %. Five years after surgery, these good results remained stable [133]. The same team repeated this procedure in two other patients this time with a decrease in symptoms of 72 and 83 %. Four other teams followed suit with a reduction of symptoms ranging from 40 to 78 % in 25 patients [112, 121, 134, 135]. Noting that the tics were similar to a movement disorder, a stereotyped form of motor, and behavioral hyperkinesia, the Viennese team led by Diederich, proposed in 2005 to target the posterior part of the internal globus pallidus devoted the sensorimotor functions [136]. A 75 % reduction in symptoms was observed after 14 months, and 66 % after 3 years. These encouraging results were found in four other patients, with a decrease in tics ranging from 75 to 88 % [123, 137–139]. One failure, however, was also recorded [140]. The same year, Houeto and the French team at the Pitié-Salpêtrière hospital conceived a procedure combining the two previous targets, thalamic and pallidal. Their procedure resulted in a 74–82 % reduction in symptoms of three patients [141]. This double implantation in the thalamus and the anterior medial part of the internal globus pallidus, containing the limbic compartment allows double-blind studies with alternating stimulation of either of these targets. The globus pallidus has the advantage, compared to the thalamic target, of allowing higher intensities of stimulation without this increase resulting in adverse effects. Given that the thalamo-cortical connections implicated in Gilles de la Tourette syndrome pass through the anterior limb of the internal capsule (ALIC), and the clinical similarities of this disease with obsessive-compulsive disorders (OCD) successfully treated by stimulation of the ALIC, Cosgrove's team in Boston implanted electrodes in this area in a 37-year-old patient [119] in a patient with symptoms of OCD as well [142]. The team justified the choice of this target, also used in the treatment of OCD, by citing the modulatory function of the nucleus accumbens in the CSTC loop. Results were slightly better for the OCD, with a Y-BOCS score decreased from 25 to 12, while tics decreased by 40 %. A similar result was obtained in a patient without OCD, but who presented the particularity of being a heavy smoker. Complete cessation of smoking was observed following stimulation [140]. The possible role of the nucleus

Table 4.5 Deep brain stimulation in the treatment of Gilles de la Tourette syndrome [111]

Study	Pts	Target(s)	Follow-up[a]	Results[b] (%)
Netherlands, 1999–2003 [122, 133]	3	Thalamus (CM-Pf)	9	82
France, 2005 [141, 144]	3	Thalamus (CM-Pf) et GPi	36	74–82
United States, 2005 [119]	1	ALIC	18	23
Luxemburg, 2005 [136]	1	GPi	14	75
Brazil, 2007 [124]	1	GPe	23	81
Germany, 2007 [142]	1	Nucleus accumbens	30	41
United States, 2007 [121]	5	Thalamus (CM-Pf)	3	44
Italy, 2008 [112]	18	Thalamus (CM-Pf)	3–18	65
Great-Britain, 2009 [118]	1	Subthalamic nuclei	12	76
Netherlands, 2011 [145]	6	Thalamus (CM-Pf)	12	49

[a] Average follow-up in months
[b] Percentage reduction in Yale Global Tic Severity Scale (*YGTSS*) and/or Rush Videotape Rating Scale (*RVRS*), *ALIC* Anterior limb of the internal capsule, *GPi* Globus Pallidus internal, *GPe* Globus Pallidus external, *CM-Pf* Centromedian and Parafascicular nuclei of the thalamus

accumbens in addictive behaviors is discussed in more detail below.[37] Finally, an 80 % decrease in tics has been reported following unilateral stimulation of the right nucleus accumbens, the two previous patients having been stimulated bilaterally [143]. A Brazilian team described in 2007 the case of two patients in whom the external globus pallidus had been targeted and whose disorders had decreased by 81 % [124]. The choice of this structure comes from animal experiments: stereotyped movements similar to tics are observed in primates after microinjections of a GABA antagonist. Finally, significant improvement in the disease was recorded in a patient also suffering from Parkinson's disease who had been implanted with an electrode in the subthalamic nucleus for the latter indication [118].

Patient Selection Criteria

The treatment of Gilles de la Tourette syndrome using deep brain stimulation remains, at present, in the research stage and only a small number of centers around the world, about 20, offer this surgery. In addition to a neurosurgical team with experience in deep brain stimulation techniques, this treatment requires a multi-disciplinary team of psychiatrists, neurologists, neurosurgeons, and psychologist specializing in this disease with at least one dedicated consultation. Given the experimental nature of this technique in this indication, inclusion criteria vary from between research protocols. However, most researchers agree on a minimum age of 18 or even 25, both for medico-legal reasons as well as due to the spontaneous evolution of the disease which can lead to significant improvement in adulthood. Some authors argue for earlier interventions, objecting that it is during the early

---

[37] Cf. p. 359.

Table 4.6 Some example inclusion criteria for a DBS protocol used in the treatment of Tourette's syndrome

	Criteria
1	Diagnosis of definite GTS established by two independent clinicians (neurologist and psychiatrist) using DSM criteria and DCI
2	Severe and incapacitating tics as the primary problem
3	Treatment refractory or intolerance to three classes of neuroleptics: (a) "classical" molecules: haloperidol, pimozide (b) modern antipsychotics: risperidone, olanzapine, clozapine (c) experimental molecules: pergolide
4	Attempt of at least 12 sessions of behavioral strategies (habit reversal training or exposure therapy)
5	Age > 25 years

years that social skills and self-esteem are developed [146, 147]. Resistance or poor tolerance to medications is also an essential prerequisite, but the duration of the trial and the type of molecules tested varies depending on the research team. Table 4.6 lists the criteria recommended by the *"Movement Disorder Society,"* but criteria can differ significantly among the various studies [148].

Conclusion

The majority of the studies mentioned above are single case reports or small series that have not been evaluated in a double-blind manner. While these studies have demonstrated good clinical tolerance technique and different targets, they struggle for now to demonstrate the supremacy of one target over another [148]. Currently, although two targets seem to be emerging, the intralaminar nuclei of the thalamus and the internal globus pallidus, it remains to be seen whether other structures or combinations of targets could be useful for specific forms of Gilles de la Tourette syndrome or psychiatric comorbidities.

Severe Depression

Abstract Depression—the most common psychiatric disorder—can sometimes be resistant to all medication and psychotherapy. Focused surgical procedures have been proposed, consisting mainly of lesions in the cingulate cortex. These irreversible procedures provide satisfactory clinical results, but can, however, lead to some permanent neuropsychological complications. With the advent of stimulation techniques, with reversible effects, new targets have emerged in the region of the nucleus accumbens and especially the subgenual cortex. Although results are satisfactory, the mechanisms of action for this stimulation is still misunderstood. Studies on the effectiveness of the stimulation of the prefrontal cortex and the vagus nerve are also underway.

From the Latin *depressio*, "lowering," depression is among the most prevalent psychiatric illness. Eight percentage of the French population is affected equalling nearly three million people, while 17 % of Americans have presented or will present a depressive episode in their lives [149]. By the number of years of disability it causes, depression is the fourth most widespread disease around the world. Two-thirds of cases are women [150]. According to the WHO, by 2020 depression will be the second leading cause of disability and premature death behind heart disease. It is responsible for the majority of suicides at a rate, according to WHO, 14 deaths per hundred thousand people in the world and 16 in France. This disease is exacerbated by certain diseases or somatic symptoms (chronic pain, myocardial infarction …) it fosters [151]. A chronic disease, approximately three-quarters of subjects are likely to develop a new depression in the 6 or 12 months following the first episode, and one in five will develop a chronic syndrome. Of all chronic diseases, depression most affects quality of life [152].

Clinical Aspects

The diagnosis of depression is often the question of normal and pathological namely that ends a normal emotional reaction to a life event—such as a separation, bereavement, illness—and that really began depressive illness. Here, the question is not, insofar as psychosurgery involves two entities with little difficulty in diagnosis: major depressive episodes (MDE) and major depressive illness (MDI). As defined by the DSM-IV [153] this is an episode lasting for at least 2 weeks marks a change from previous functioning [153]. Among the following nine symptoms, at least five must be present including the first or second:

1. depressed mood or irritability;
2. marked reduction of interest or pleasure in all or most activities;
3. significant weight loss or gain or decrease or increase in appetite;
4. insomnia or hypersomnia;
5. psychomotor agitation or retardation;
6. fatigue or loss of energy;
7. feelings of worthlessness or excessive or inappropriate guilt;
8. difficulty concentrating or indecisiveness;
9. recurrent thoughts of death or suicide or suicide attempt.

These symptoms must be present nearly every day and cause distress or impairment of normal functioning. Major depressive illness involves the occurrence of one or more of these MDEs without manic or hypomanic episode.[38] If the latter are present it is no longer a MDI but a bipolar disorder.

---

[38] Some aspects of mania suggest that it is akin to an "inverse depression:" the patient, who manifests excessive confidence, is agitated by a euphoric that translates to feelings of excitement,

Assessment

The assessment of the severity of a major depressive episode occurs, in clinical studies, using scales. These assessment instruments have the advantage of such a rigorous as possible collection of clinical information to compile statistics necessary for scientific work. It should nevertheless be wary of a fetishistic belief in these figures, which only approximately reflect the psychic reality. On the other hand, the proliferation of versions and differences in coding according to the examiner may limit the scope for comparison. Several scales are available, some, self-evaluation, are performed by the patient himself[39] while those of hetero-evaluation are the practitioner. We will discuss those commonly adopted in psychosurgery.

Self-Assessment Scale

The most used is the *Beck Depression Inventory* (BDI) measuring depressive effects mainly in their dysphoric dimensions (Table 4.7) [154]. The inventory provides, for each item, a series of four statements representing increasing degrees of symptoms from zero to three. A score above 16 denotes severe depression.

Hetero-Assessment Scale

The *Hamilton Rating Scale for Depression* (HRSD), abbreviated as HAM-D, is one of the most commonly used multiple choice questionnaires to measure the severity of symptoms observed in depression (Table 4.8). The clinician selects one of the provided responses after questioning the patient or observing her symptoms. Several types of questionnaires are available from 17 (HRSD$_{17}$) to 29 questions (HRSD$_{29}$). The higher the score the more severe the depression [155]. Following treatment, the term *"remission"* is used if the depression[40] *"response"* score is reduced by more than 50 %, and "response" when the score falls below ten.

(Footnote 38 continued)
exaltation and sometimes irritability or even emotional lability leading to alternating bouts of laughter and tears. Sexual disinhibition, distractibility, fleeting ideas, and overcrowded thoughts may be present. In general, the subject doe not feel the need for much sleep. They may experience altruistic feelings like wanting to help someone and are likely to feel the emotions of others.

[39] The correct use of these scales requires that a number of rules be followed and a training session in proper grading. Among the precautions there has to be for example an interval of 4–8 days between two evaluations to avoid a "test-retest" effect. The assessor must have enough time for the evaluations, which must follow identical schedules to control for day/night cycle variations.

[40] This definition can vary depending on the study.

Table 4.7 Self-evaluation scale for depression (Beck Depression Inventory)

0	I do not feel sad
1	I feel sad
2	I am sad all the time and I can't snap out of it
3	I am so sad and unhappy that I can't stand it
0	I am not particularly discouraged about the future
1	I feel discouraged about the future
2	I feel I have nothing to look forward to
3	I feel the future is hopeless and that things cannot improve
0	I do not feel like a failure
1	I feel I have failed more than the average person
2	As I look back on my life, all I can see is a lot of failures
3	I feel I am a complete failure as a person
0	I get as much satisfaction out of things as I used to
1	I don't enjoy things the way I used to
2	I don't get real satisfaction out of anything anymore
3	I am dissatisfied or bored with everything
0	I don't feel particularly guilty
1	I feel guilty a good part of the time
2	I feel quite guilty most of the time
3	I feel guilty all of the time
0	I don't feel disappointed in myself
1	I am disappointed in myself
2	I am disgusted with myself
3	I hate myself
0	I don't have any thoughts of killing myself
1	I have thoughts of killing myself, but I would not carry them out
2	I would like to kill myself
3	I would kill myself if I had the chance
0	I have not lost interest in other people
1	I am less interested in other people than I used to be
2	I have lost most of my interest in other people
3	I have lost all of my interest in other people
0	I make decisions about as well as I ever could
1	I put off making decisions more than I used to
2	I have greater difficulty in making decisions more than I used to
3	I can't make decisions at all anymore
0	I don't feel that I look any worse than I used to
1	I am worried that I am looking old or unattractive
2	I feel there are permanent changes in my appearance that make me look unattractive
3	I believe that I look ugly

(continued)

Table 4.7 (continued)

0	I can work about as well as before
1	It takes an extra effort to get started at doing something
2	I have to push myself very hard to do anything
3	I can't do any work at all
0	I don't get more tired than usual
1	I get tired more easily than I used to
2	I get tired from doing almost anything
3	I am too tired to do anything
0	My appetite is no worse than usual
1	My appetite is not as good as it used to be
2	My appetite is much worse now
3	I have no appetite at all anymore

Table 4.8 Example hetero-evaluation scale for depression

Depressed mood (sadness, hopeless, helpless, worthless)

0 Absent

1 These feelings states indicated only on questioning

2 These feelings states spontaneously reported verbally

3 Communicates feeling states non verbally—i.e. through facial expressions, posture, voice and tendency to sleep

4 Patient reports these feeling states in his spontaneous verbal and non verbal communications

Feelings of guilt

0 Absent

1 Self reproaches, feels he has let people down

2 Ideas of guilt or ruminations over past errors or sinful deeds

3 Present illness is a punishment. Delusion of guilt

4 Hears accusatory or denunciatory voices and/or experiences threatening visual hallucinations

Suicide

0 Absent

1 Feels life is not worth living

2 Wishes he were dead or any thoughts of possible death of self

3 Suicidal ideas or gestures

4 Attempts at suicide

Insomnia early

0 Absent

1 Complains of occasional difficulty falling asleep—i.e. more than ½ h

2 Complains of nightly difficulty falling asleep

Insomnia middle

0 No difficulty falling asleep

1 Patient complains of being restless and disturbed during the night

2 Waking during the night

Insomnia late

0 No difficulty

1 Waking in early hours of the morning but goes back to sleep

2 Unable to fall asleep again if he gets out of bed

(continued)

Table 4.8 (continued)

Work and activities

0 No difficulty

1 Thoughts and feelings of incapacity, fatigue or weakness related to activities; work or hobbies

2 Loss of interest inactivities, hobbies or work—either directly reported by patient, or indirect in listlessness, indecision and vacillation (feels he has to push self to work or activities)

3 Decrease in actual time spent in activities or decrease in productivity

4 Stopped working because of present illness

Retardation: psychomotor (slowness of thought and speech, impaired ability to concentrate, decreased motor activity)

0 Normal speech and thoughts

1 Slight retardation at interview

2 Obvious retardation at interview

3 Interview difficult

4 Complete stupor

Agitation

0 None

1 Fidgetiness

2 Playing with hands, hairs, etc.

3 Moving about, can't stand still

4 Hand wringing, nail biting, hair pulling, biting of lips

Anxiety (psychological)

0 No difficulty

1 Subjective tension and irritability

2 Worrying about minor matters

3 Apprehensive attitude apparent in face or speech

4 Fears expressed without questioning

Anxiety somatic (dry mouth, stomach cramps, palpitations, headaches, paresthesia, hyperventilation, sweating, tremor)

0 Absentee

1 Mild

2 Moderate

3 Severe

4 Incapacitating

Somatic symptoms (gastro-intestinal)

0 None

1 Loss of appetite but eats without encouragement from others

2 Difficulty eating without urging from others. Marked reduction of appetite and food intake

Somatic symptoms general

0 None

1 Heaviness in limbs, back or head. Backaches, headaches, muscle aches. Loss of energy and fatigability

2 Any clear cut symptoms rate 2

Genital symptoms (loss of libido, menstrual disturbance)

0 Absent

1 Mild

2 Severe

(continued)

Table 4.8 (continued)

Hypochondria
0 Not present
1 Self absorption (bodily)
2 Preoccupation with health
3 Frequent complaints, requests for help
4 Hypochondriacal delusions
Loss of weight
0 No weight loss
1 Probably weight loss associated with present illness
2 Not assessed
Insight
0 Acknowledges being depressed and ill
1 Acknowledges illness but attributes cause to bad food, climate, overwork, virus, need for rest etc.
2 Denies being ill at all

As with Y-BOCS[41] in the assessment of OCD, this scale is frequently associated with the GAF scale[42] that quantifies the impact of the disease on the subject's life.

Physiopathology

The different emotional, cognitive, and autonomic symptoms observed in depressive illness are dependent on many brain regions. Thus depression appears to result from a network anomaly rather than a dysfunction of any one anatomical structure or neurotransmitter (Fig. 4.4).

Data from functional imaging and clinical outcomes, including ablative psychosurgery or neurostimulation, indeed point to a set of structures. Thus, in depressed patients, there is a hypoactivity of the dorsolateral prefrontal cortex, which is manifested clinically by psychomotor, apathy, memory disorder, and attention deficit Hyperactivity encountered in the orbitofrontal cortex and the amygdala may result in greater sensitivity to pain and increased anxiety. Faced with a negative emotional stimulus, this hyperactivity is further accentuated in the two structures, but also the ventral striatum. However during a pleasant stimulation the ventral striatum appears abnormally hypoactive. Thus Rauch [157] and Mayberg [158] draw a distinction, in patients with severe depression between a "*dorsal*" hypoactive contingent which includes the dorsolateral prefrontal cortex[43] [15, 159], and the dorsal part of the cingulate gyrus [160] and a "*ventral*" hyperactive contingent composed of the orbitofrontal cortex [161–163], the anterior part of the insula and subgenual cortex [164–167]. In patients successfully

---

[41] Cf. description of the scale p. 273.

[42] Cf. idem p. 276.

[43] Cf. p. 92.

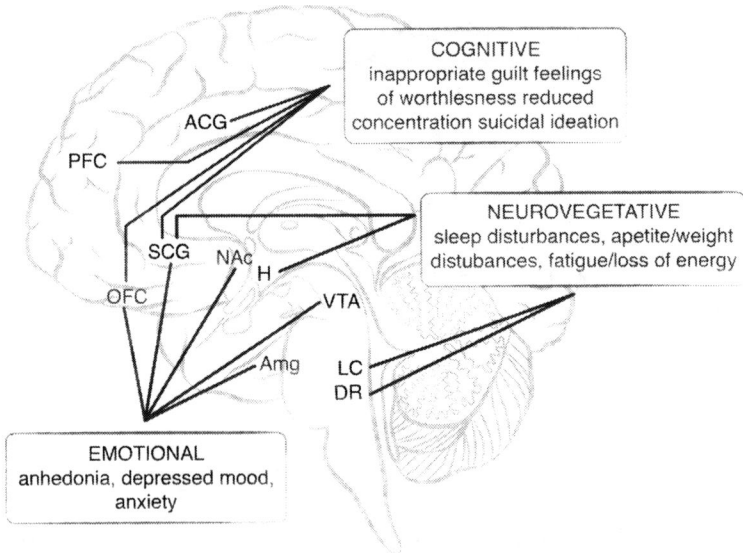

Fig. 4.4 Brain structures involved in symptoms of severe depression. *A* Amygdala, *VTA* Ventral Tegmental Area, *ACC* Anterior Cingulate Cortex, *DLC* Dorsolateral Cortex, *OFC* Orbitofrontal Cortex, *H* Hypothalamus, *LC* Locus Coeruleus, *AN* Nucleus Accumbens, *RN* Raphe Nuclei, according to [156]

treated with antidepressants, activity in these regions tends to return to normal including in the subgenual cortex [168–172].

Therapeutic Management

Management of a major depressive episode is based primarily on psychotherapy and medication. This psychotherapy is built on a supportive attitude consisting of listening and understanding, whose inspiration may be psychoanalytic or cognitive-behavioral. In adults, medication is often associated with this therapy. The choice of drug among a group of about twenty molecules depends on the risk factors of the subject vis-à-vis side effects, the severity of the table, the presence of anxiety, agitation or of insomnia. It is estimated that about half of patients respond to this combination therapy. Among them, two-thirds will be considered in remission [173, 174]. Some items may predict a disappointing response such as a family history of depression, the presence of psychiatric comorbidities such as addiction or an anxiety disorder, the time between onset of symptoms and treatment, chronic disorder, or even pathological personality: histrionic, dependent, obsessive… [173–176]. In the absence of clinical response, the dose may be increased or a different class of molecule may be used. The notion of pharmacological treatment failure is debated by

Table 4.9 Example of a classification of the severity of depression based response to medication. (according to [180])

Stage	Treatment response
0	No single adequate trial of medication
1	Failure to respond to an adequate trial of one medication
2	Failure to respond to two different monotherapy trials of medication with different pharmacological profiles
3	Stage 2 plus failure to respond to augmentation of 1 of the monotherapy
4	Stage 3 plus failure of a second augmentation strategy
5	Stage 4 plus failure to respond to ECT

psychiatrists: at what point in the treatment, at what dosage, after "testing" how many molecules can it be considered depression? Classifications exist to assess the severity of the drug-resistance but are often controversial (Table 4.9) [177, 178]. To these questions may be added the question of therapeutic compliance [174, 176, 179].

Non-Invasive Techniques

Electroconvulsive Therapy

With its undeniable clinical results in the treatment of severe depression [181] electroconvulsive therapy (ECT) remains the only technique that survived the *"studies establish comparable efficacy between convulsive therapy and antide-pressants. Despite recent therapeutic advances [...], ECT remains an important treatment for depression. His place is unique in severe depression and ECT can still improve patient survival"* noted Fossati Shusha et Fossati from the Pitié-Salpêtrière [182]. It is reserved for patients with severe depression, delusional melancholy, or catatonia. As before with camphor or cardiozol, ECT triggers widespread epileptic seizures which have indisputable antidepressant effects although the mechanism is still poorly understood. This epilepsy induced by transcranial administration of an electric current is performed under general anesthesia with EEG recording to confirm the occurrence of a crisis of a few tens of seconds. The paralysis in this gesture can limit motor seizures and possible joint or dental consequences. Several sessions spaced over time is often necessary Because of the constraint and risks of ECT, pharmacological treatment must be prefer, except where fast and powerful improvement is required (risk of suicide, malnutrition, and severe dehydration). ECT has demonstrated antidepressant efficacy, with 50–60 % of responders in patients for whom antidepressants have not been successful Melancholy is, also, an excellent indication with 80–90 % of responses. This treatment may also be useful in elderly patients or those with cons-indications to pharmacological treatments. The convulsive therapy, or ECT, however, has two drawbacks. On the one hand, the rate of depressive relapse between 35 and 80 % in the year following the end of the ECT sessions. In this case, a consolidation treatment is needed can call on antidepressants or new ECT sessions [183]. On the other hand, side effects may occur as a brief confusion, but also disorders, frequent, memory,[44] muscle pain, headache, or hypomanic excitement.

Repeated Transcranial Magnetic Stimulation[45]

Based on a different mechanism from ECT (it is no longer intended to induce a seizure), but with similar efficacy [184–187], repeated transcranial magnetic stimulation (rTMS) offers greater flexibility of implementation and no side effects. This non-invasive technique involves applying a regularly alternating magnetic field to alter neuronal activity in the region being targeted (Fig. 3.21, p. 156). It is usually the left dorsolateral prefrontal cortex and sometimes right [188]. However, given that its effectiveness is delayed it is not intended for vital emergency treatment such as reducing the risk of a suicide. The other more frequent drawback is the transient nature of the mood improvement obtained, which requires regular sessions to consolidate the gains. The establishment of cortical stimulation electrodes facing the dorsolateral prefrontal regions covered by rTMS could be a solution to this pitfall. These permanent electrodes, whose effects appear close to rTMS, can permanently maintain the antidepressant effect. Although the implementation of a sustainable system of cortical stimulation is the logical next step for rTMS, confirmation of clinical efficacy is still in its infancy, with only two teams in the world have published their experiences on this subject [189, 190].

Magnetic Seizure Therapy

Rarer than the two techniques mentioned above, but they are derived from the convulsive transcranial stimulation or *"Magnetic Seizure Therapy"* (STDs) remain a cause intended effects of ECT experimental technique—seizure—a technique Transcranial magnetic stimulation close to rTMS. The originality of this procedure against the ECT would cause more focused seizures that would reduce the cognitive side effects experienced with ECT. In 2001, Lisanby of Columbia University in New York for the first time describes this procedure in animals and in humans with refractory depression [191, 192]. Studies about this still relatively confidential technique report equivalent efficacy to ECT while others confirm the supremacy of the latter [193–195]. A recent work on 20 patients showed no obvious difference between the ECT and MST both from the point of view of clinical findings—satisfactory—as good cognitive tolerance, EEG tracings were collected for comparable elsewhere [193]. The mechanisms of action of the MST are unknown as are, moreover, those of ECT. It can still be imagined that the results of this

---

[44] Anterograde amnesia is a partial or even total loss of memory following the disease, accident, or intervention that provoked it. The subject becomes incapable of making new memories. We can compare the situation to the hard-drive of a computer that is able to read all the data but has a defective writing mechanism which prevents it from recording new information.

[45] This technique and its results are discussed p. 230.

fledgling technology can be improved by specifying the criteria for selection of patients while refining parameters and the location of this convulsive magnetic stimulation [196].

Invasive Techniques

Despite the treatments discussed above, 5–10 % of patients with severe drug-resistant depressions remain refractory to any treatment. This category of patients in large mental suffering, unable to work and linking hospitalization stays, is a therapeutic challenge. Lesional surgery on anatomical targets, like the anterior limb of the internal capsule[46] and the anterior cingulate cortex,[47] had proven their efficacy (Fig. 4.5). These irreversible gestures are increasingly being abandoned today in favor of new stimulation techniques. Three invasive neurostimulation techniques are currently under study: deep brain stimulation, vagus nerve stimulation, and cortical stimulation (Fig. 3.12, p. 130). Before detailing the methods and results of each of these techniques, we will review the clinical criteria commonly accepted that justify the use of these gestures.

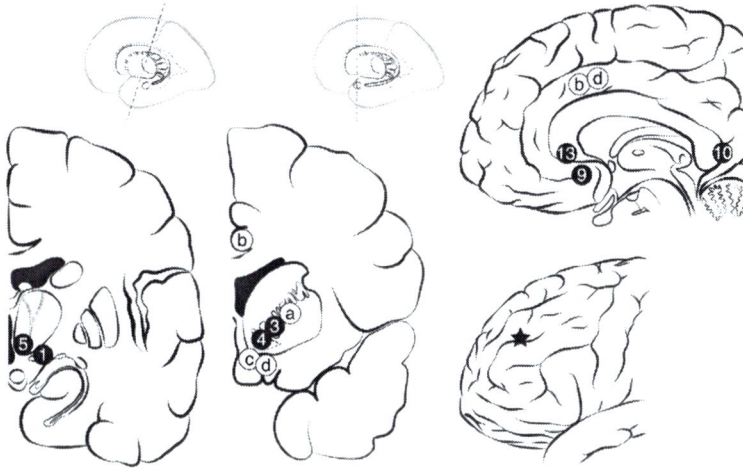

Fig. 4.5 Lesional or deep brain stimulation (*DBS*) targets for the treatment of depression. (*a*) Anterior capsulotomy [197], (*b*) cingulotomy [48, 198, 199], (*c*) subcaudate tractotomy [200], (*d*) limbic leucotomy [201], (3) *DBS* of the ventral striatum (*VC/VS*) [202, 203], (4) *DBS* of the accumbens nucleus [204–206], (5) *DBS* of the inferior thalamic peduncle [207], (9) *DBS* of the subgenual cortex [208–213], (10) *DBS* of the habenula [214], (13) *DBS* of the medial forebrain bundle [215], (*Filled star*) stimulation of the dorsolateral cortex [189, 190]. Stimulation of the vagus nerve is not represented

---

[46] Cf. p. 125.

[47] Cf. p. 95.

Library
College of Physicians & Surgeons of B.C.
300 - 669 Howe St.
Vancouver, BC V6C 0B4

Inclusion and Exclusion Criteria

The inclusion criteria for research protocols to assess the effectiveness of these invasive procedures, although very restrictive, may significantly differ from one study to another, particularly as regards the criteria for drug-resistance [189, 216, 217]. The disease must, of course, meet the diagnostic items of major depressive episode (EDM) to severe intensity according to DSM-IV.[48] Major depressive illness involves the occurrence of one or more of these EDM concept of manic or hypomanic episode. Otherwise, with the exception of a few studies [190, 218–220], in case of bipolar disorder, clinical research protocols usually exclude, these patients, mainly for fear of a "*turn maniac*". These patients must be adults or sometimes be older than 30 years and suffer from symptoms whose severity is reflected by a score higher than 20 on the $HRSD_{17s}$ scale[49] and than 30 on the self-administered BDI^{50} questionnaire. These symptoms must have a strong impact on the lives of the subject with a score of less than 50 GAF.[51] The disease must evolve from a minimum of 2 years, this period may sometimes be shortened when the disease is chronic with at least four episodes in the past. The failure of psychotherapy and medication must be formally established with, in general, resistance to at least two or three different mechanisms of antidepressant pharmacological action (IRS, SNRIS et tricyclics), one of which has been a imipramique tricyclic or phosphate iproniazid, prescribed at effective doses for a minimum of 6 weeks. The failure of ECT or rTMS sessions is required except in studies of cortical stimulation for which we shall see, the efficacy of rTMS may become, instead, an inclusion criterion. Cognitive deterioration,[52] personality disorders, or other psychiatric disorders such as schizophrenia or addictive behavior are exclusion criteria common to all studies. All procedures except for the stimulation of the vagus nerve, requiring the completion of an MRI, the subject must not have any cons-indication for this examination and the surgical act itself, like for example, clotting disorder or a brain abnormality that may deflect the electrodes during their descent into the brain parenchyma. The precautionary principle requires that women who are pregnant or trying to conceive be excluded from these studies.

---

[48] Cf. Description of the DSM-IV for the diagnosis of major depressive episodes p. 309.

[49] Cf. description of the $HRSD_{17}$ scale p. 313.

[50] Ibid.

[51] Ibid.

[52] The MATIS neuropsychological scale is used and the score must be inferior to 130.

Lesional Surgery

Only the results of current surgical techniques are being exposed. As with OCD and other disorders, analysis of technical articles on lesional faces the same obstacle[53]: publications, including a large number of patients are older, usually before the eighties, and do not use standardized scales. The most recent work do use a better methodology, but often relate to small numbers.

Capsulotomy[54]

Few teams have targeted the anterior limb of the internal capsule in this indication. Indeed this procedure is typically reserved for the treatment of OCD, and the occurrence of depression has even been described as a complication in this indication [221, 222]. However let us consider the British prospective study of 20 patients [197]. Its author, Christmas, reported in 2011 50 % response and 40 % remission among these patients after an average follow-up period of 7 years. No neuropsychological deterioration was reported.

Cingulotomy[55]

Cingulotomy lesions appear to guarantee the best results. A review of the literature monitoring more than 400 patients pointed the supremacy in terms of efficacy of the anterior cingulotomy in ablative surgery treatment of depression [223]. In 1996, the Boston team proceeded lesion of the anterior cingulate gyrus on 15 patients and witnessed a decrease of more than half of the BDI score in 60 % of patients, while 12 % were "partial responders"[56] [53]. In 2008, the same team achieved similar results in 33 patients with 30 % of responders[57] and 43 % "*partial responders*" [224]. A year after the cingulotomy, in the absence of clinical improvement, a subcaudate tractotomy was performed in 6 patients, among them one quarter responded and half partially. All complications observed were transient: urinary incontinence (3 patients), temporarily impaired memory (1), one seizure, one abscess resolved after surgical drainage and antibiotic therapy. Other older studies using different scales, making comparisons difficult, showed improvement in 44–92 % of patients. Weight gain, urinary incontinence, and rare cases of personality changes were reported [225].

---

[53] Cf. p. 184.

[54] Cf. also p. 167.

[55] Ibid. p. 173.

[56] Patients are partial responders if their CGI score decreased by at least 35 %.

[57] Patients are responders if their CGI score decreased by at least 50 %.

Subcaudate Tractotomy

Rarely performed, the subcaudate tractotomy developed by Knight is almost always used in conjunction with a cingulotomy when the latter has yielded insufficient benefit: the combination of the two procedures is called a limbic leucotomy. In 1995, the team at *Brook General Hospital* in London published the results of a series of 183 patients operated from 1971 to 1991. After a year of monitoring, 63 patients showed no symptoms of depression, 53 had improved while 57 had not changed or had deteriorated. A 3 % mortality rate was reported while marked fatigue, weight gain and seizures (2 %) were the most frequent complications [61].

Limbic Leucotomy[58]

The limbic leucotomy, a combination of the two previous interventions, was developed in 1973 by, but is hardly ever practiced today. It was commonly indicated alongside cingulotomies for the treatment of depression [94]. Older studies or those using nonstandard scales show improvements ranging from 39 to 78 % [35, 226, 227]. One of the latest studies, conducted by R. Cosgrove in Boston in 2002, involved a small sample of six patients [201]. After a follow-up ranging from 6 to 60 months, three patients were classified as responders by psychiatrists but only one of these patients considered himself truly improved. The authors only give the overall percentages of adverse effects for all 21 patients including those operated for OCD. Definitive complications included 14 % urinary incontinence, 9 % impaired short-term memory, and 5 % epilepsy.

Deep Brain Stimulation

The benefits of deep brain stimulation over ablative surgery have already been presented: reversible and adjustable action, the possibility of varying the site of the stimulation and the possibility of conducting double-blinded studies. The first reference in the literature to deep brain stimulation in the treatment of depression appears in 1968. The Norwegian psychiatrist Sem-Jacobsen implanted intracerebral electrodes in 65 patients with schizophrenia or Parkinson's disease. In his controversial book, Delgado recounts seeing a film recorded during the study: "*we see a patient with a sad expression and slightly depressed mood smiling whenever a brief stimulation is applied to the rostral part of the brain* [septal area] *and then returning quickly to his usual depressive state before smiling again when a new stimulation occurs. Then, a ten-second stimulation completely changed his behavior and facial expression and gave him a happy and pleased appearance that lasted for the ten seconds*". Delgado adds, "*some mentally ill patients were fitted*

---

[58] Cf. p. 182.

with portable stimulators which they used to self-treat depressive states with clear clinical success" [228]. These patients remained dependent on a bulky external device which, in addition to the obvious discomfort, became over time an entry point for infections. This study, which was hard to reproduce and made under questionable ethical and methodological conditions, was an isolated trial. Since 1987, thanks to technological breakthroughs and advances in neuroscience thousands of patients have benefited from Parkinson's treatments with brain stimulation of the subthalamic nucleus. Right from the start of this technique, manic episodes [229–233] as well as depression [234–239] or suicide [232, 237–243] were observed. These clinical effects point to the involvement of this structure, in particular the limbic portion[59] (Fig. 2.20, p. 79) [244, 245], in the modulation of mood. Conflicting effects on mood that subthalamic stimulation are that if this target has sometimes been considered [246] it has, for now, never been adopted in this indication. In 1987, during stimulation of the thalamus in a patient with intractable pain, the team observed a regression of symptoms of reactive depression associated with pain. A similar efficiency was obtained by the Mexican team led by Jiménez after implantation at the base of the thalamus [207]. In the latter case, in 2002, the authors envisaged initially to achieve a subcaudate tractotomy by thermocoagulation. However, before performing the intervention, they performed electrical stimulation along the route of the tractotomy. After obtaining a decrease in anxiety and the occurrence of pleasant sensations, researchers ultimately decided to leave the electrode in. This stimulation was applied to the lower thalamic peduncle, a region through which pass connections between the thalamus and orbitofrontal cortex. The functional imaging studies have revealed that the lower stem and the orbitofrontal cortex were hyperactive in depressed subject. High frequency, and thus inhibitory, electrical stimulation of a part of the network tends to normalize its operations and reduce depressive symptoms [180, 247]. Still based on functional imaging data, the Canadians H. Mayberg and A. Lozano explored the subgenual gyrus, Brodmann area 25 (CG25), an area in front of the cortex of the cingulate gyrus (Fig. 2.4, p. 56), as a potential target in the treatment of depression. The Toronto team based their decision on imaging studies showing hypermetabolism of this region during states of depression or sadness [158, 171, 248–251]. Conversely, normalization was observed following an effective treatment, whether cognitive-behavioral therapy [170], antidepressants [252], rTMS [253], ECT [254] or lesional surgery [198, 255] Thanks to tractography studies, it is known that this region has close connections with the ventral striatum,[60] the shell of the nucleus accumbens[61] and the orbitofrontal,[62] prefrontal, anterior

---

[59] The motor zone of the subthalamic nucleus is usually targeted in the treatment of Parkinson's disease.

[60] Cf. p. 128.

[61] Cf. p. 129.

[62] Cf. p. 93.

cingulate[63], and dorsolateral cortices [172, 256]. Reciprocal connections also exist between this area 25 and the centromedian nucleus of the amygdala (Fig. 2.7, p. 59), hypothalamus, and serotonergic circuit (Fig. 2.31, p. 94). These various anatomical regions are each in their own way involved in the symptoms of depression. Sleep, endocrine, appetite, and libido disorder are attributable to the hypothalamus, while psychomotor retardation, concentration, and memory deficits are rather attributable to the prefrontal cortex. Anhedonia, the inability to feel pleasure, is a dysfunction of the dopaminergic reward system,[64] which is part of the nucleus accumbens while anxious episodes are attributable to the amygdala. This long list of anatomical structures and neurotransmitters involved in depression shows that this pathology is a *"system dysfunction,"* to borrow H. Mayberg's expression, rather than a dysfunction in an isolated structure. Researchers from the University of Toronto, noting the central role of this subgenual area, proposed curbing activity in this structure to modulate the dysfunctional activity throughout the system [208, 221]. The results obtained in the first six patients implanted in area 25 were very encouraging and have opened the door for further studies. A different approach to the treatment of severe depression attempts to modulate the activity of the nucleus accumbens or the surrounding ventral striatum. The Bordeaux team of Aouizerate and Cuny observed in 2004 in a patient with OCD that modulation of this region of the ventral striatum mitigated not only obsessive symptoms but also depressive ones [78]. In 2008, German neurosurgeons and psychiatrists, based on previous data, targeted the nucleus accumbens in three patients suffering from depression only. The team led by T. Schlaepfer and V. Sturm achieved satisfactory clinical results. The anterior cingulate cortex, i.e., Brodmann area 24, is a well-known target for ablative surgery in the treatment of depression, but it has, so far, not been the subject of clinical research in deep brain stimulation. Functional imaging shows, however, that this region is overactive in depressed subjects [164–166]. Mayberg, however, showed that this hyperactivity was present in responders to drug treatment, while it did not exist in nonresponders [165]. More anecdotally, the habenula has been proposed as a possible target because of its increased activity in depressed patients [257]. It is a group of small nuclei which borders the back of the thalamus and projects connections to structures in three neurotransmitters circuits: dopaminergic, noradrenergic, and serotonergic, in order to curb their production. The psychiatrist Sartorius and his team in Mannheim suggested this target for the treatment of depression [258] but for now, only one patient has undergone treatment. Results of the procedure were considered satisfactory [214] (Table 4.10).

---

[63] Cf. p. 95.

[64] Cf. p. 146.

Table 4.10 Results of deep brain stimulation for treatment-refractory depression

Study	Pts	Target	Follow-up	Results[a]
Mexico, 2005 [207]	1	Inferior thalamic peduncles	16	Remission
North America, 2008–2011 [210, 212]	20	Subgenual cortex	36	75 and 50 %
USA, 2009 [203]	15	VC/VS[b]	23	53 and 43 %
Germany, 2009 [204]	10	Nucleus accumbens	12	50 and 30 %
Spain, 2011 [209]	8	Subgenual cortex	12	62 and 50 %
Germany, 2010 [214]	1	Habenula	14	Remission

[a] Response and remission in percent
[b] *VC/VS* ventral portion of the anterior limb of the internal capsule and ventral

The Subgenual Cortex (CG 25)

Lozano's team in Toronto was the first to target the most anterior part of the cingulate cortex. Recruitment of 14 new patients after the pilot study of 2005 [208] has led to a new series of 20 patients with severe drug-resistant depression. A decrease of half the HRSD17 score was achieved in 11 of them (55 %) after 1 year of follow-up [210]. Improved scores on neuropsychological tests were also recorded, as is generally the case after regression of depressive symptoms [259]. These results held at 3 and 6 years [212]. A second, multicenter study, involving centers in Montreal and Vancouver, brought together 21 patients [216]. The results published in 2012 revealed 57 % response after 1 month, 48 % at 6 months, and 29 % at 1 year. This percentage rises to 62 % if response is defined as an HRSD17 score decrease of 40 %. Among the complications, the authors reported one suicide by drug intoxication and one attempted suicide. In nine patients, episodes of nausea and vomiting were deplored, but no causal relationship was formally established with the stimulation. These encouraging results were confirmed in eight patients by a Barcelona team. After 1 year of stimulation, half were in remission [209].

The Nucleus Accumbens

The nucleus accumbens can be seen as an interface between the limbic system responsible for emotions and the motor system responsible for our actions. Its central role in the reward pleasure circuit makes it a kind of *"motivational gate-way"* between emotion and action. In other words, the nucleus modulates behavior seeking a reward. Anhedonia as well as decline in motivation are important symptoms of depression. Functional imaging studies also show decreased activity of the nucleus accumbens in the process bringing into play the concept of reward in these patients with severe depression [260]. Therefore, some authors as Schlaepfer hypothesized that modulation of this structure could alleviate depressive symptoms [206]. In 2010, Denys, in Amsterdam observed mood improvement following stimulation of the nucleus in patients treated because of OCD [261]. The same year, Bewernick and colleagues in Bonn have published the results of a series of 10 patients with severe drug-resistant depression and the nucleus accumbens [204]. One year after the onset of stimulation half of the patients saw their HDRS scores cut in half. A decrease in anxiety for the whole group, including those who did not have a mood response, was also noted.

The Ventral Part of the Internal Capsule and of the Striatum (VC/VS)

The ventral parts of the anterior limb of the internal capsule (VC) and striatum (VS) border the nucleus accumbens such that any distinction may seem artificial. When an electrode is implanted in one of these structures, it becomes difficult to know exactly which structure is responsible for the observed clinical effects. This uncertainty grows as the electrical intensity of the stimulation electrode increases, because as it increases its effective range is expanding and "recruiting" new anatomical regions. The American teams of Malone, Dougherty, and Greenberg targeted this VC/VS area in 17 patients [202, 203]. Six months after the stimulation, 47 % of patients were responders, 29 % in remission, and after a year these numbers increased, respectively, to 53 % and 41 %. After a mean follow-up of 37 months, 71 % of patients were responders and 35 % were in remission. These researchers from the *Cleveland Clinic, Brown University,* and *Harvard University* increase in depressive symptoms. These events were corrected by adjusting the parameters of stimulation as well as by changes in medication. Neuropsychological tests given to a majority of the patients did not reveal any cognitive impairment. As with previous studies, methodological problems remained, namely that the study was not double-blinded and did not include a control group.

The Inferior Thalamic Peduncle

The inferior thalamic peduncle contains bundles connecting the intralaminar nuclei of the thalamus to the orbitofrontal cortex. A cortex involved in emotional and motivational processes [262] which is hyperactive in depression [263]. According to the Mexican team led by the neurosurgeon Jiménez z, these bundles transmit the inhibitory action of the orbitofrontal cortex to the deep structures of the brain [207, 247]. Stimulation of the thalamic peduncle would, therefore, curb this exacerbated inhibition in order to reduce emotional and motivational manifestations. To date, only one patient underwent surgery for this target, and a marked improvement in his symptoms occurred (HAM-D score of 42 decreased to three) even before stimulation. This effect was maintained during stimulation of 2.5 V to 130 Hz for 8 months. During the double-blind phase, in which the stimulation was stopped, a worsening in mood was observed but only 10 months after cessation of the stimulation. The symptoms disappeared after a few days of renewed stimulation.

The Habenula

In depressed subjects, the lateral portion of the habenula shows an increase in activity which can curb activity in the dopaminergic, noradrenergic, and seroto-nergic circus but to which it is connected [257]. In animal, electrical inhibition of the habenula results in an increase in the release of norepinephrine in the prefrontal cortex and serotonin in the striatum [258, 264]. A German team has targeted the habenula in 1 patient, and one month after the onset of stimulation, remission was obtained. Symptoms returned soon after the sudden and unexpected shutdown of the neurostimulator. After the device was repaired, the symptoms disappeared again after 1 month. The psychiatrists from Manheim highlighted this incident as evidence that the results of this "open" study were not due to the placebo effect [214].

The Medial Forebrain Bundle

This bundle,[65] which is part of the reward circuit connects the ventral tegmental area to the nucleus accumbens (Fig. 2.30, p. 93) [265]. In 2012, the team of Coenen and Schlaepfer in Bonn announced preliminary results for seven patients suffering from severe depression treated with bilateral stimulation of the medial forebrain bundle (MFB) [215]. The average MADRS score for this cohort decreased from 30 to 25 after 12 weeks of stimulation. At the time of the last observation, somewhere between the 12th and 33rd week, six patients were responders including three in remission. These preliminary results suggest that stimulation of the bundle can significantly reduce the symptoms of severe depression. Unlike previous studies and targets, the onset of the antidepressant effect was very rapid, and patients responded to relatively low intensities of stimulation.

Conclusion

The successes of deep brain stimulation in the treatment of depression appear undeniable. However, a significant methodological shortfall in a majority of studies is the absence of a double-blind component to eliminate any placebo effect. The frequent visits to the psychiatrist dictated by the research protocol, the feeling of being "useful" in this experimental context or of being closely observed can contribute to enhanced mood independently from the stimulation. Unlike with OCD, symptoms respond less rapidly to stimulation and are more prone to

---

[65] Cf. p. 146.

fluctuations. These mood swings increase the risk of suicide, as psychiatrist J. Luigjes notes, making close monitoring of patients absolutely necessary [261].
Cortical Stimulation[66]

For 10 years, repeated transcranial magnetic stimulation (rTMS) sessions have been available for patients with severe treatment-resistant depressions. rTMS presents the disadvantage of having to be repeated and having in most cases only a temporary effect. In order to sustain beneficial effects, some teams have implanted electrodes under the skull near.[67] The dorsolateral prefrontal cortex, the region commonly targeted by rTMS, to provide ongoing stimulation (Fig. 3.22, p. 160). So far, only two American studies have been conducted. The first, a multicenter study in 2008 led by Kopell included a dozen patients [189, 266, 267]. During the first 2 months, a double-blind phase was conducted showing no difference between stimulated and unstimulated groups. During the open phase lasting 21 months, five patients were, at one time or another, responders, including four in remission. The second study, led by Nahas [190], included five patients. On average, patients saw their HRSD24 score go from 28 before surgery, to 25 after 15 days, 19 after 4 months, and 13 after 7 months. At that time, four of the five patients were responders including three in clinical remission.

Vagus Nerve Stimulation[68]

Stimulation of the vagus nerve (Fig. 3.24, p. 165) has been used for decades in the treatment of some forms of refractory epilepsy. Observations in this indication have shown that the procedure had antidepressant properties, but the mechanism of action remains unclear. Surgical details and complications are discussed in another chapter.[69] Attention is given here to the results of the extracranial technique. Vagus nerve stimulation has the advantage, unlike the interventions discussed above, of not requiring perforation of the skull or brain parenchyma. The first nonblinded clinical studies, conducted in the United States by Rush and George [218, 268, 269] showed that a third of patients saw their symptoms clearly decrease 3 months after the onset of stimulation. Presented with these results, the *Food and Drug Administration* (FDA) decided,[70] to authorize commercialization of the implantable device in 2005. However, no insurance company agreed to reimburse the intervention due to insufficient proof of efficacy [270]. The only study undertaken, lasting only 10 weeks, was a double-blinded comparison of 119 stimulated patients versus 116 patients who were implanted with the device but not

---

[66] For a description of the technique cf. p. 230.

[67] Cf. p. 236.

[68] For a description of the technique cf. p. 244.

[69] Cf. p. 241.

[70] Conflict of interest and pharmaceutical industry cf. p. 432.

stimulated. It did not reveal any significant difference in the evolution of depressive symptoms. After 3 months, 15 % of stimulated patients had some improvement versus 10 % for the placebo group [271]. Observation of this cohort of patients continued during an open phase involving 59 of the patients. After 1 year 30 % were responders and 17 % were in remission [272]. In 2008, a European multicenter study of 74 patients reported 37 % response and 17 % remission after 3 months of stimulation. After 1 year, the rates were 53 and 44 %, respectively [217]. Overall, a critical review of the 13 papers published to date evaluating the effectiveness of vagus nerve stimulation in depression reveals that 32 % of the almost 500 patients who participated in "open" studies responded to the technique [273]. Statistical meta-analysis of these open studies and the single randomized double-blind study does not yet give incontestable proof of the efficacy of vagal stimulation in the treatment of depression.

Conclusion

Techniques involving implanted stimulation devices for the treatment of severe and refractory depression remains under evaluation both in terms of effectiveness and safety. Although the benign nature of these techniques is in the process of being established, their effectiveness remains difficult to demonstrate. Clinical studies of the effectiveness of implantable stimulation device techniques in depression virtually all present the same weaknesses. Namely, a limited number of patients significantly reduce their statistical reach. Second, for the most part these studies are "open" and do not control for a placebo effect.[71] Experts on this topic remain divided on the importance of this phenomenon. Researchers have evaluated its impact in depression at 30–40 %, or even 70 % for less severe symptomologies [274]. However, this effect tends to diminish with the severity of symptoms and abates over the duration of the test [275]. Studies with double-blinded phases lasting 10 weeks, such as the randomized study by Rush in 2005 [271], appear too short to demonstrate the effectiveness of vagus nerve stimulation. However, the inclusion criteria used in each study selected patients with severe, drug-resistant depression, who were thus *a priori* less susceptible to the placebo effect. However, these reflections on the placebo effect must be considered with caution since this

---

[71] Work by H. Mayberg using metabolic imaging (TEP-scan) has shown that placebo response was associated with activations in the prefrontal, premotor and parietal cortices, posterior insula and the cingulate gyrus and concurrent decreases in the subgenual cingulate gyrus, parahippocampic gyrus and thalamus. These regions show the same modifications in patients who respond to antidepressants (fluoxetine). These modifications common to placebo and antidepressant responders, suggest that these changes are necessary for remission of the depression regardless of the treatment modality (in Vallance, A.K. 2007. A systematic review comparing the functional neuroanatomy of patients with depression who respond to placebo to those who recover spontaneously: is there a biological basis for the placebo effect in depression? J Affect Disord 98:177–185).

Table 4.11 Evolution of the HAM score after 1 year according to the stimulation technique and target

Target	Center(s)	Patients	Percentage of responders (1 year)
Area 25	Toronto [210]	20	55
	Toronto, Montréal, Vancouver [216]	21	29
Nucleus accumbens	Bonn, Baltimore, Cologne [204]	10	50
VC/VS	Cleveland, Boston, Rhodes-Island [203]	17	53
Inferior thalamic peduncle	Mexico [207]	1	100
Habenula	Manheim [214]	1	100
Medial forebrain bundle	Bonn [215]	7	86 (12 weeks)
Vagus nerve	Multicentric [276]	181	30
	Londres, Dublin [277]	11	55
	Multicentrique (Europe) [217]	59	53
Prefrontal cortex	Multicentric [190]	11	18

effect has been studied for drugs and not for implanted devices. However, it is known that the effect increases proportionally to the invasiveness of the technique. To these methodological difficulties is added the search for optimal stimulation parameters for each target. Although Table 4.11 summarizes these trials in terms of anatomical targets, the small patient populations and different inclusion criteria make direct comparisons difficult. In addition to optimizing stimulation parameters, determining the optimal electrode placement for each treatment-resistant target, the evolution of the disease and its characteristics should improve clinical outcomes. Mapping of functional imaging data should also lead to a treatment map for depressive and OCD patients where the stimulation parameters can be calculated from the symptoms and anomalies visible in functional imaging.

Aggressive Behavior Disorders

Abstract Aggressive behavior disorders, except for rare diseases such as Lesch–Nyhan syndrome, are a hard to define family of diseases with social and political implications. Some lesional techniques such as amygdalotomies, the hypothalamotomies were once indicated but have now been replaced by capsulotomies or cingulotomies—used much more rarely but still contested. Deep brain stimulation now offers a reversible and therefore more acceptable treatment for these patients.

The treatment of aggressive behavior by a surgical treatment remains controversial from medical and ethical perspectives (Fig. 4.6, p. 231). First off, this nosological "entity" must be given a medical definition. It can be defined as recurrent states of

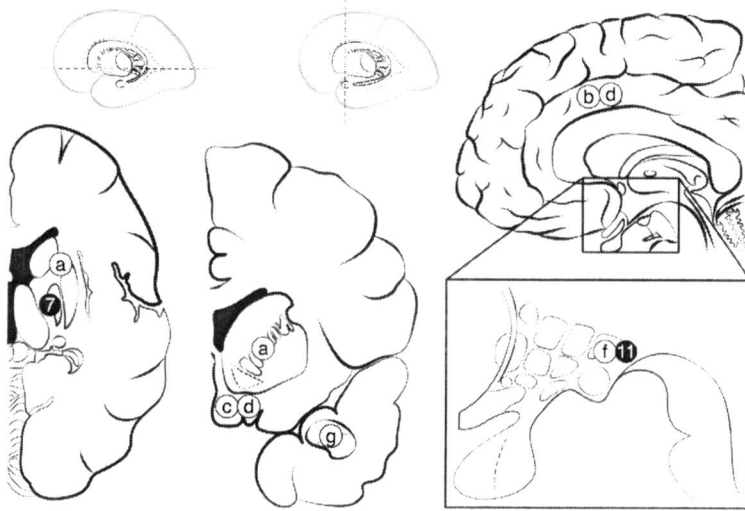

Fig. 4.6 Lesional or deep brain stimulation (*DBS*) procedures for the treatment of aggressive behavior disorders. (*a*) Anterior capsulotomy [279–282], (*b*) cingulotomy [281, 282], (*c*) subcaudate tractotomy [280], (*d*) limbic leucotomy [279, 280], (*f*) posterior hypothalamotomy [283], (*g*) amygdalotomy [284], (7) *DBS* of the internal globus pallidus [285, 286], (11) *DBS* of the posterior hypothalamus [287]

rage or uncontrollable furor followed by verbal or physical violence [278]. The World Health Organization (WHO), extends this definition to "*the deliberate use or threat of deliberate use of physical force or power against oneself, against another person or against a group or community, which results or may result in injury, death, psychological harm, maldevelopment or deprivation*" This highlights the risk of self-mutilation, aggression of others, and incarceration inherent in such behavior. The first of this psychiatric dangerousness must be accompanied by a historical and political view, the definition of this concept and its references to the law may reflect social concerns, or security of a society. It is understood that these concepts may vary through space and time. The therapeutic management of these disorders has evolved considerably over the last 4 years due mainly to pharmacological progress but also the evolution of the concept of *aggressive behavior disorder*. Bioethics raises questions: first, the crucial issue of informed consent in these patients and, second, the problem of conflict of interest. Surrounding these patients with aggressive behavior and society have an interest in normalizing potentially criminal behavior.[72] Today, psychosurgery is concerned almost exclusively with severe drug-resistant hetero and autoaggressive behavior disorders most commonly resulting from brain lesions or Lesch–Nyhan syndrome, a rare genetic disorder characterized by mental retardation, abnormal movements,

---

[72] Cf. p. 428.

Table 4.12 Amygdalotomies performed in patients with aggressive behavior

Country/Date	Number of pts	Target	Complication	Immediate results (%)	Long term results
Switzerland, 1966 [295]	85	Medial amygdala[b]	None	100	Unknown
USA, 1966 [296]	20	Antero-medial amygdala	None	75	Unknown
Japan, 1966 [297]	98[a]	Lateral amygdala[b]	1 synd. de Klüver-Bucy[c]	85	67 % (after 3 years)
Switzerland, 1972 [298]	45[a]	Amygdala §§	Unknown	100	Unknown
Great-Britain, 1973 [294]	18	Medial amygdala §§	None	33	Unknown
Australia, 1974	18	Central amygdala[b] or §	5 % hemiparesis	50	39 % (27 months to 6 years)
India, 1975 [295]	235	Central amygdala[b] or §§	3.8 % mortality	75	Unknown
USA, 1977 [299]	58[a]	Antero-medial amygdala §§	Transient polydipsia (% not specified)	33	Unknown
Poland, 1980 [300]	70	Medial Amygdala	None	83	Unknown
India, 1988 [284]	481	Central amygdala[b] or §§	6 % hemiplegia	76	42 % after 3 years

[a] Group includes patients also treated for refractory epiplepsy
[b] lesion created by injection of a mix of olive oil and beeswax [295]
[c] In 1937 two American researchers, H. Klüver and P. Bucy, observed that patients presenting bilateral temporal lobe lesions had decreased levels of fear and emotions in general, loss of social interactions, visual agnosia and hypersexuality. This association of symptoms has become known as Klüver and Bucy syndrome. Cf. definition p. 98
§ Lesion created by cryotherapy ($-60°$ à -120 °C)
§§ Lesion created using stereotaxy and thermo/electrocoagulation

and a tendency to self-mutilate. In the past and in some countries, these indications have been less strictly enforced, as was the case with amygdalotomies performed in India up to the end of the 1980s.

Amygdalotomy: An Obsolete Technique

In the late 1960s, following animal studies by Klüver and Bucy [288], Thomson and Walker [289], and Kling showed that the removal of the inner portion of the temporal lobe made monkeys and cats more docile. Terzian [290] showed that bilateral ablation in humans of the amygdala contained within this lobe, decreased aggressiveness. At the same time, Ursin [291] observed that electrical stimulation of the amygdala in animals and humans could provoke intense anger. It is from this data that the Japanese team led by Narabayashi [292] realized stereotactic lesions in the amygdala of 60 individuals with severe aggressive behavior and sometimes hyperactivity. Forty of these patients were under the age of 14. Thirty-nine amygdalotomies were performed unilaterally the remainder bilaterally. The authors reported an immediate "good result" in 85 % of cases. This result was maintained after 3–6 years for 68 % of patients. Following this series, a little over 1,000 patients with aggressive behavior, sometimes associated with seizures, were operated on around the world, mostly in Japan, India, and the United States [293, 294]. Published series with a minimum of 10 patients are summarized in Table 4.12. However, the comparison of these publications has little value as patient groups are heterogeneous, variable, and received uneven technical monitoring. However, we note that the majority of these interventions were guided by an EEG recording and stimulation of the amygdala. This type of stimulation, performed while the patient is awake, allows the analysis of his reactions—often fear or rage—to ensure that the tip of the instrument is positioned at the desired location before creating a lesion. Moreover, some patients also suffering from intractable epilepsy, had fewer or no subsequent exacerbations after the intervention since the amygdala–hippocampal complex is one of the sources of these episodes.

The use of amygdalotomies to treat aggressive behavior has virtually disappeared [301]. Advances in psychosocial management and neuropharmacology have reduced the indications for this surgery. Growing concerns in the West over psychosurgery in the 1970s and 1980s also contributed to this decline. The publication in 1970 of the book *"Violence and the brain"* by Mark and Ervin awakened public opinion [302]. The philosopher and historian JN Missa explains that, *"after the publication of Mark and Ervin, the debate focused on the possibility of society controlling violence through psychosurgical methods. Mark and Ervin suggest in their book that many Americans suffer from a dysfunction of the amygdala which may lead to aggressive behavior. According to them, these behavioral disorders can be treated by manipulation of the brain. At a time when revolt was brewing in the black ghettos, the dissemination of* 'Violence and the Brain' *fostered fears over the large-scale application of surgical techniques for treating violent behaviors stemming from social causes"* [303]. During the same period, the press widely reported on Delgado's experiments in the Seville arena remote control of a bull using implanted chips. This "first" by the Spanish-American researcher was widely publicized and increased awareness of the potential for abuse in these interventions intended to correct antisocial behavior [304]. In 1977, the potential for abuse became even clearer after a Senate inquiry revealed the existence of a secret CIA program, *"Project MK-Ultra"*. Although ultimately the program had little to do with psychosurgery, it did investigate the possible uses of psychotropic drugs as police and military tools [305]. For these many reasons—in spite of technical refinements in imaging and stereotaxy—with few exceptions, amygdalotomies are no longer practiced [301].

Cingulectomy, Cingulotomy, and Capsulotomy

Until the early 1960s, before amygdalotomies and hypothalamies, frontal lobot-omies and cingulectomies were prescribed in the treatment of *"reactions stemming from dangerous aggressiveness and impulsivity likely to cause antisocial acts"* [306]. The literature preserves, however, little evidence of these interventions. Purple and David, two Parisian neurosurgeons, believed in 1961 that *"positive results are rare. The existence of some hereditary or family traits is a factor generally unfavorable to psychosurgery. There is a risk of causing intellectual impairment which, by reducing the mental control faculties of the patient, wastes what could have been achieve with regards to the hyper-emotionality. Under these conditions psychosurgery seems reserved to a few patients in whom one can discover a marked anxiety contributing to the antisocial release of the emotional tendencies. Brousseau, Rylander, Mugica report some good results in repeatedly offending delinquent perverts with anxiety, a state of permanent instability. But it would seem that psychosurgery is generally not recommended"* [306]. Nonethe-less, in the late 1960s, the Italians Schergna and Mingrino performed cingulotomy interventions in this indication [307]. Despite being a more targeted procedure, the results the team presented in 1970 at the *Congress of Psychosurgery* in Copen-hagen were relatively disappointing [308]. Only 2 of the 10 patients showed a marked decrease in their aggressive symptoms 27 months after the stereotactic cingulotomy intervention. Despite poor results in this indication, the procedure is still practiced. In 2006 a Mexican team reported that a 13-year-old patient who, in addition to symptoms of OCD, presented significant aggression had received an open-surgery cingulotomy. The operation was a failure. A subsequent radiosurgery of the anterior capsule attenuated the aggressive symptoms [279, 280]. These articles also mention six other individuals with hetero or self-aggression behaviors who received Gamma Knife radiosurgery treatments: anterior capsulotomy (2 patients), limbic leucotomy (3), and subcaudate tractotomy (1). For five of these patients, the authors alleged an improvement in symptoms but did not provide any details on the neuropsychological follow-ups. In 2011, another Mexican team presented the clinical results of combined cingulotomy and capsulotomy procedures using stereotactic thermocoagulation for 12 patients with aggressive behavior [281]. Nine of them suffered from mental retardation and three from schizophrenia. The authors argued that 6 months after each of these combined interventions there was a significant improvement, for the group overall, in "functional scores."[73] Still reporting on the group as a whole, they noted complications including four cases of hyperphagia, three of drowsiness, two disinhibition or hypersexuality, and one infection and one paraparesis.[74] The same team in 2012, without stating clearly whether or not it was reporting on the same cohort or not, gave similar results in 10 patients aged 15–58. This time, follow-up lasted 4 years. They reported

---

[73] Mayo-Portland Adaptability Inventory (MPAI) and Global Assessment of Functioning (GAF).
[74] Incomplete paralysis of the inferior limbs.

the same number of complications with the addition of one death [282]. These studies are discussed further in chapter on ethics.

Lesioning and Stimulation of the Posterior Hypothalamus

In the 1970s, the Japanese neurosurgeon Sano suggested treating hyperaggressivity through lesions of the posterior hypothalamus. This region[75] is involved in the regulation of sympathetic manifestations of the autonomic nervous system. As with amygdalotomies, the creation of these lesions is preceded by electrical stimulation of the hypothalamus to locate the ergotropic region. This *posterior hypothalamotomy* procedure was performed in more than 40 patients leading to significant benefit in 95 % [283, 309]. Arjona [310], Schvarcz [311], Ramamurthi [284]. For reasons similar to those that ended the use of amygdalotomies, hypothalamotomies disappeared in the late 1980s. Since 2002, the Milanese team of Franzini and Broggi [312], based on previous work, has taken this anatomical target using a technique of deep brain stimulation for the treatment of patients with severe aggression resulting from brain damage (perinatal toxoplasmosis, brain injury, cerebral anoxia ...). Six patients, aged 20–64, received the operation, and all had an IQ less than 40. In three of them the authors observed a marked reduction, or disappearance in two patients, of episodes of hetero-aggressive violence, allowing the resumption of socialization. Patients with little or no response all presented lesions in the prefrontal cortex. In Spain, the team of Hernando and Sola performed the same procedure in a 22-year-old patient with severe idiopathic mental retardation and violent episodes of autoaggression [313]. Again, the clinical course, under stimulation, was excellent with a very sharp decrease in violent outbursts allowing a resumption of social activities. Curiously, these satisfactory results were obtained, not by high frequency stimulation (SHF) (>100 Hz), as was the case with the Italian team, but at low frequency (15 Hz). In this patient, HFS caused a series of sympathetic signs without reducing the manifestations of aggression. This unexpected clinical finding goes against the widely accepted and verified[76] notion that HFS has an inhibitory effect on the surrounding anatomical structures. Some authors compare its *functional effects to a lesion* [314]. Meanwhile low frequency stimulation reportedly has an activating effect. This case shows once again that the mechanisms of action of DBS remain unclear.[77] In 2002, during an operation, the Parisian team Agid found the occurrence, also unexpectedly, to aggressive outbursts during deep brain stimulation at high frequency in a patient with Parkinson's disease [315]. The team at the Pitié-Salpêtrière hospital concluded that the electrodes were not located within the

---

[75] Cf. p. 123.

[76] Cf. p. 198.

[77] Ibid.

subthalamic nuclei as the procedure calls for but in the neighboring region, the posterior part of the hypothalamus. Again, this observation seems to contradict those made by Franzini and Broggi. Even though the patient was not suffering from an aggressive disorder, HFS at 140 Hz applied to this region should have had an inhibitory effect.

Pallidal Stimulation in Lesch–Nyhan Syndrome

Lesch–Nyhan syndrome is a rare genetic disease that affects one in a little under 400,000 individuals [316]. It is characterized by a deficiency of hypoxanthine-guanine phosphoribosyltransferase (HGPRT), an enzyme involved in the metabolism of purines [317]. Described in 1964 [318] by the pediatrician Nyhan and his young intern, Lesch this syndrome involves abnormal movements and self-mutilation behavior.

Clinical Aspects

These patients are usually normal at birth and developmental delay only becomes apparent at 6 months [319]. The diagnosis is usually made during early childhood when compulsive self-mutilation disorders become manifested in the child biting his lips, cheeks, or fingers. It is not uncommon for these mutilations to lead to severe infection or even amputation [320]. This aggressive behavior can also turn outwards and lead to striking or insults. Delayed motor development appears quickly and is manifested initially by hypotonia and gradually by disabling generalized dystonia and dyskinesia. Mental retardation is common [321].

Physiopathology

Lesch–Nyhan syndrome is one of the recessive genetic disorders linked to the X chromosome, which means that women transmit this anomaly without being affected. This disorder is caused by a deficiency of the enzyme HPRT, involved in purine metabolism, leading to increased blood levels of uric acid and the formation of crystal deposits in the kidney, skin, and joints. Even if this hyperuricemia helps explain joint (gout) and skin (tophus) symptoms, the pathophysiology of neurological manifestations remains unexplained. Based on models developed in animal, self-mutilation behavior may be related to hypersensitivity of the D1 subclass of dopamine receptors in the basal ganglia [104, 322, 323].

Pharmacological Treatment

Self-inflicted injuries can be prevented by wearing a helmet, gloves, or a mask. In the most severe cases, tooth extraction is necessary. Currently, there is no causative drug treatment but some molecules are used to limit symptoms: Allopurinol reduces the uric acid and prevents kidney or joint manifestations. The use of psychotropic drugs reduces behavioral disorders while some classes of drugs used in the treatment of spasticity or Parkinson's disease have a limited effectiveness on dystonia.

Stimulation of the Internal Globus Pallidus

In 2000, Taira and Hori in Tokyo implanted electrodes for deep brain stimulation in the internal globus pallidus (GPi) of a 19-year-old patient with Lesch–Nyhan syndrome with extremely debilitating dystonia for over 10 years [286]. This anatomical target was previously proposed in deep brain stimulation treatment of certain forms of dystonia [324–327]. In the aftermath of this intervention, the Japanese neurosurgeons were surprised to observe, along with the regression of abnormal movements, disappearance of self-injurious behavior. This first observation agrees with the hypothesized involvement of, on the one hand, the CSTC motor loop causing dystonia, and on the other hand, the limbic loop causing aggressive behavior disorders. As with Gilles de la Tourette syndrome, the neurobehavioral manifestations are probably a result of an alteration in the interaction between the motor and limbic loops [92, 104, 105]. Based on this hypothesis, as well as on electrophysiological recordings [328], Coubes' team in Montpellier, France, implanted two electrodes in a 16-year-old patient with a severe form of the syndrome: one in the posterior part of the GPi,[78] corresponding to the motor area, and the other in the anterior ventral portion, containing the limbic area. When the posterior electrode was stimulated at high frequency (130 Hz), the Montpellier team found that dystonia disappeared in less than a week. Meanwhile, 3 days of stimulation of the anterior ventral electrode led to the disappearance of aggressive behavior [285]. The 28 month follow-up period demonstrated the stability of the results in this patient. Using an identical follow-up procedure, a team in Chicago also reported excellent clinical results for a 7-year-old child using only a single electrode in the GPi [329].

---

[78] Cf. p. 128.

Conclusion

Advances in psychopharmacology, unfavorable public opinion, and bioethics have restricted the use of amygdalotomies and hypothalamotomies, used in the 1970s in the treatment of severe aggressive behavior disorders, or the internal globus pallidus in Lesch–Nyhan syndrome, cerebral stimulation offers encouraging results. The reversibility of stimulation provides better ethical safeguards than are possible with lesional techniques. In these patients, the vast majority of whom have some form of mental retardation, the burden of consent is lighter if the treatment is not permanent. These treatments of aggressive disorders by surgery, either lesional or stimulation, demand extreme caution as the contour of the disease can be dependent on "politics." This warning is not directed only at researchers and doctors, but at society as a whole. It is hard to imagine that "practitioners" in a totalitarian regime would publish clinical results in international journals for a series of *patients treated* under conditions that bioethicists reject. These considerations are also valid for the treatment of addiction[79] and sexual behavior.[80]

Addiction

Abstract The socioeconomic consequences of addiction and failures of detoxification, notably to opiates, encouraged clinicians to turn to surgical treatment starting in the 1970s. The cingulotomy the hypothalamotomy and, more recently, the removal of the nucleus accumbens have been proposed. The results of these actions remain methodological therapeutically, and ethically controversial. The effectiveness of these techniques has rarely been compared to other therapies like substitution techniques. Additionally, the conditions for obtaining informed consent in these vulnerable populations are even more problematic since the effects of these interventions are irreversible. Recently, the research is directed toward brain stimulation techniques, including nucleus accumbens, in the treatment of chronic forms of rebels alcoholism or drug addiction to opiates.

The term addiction comes from the Latin *addicere* to assign. Under the Roman Empire, slaves did not have a proper name and were *addicere* their *Pater familias*. As is apparent, addiction is manifested by a lack of freedom and is characterized by a physical or psychological addiction to a substance like alcohol, tobacco, cocaine, or excessive practices like gambling or sex. WHO estimates, depending on the country, the consumption of prohibited substances to be from 0.1 to 3 % of the population [330]. The prevalence of alcohol dependence is around 7 % of the population, while tobacco affects one in three adults [331]. Addictions are

---

[79] Cf. p. 426.
[80] Cf. p. 425.

therefore a public health concern as well as an economic and social problem. The goal of treatment by medication or psychotherapy, is to achieve cessation but failure is frequent. If we take the example of severe chronic alcoholism, it is estimated that the relapse rate is nearly 80 % [332]. Recent data from neurobiology sheds light on the mechanisms involved in the genesis and perpetuation of addiction and paves the way for new treatments, including surgery, of severe forms.

Clinical Aspects

According to WHO, addiction is defined as a syndrome in which the consumption of a product becomes a necessity at the expense of other behaviors which previously had greater importance. The definition of this disorder in the DSM-IV is more stringent and requires at least three of the following seven signs with an evolution of over 1 year [153]:

1. Tolerance, as defined by either of the following: (a) A need for markedly increased amounts of the substance to achieve intoxication or the desired effect or (b) markedly diminished effect with continued use of the same amount of the substance;
2. Withdrawal, as manifested by either of the following: (a) The characteristic withdrawal syndrome for the substance or (b) the same (or closely related) substance is taken to relieve or avoid withdrawal symptom;
3. The substance is often taken in larger amounts or over a longer period than intended;
4. There is a persistent desire or unsuccessful efforts to cut down or control substance use;
5. A great deal of time is spent in activities necessary to obtain the substance, use the substance, or recover from its effects;
6. Important social, occupational, or recreational activities are given up or reduced because of substance use;
7. The substance use is continued despite knowledge of having a persistent physical or psychological problem that is likely to have been caused or exacerbated by the substance.

Physiopathology

The physiopathology of addiction is better understood than that of psychiatric disorders discussed elsewhere in this chapter; thanks to the fact that many aspects of addictive behavior are reproducible in laboratory animals. These experiments have shown that all addictive substances, whatever their nature, cause a release of

Orbitofrontal cortex ——————

Anterior cingulare cortex ——————

Nucleus accumbens ——————

Ventral tegmental areas ——————

Amygdala ——————

Hippocampus ——————

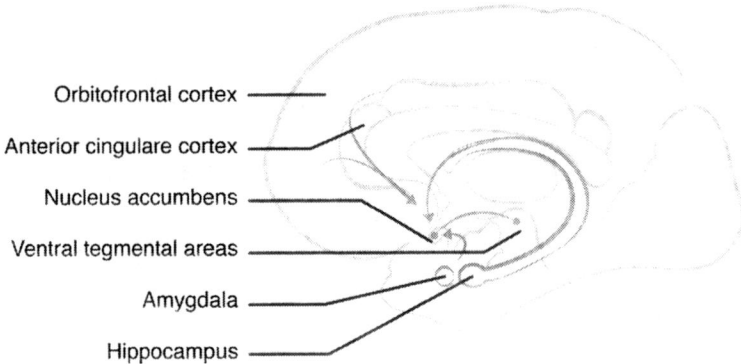

Fig. 4.7 Some of the neuroanatomical structures involved in addiction, according to [336]

dopamine in the nucleus accumbens[81][333]. This release is the cause of the feeling of well-being, the *high* [334], felt when taking the product which generates a *positive reinforcement* [335]. This nucleus is part of the *mesolimbic* dopaminergic[82] reward circuit. This circuit is a network of neurons in the ventral tegmental area (VTA) whose dopaminergic axons project to the ventral striatum notably its basal portion, the nucleus accumbens via a bundle of axons, the medial forebrain bundle (MFB) (Fig. 2.30, p. 93) [336–338]. This nucleus belongs not only to the reward circuit but also to the system of cortico-striato-thalamo-cortical (CSTC) loops[83] [339] This dual membership makes it an interface between the reward system and the functions, including motor, of these CSTC loops. In other words, it contributes to the transformation of desire into action. The second, *mesocortical* dopaminergic pathway, is formed by projections of neurons from the VTA via the MFB also to the prefrontal and cingulate[84] cortices, the amygdala[85] and the hippocampus[86] (Fig. 4.7, p. 240).

These structures influence, in turn, the nucleus accumbens. If we take the example of nicotine or heroin, these molecules trigger the release of dopamine in the VTA by nicotinic and opioid receptors. In response cocaine, dopamine is released directly to the nucleus accumbens by selective inhibition of the reuptake of the neurotransmitter in the synaptic gap. The released dopamine produces *positive reinforcement* [340]. During habitual use, these substances cause progressive adaptations in the reward circuit, which will be lead to habituation and dependency. The addict requires more frequent doses of the drug to have the same

---

[81] Cf. p. 129.

[82] Cf. p. 146.

[83] Cf. p. 139.

[84] Cf. p. 103.

[85] Cf. p. 98.

[86] Cf. p. 103.

effect on mood and concentration. It is addictive. This rise in consumption leads to addiction, a need resulting in psychological distress and physical pain that only the drug can relieve. This is a *negative reinforcement* that can result in a feeling of depression, tremors, pain, and sweating [341, 342]. This condition creates the avoidance and criminal behavior of the withdrawal syndrome. Koob suggested that in dependent individuals, repeated administration resulted in *alternating positive and negative reinforcements* that led to dysfunctional of the reward system [343]. Besides the feeling of well-being, self-administration of the product causes an influx of dopamine in the amygdala[87] and hippocampus,[88] which would strengthen the associations between the rewarding qualities of the substance and the memories of the associated environment [344, 345]. The drug highlights the context associated with the reward. Confrontation with an identical emotional environment in turn creates the irrational need the product, *"craving"*, This is particularly true for alcoholics, smokers, and heroin addicts in whom the environment becomes a powerful conditioning. Tassin, a neurobiologist specializing in addictions, cites the example of *GIs in Vietnam who had such high rates of heroin addiction that the U.S. government began to consider a special detoxification program. To the relief of the authorities, once the soldiers returned to their families, the percentage of drug addicts dropped to a level barely above that of the general population: the environment had changed* [346]. Likewise, stories of heroin or cocaine addicts who relapse when they see syringe or talc abound. The dysfunction of the dopaminergic system affects, via the mesocortical circuit, the prefrontal cortex[89] and the anterior cingulate cortex[90] [334, 347]. This dysfunction of the cortex leads to a reduction of cortical inhibitory control on the craving mesolimbic pathway and may explain the difficulty addicts have resisting substance abuse while at the same time being aware of the harmful consequences of their behavior [334, 347, 348]. The amygdala, which gives positive emotional coloring to an environment through its connections with the nucleus accumbens [349], could also contribute to this phenomenon causing relapses during confrontation with a situation associated with the use of opiates [350]. Some authors see this as a potential target in the treatment of addiction [351, 352].

Procedures

Medical complications, social consequences, and the cost of addiction led many teams in the 1960s to prescribe stereotactic cingulotomy and hypothalamotomy interventions or ablation of the nucleus accumbens (Fig. 4.8). The same concerns

---

[87] Cf. p. 98.
[88] Cf. p. 103.
[89] Cf. p. 90.
[90] Ibid.

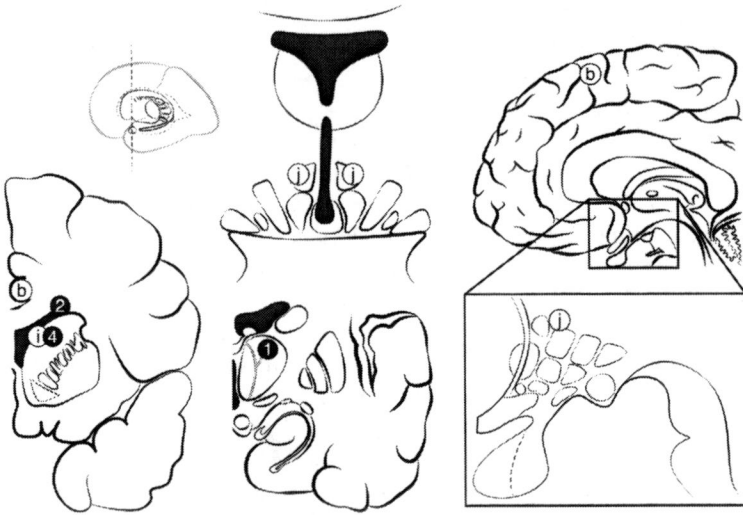

Fig. 4.8 Lesional or deep brain stimulation (*DBS*) targets explored, some fortuitously (*1*), in addiction treatment. (*b*) Bilateral anterior cingulotomy [360, 361], (*i*) ablation of the nuclei accumbens [354], (*j*) uni/bilateral ventromedial hypotalamotomy [362], (1) *DBS* of the subthalamic nuclei [363], (2) *DBS* of the dorsal part of the anterior limb of the internal capsule [358], (4) *DBS* of the nuclei accumbens [358, 364]

which ended the use of amygdalotomy and hypothalamotomy interventions in the treatment of aggressive behavior disorders, led to the cessation of these interventions for addiction in the early 1980s, with the notable exception of teams in Russia and China[91] [353, 354]. Advances made in deep brain stimulation make it possible to now consider applying the technique to structures formerly targeted with lesional surgery such as the nucleus accumbens [355–359].

Cingulotomy

The *craving* of addicts has been likened to a form of obsessive-compulsive disorder. Pursuing this hypothesis, Balasubramaniam put forward the idea of a cingulotomy,[92] intervention, also used in the treatment of patients suffering from severe OCD [360, 361, 365] in the treatment of addicted patients. The Indian neurologist also based this choice on the work of Foltz, and White who in 1962 had performed this procedure in patients with chronic intractable pain [366]. Fourteen out of the 16 subjects had developed an addiction to narcotics. Besides pain relief achieved in 12 patients, these Seattle-based neurosurgeons noted that

---

[91] The bioethical questions raised by these procedures are discussed separately p. 426.

[92] Cf. p. 49 for the history of this procedure and p. 173 for the technique itself.

none of the previously drug-dependent patients had resorted to morphine after surgery, and only five had shown moderate signs of withdrawal. The Indian team in Madras performed cingulotomies on 73 patients suffering from alcohol or morphine addiction. Weaning, after a period of 1 to 6 years, was obtained in 80 % of morphine and 68 % of alcohol dependent patients. This intervention, which was no longer used for this indication, was adopted at the end of 1990s by Medvedev and his team in St. Petersburg for heroin-addicted patients. Before this program was criticized interrupted in 1998 by the Russian authorities, 348 patients were operated by bilateral cryo-cingulotomy a variant of stereotactic cingulotomy a cold source at the end of an instrument: the cryoprobe -70 °C for 5 min Monitoring of this cohort has shown, with a follow-up of 2 years, 45 % complete cessation and 17 % cessation after one or two relapses [353]. Curiously, these major Indian and Russian studies did not report on neuropsychological alterations. This contrasts with the work of much smaller studies which reported attention deficit or executive function disorders[93] [367, 368]. Anecdotally, it has been observed by the French team Jarraya and Palfi that a lesion in the posterior part of the cingulate cortex could result in tobacco-use cessation [369].

Hypothalamotomy

In 1973, Müller assuming that the somatic symptoms of withdrawal—fever, tremors, hypertension, sweating, or dehydration—were manifestations of hyperactivity of the hypothalamus, led a team from Göttingen which performed a unilateral ventromedial hypothalamotomy intervention in an alcoholic patient of about 30. Initial results were encouraging, but relapse occurred in the eleventh month [370]. Müller concluded that the intervention should be performed bilaterally. Five years later, Dieckmann and Schneider in Homburg, treated 6 out of 13 patients with alcoholism and addiction by stereotactic bilateral hypothalamotomy [362]. Four of the six developed memory problems, visual disturbances, or apathy. However, the authors concluded that this intervention enabled patients to increase their *self-control* over the 1–3 years of monitoring. They indicated that all patients complained of a marked decrease in their libido. It should be noted that this effect had been "used" in West Germany from 1962 to 1979, by Müller among others [298, 370], in the controversial, to say the least, "treatment" of 75 offenders and 59 sexually "deviant" individuals[94] (Fig. 5.1) [371–373].

---

[93] Cf. p. 179.

[94] Cf. p. 425 for the ethical questions raised by such interventions.

Ablation of the Nucleus Accumbens

The nucleus accumbens plays a central role in the pathophysiology of addiction and according to Li and Gao "removal of this structure lead to a blockage of the dopamine mesocorticolimbic circuit, preventing cravings for drugs after detoxification and in this way would prevent relapses" [354]. Studies in animal exploring this link were conducted by physicians at the military hospital in Xi'an. They showed that a lesion in the heart of the nucleus halts self-administration of opioids [374]. Given these encouraging preliminary results, the team practiced stereotactic interventions in 28 heroin patients and followed them for 15 months [375]. According to the authors, 11 patients did not relapse during this period, with psychological assessments showing a reduction in impulsivity and depression and anxiety symptoms. The Chinese team reported personality changes in two patients and transient memory disorders in four. It should be noted that seven patients were not included in the analysis results and contact was lost with two patients. It is estimated that "over one thousand addicts in nearly twenty hospitals were operated in 2004" by lesional surgery [354]. Interventions have not only targeted the nucleus accumbens but also the amygdala and cingulum. The Chinese Medical Journal reports that "the Chinese Ministry of Health announced in November 2004 (381) a ban on this practice [in the treatment of opiate addiction, Author's note] given the limited effectiveness of the operation, safety, and ethical implications, but it encouraged the scientific evaluation of this practice" [352]. Subsequently, studies evaluating this surgery estimated the relapse rate after 6–12 months between 15 and 54 % [376–378]. In 2012, Gao and colleagues published the results of a cohort of 272 heroin patients operated before 2004, with 69.5 % weaning after on year, and for 93 of them, 58 % cessation after 5 years [354, 379]. From 2007 to 2009, the Chinese team continued this surgery in twelve patients with a severe addiction to alcohol [380]. During a monitoring period lasting from 6 months to 2 years following the intervention, only two patients appeared to have relapsed. The authors mention that an average improvement in IQ was observed as well as decreased irritability and depressive symptoms. A team at another military hospital in Chengdu, conducted stimulation of the nucleus accumbens and amygdala prior to stereotactic ablation in 70 heroin patients. This study conducted from August to November 2004 does not mention results or monitoring practices and simply indicates that these experiments showed that stimulation of these regions (50 Hz à 2–4 V) could induce states of euphoria similar in intensity to the "high" of heroin use [352].

Deep Brain Stimulation of the Nucleus Accumbens

In 2005, Witjas et al. reported on two patients with Parkinson's disease also suffering from a *dopamine dysregulation syndrome,* which is a severe addiction to dopamine resulting in dopaminergic drug bulimia [363]. Both patients were treated by stimulation of subthalamic nucleus. The first patient, who suffered not only from this syndrome but also chronic alcoholism was weaned both off the syndrome and alcohol. The second patient was able to reduce his dopamine medication intake by three-quarters. The Marseille team suggested that this dependence could be counteracted by a direct stimulation of the reward circuit. The German team of Kuhn and Sturm reported the story of a 54-year-old man with severe agoraphobia associated with secondary depressive disorder and chronic alcoholism [381]. He was treated by bilateral stimulation of the nucleus accumbens (130 Hz, 3 V) for the treatment of severe anxiety. In the study, only a slight reduction in anxiety and depressive disorder was noted. However, the Cologne team did observe a drastic decrease in alcohol consumption. Based on this unexpected discovery and con-clusive results in animals for cocaine [382] and alcohol [382–384], withdrawal following stimulation of the nucleus accumbens, these researchers and students of the University Magdeburg turned to humans. Three patients addicted to alcohol for over 20 years who had failed all detoxification treatments were treated by stim-ulation of the nucleus accumbens. With a follow-up of 14 months, they showed that this stimulation, the electrodes located at the *shell*[95] of each of the cores, allowing a complete withdrawal in two of these patients while the third presented a single episode of relapse [385, 386]. The German team won, after a year of stimulation in a patient sixty nine consuming, on average, half a bottle of vodka a day for over 30 years, a complete withdrawal [387]. According to electrophysi-ological studies in the fourth chronic alcoholic patients, the effectiveness of deep brain stimulation would be based on a normalization of the activity of the anterior cingulate cortex made possible by modulating the activity of the nucleus accum-bens. We saw earlier, this is dysfunction of the dopaminergic system affecting the operation of anterior cingulate cortex [334, 347]. This failure causes a reduction of cortical inhibitory control explaining the difficulty resisting a refill [388]. After a new German study has come to confirm these results in five patients [359] ran-domized prospective studies, double-blind, this time, are now conducted in Ger-many in this indication. Following stimulation of the nucleus in a patient with severe OCD, a team from the Netherlands also found, in addition to the healing of OCD, tobacco cessation and morbid obesity overeating [356]. In 2011, a team from the University Hospital of Shanghai, led by Zhou and Jiang, published clinical results made 7 years ago by implantation of electrodes in the nucleus accumbens in a heroin addict patient, consuming an average of 1–2 g per day for 5 years [356]. This observation reinforces the hypothesis of close entanglements between CSTC circuits—including deregulation explains compulsive behaviors—and reward involved in addiction [356]. In 2011, a team from the University Hospital of Shanghai, led by Zhou and Jiang, published clinical results made 7 years ago by implantation of electrodes in the nucleus accumbens in a heroin addict patient, consuming an average of 1–2 g per day for 5 years [364]. Stimu-lation (145 Hz, 0.8–2.5 V) led to complete withdrawal allowing the removal of the neurostimulator 3 years later. The patient has not relapsed since. This Shanghai-based team has since operated on a new heroin patient but with a disappointing

---

[95] Cf. p. 129.

Table 4.13 Results of deep brain stimulation in the treatment of addiction

Study	Pt(s)	Addiction/target of DBS	Follow-up in months	Results
France, 2005 [363]	2	Dopamine/Subthlamic nucleus (Parkinson's)	18	Weaned
Netherlands, 2010 [356]	1	Tobacco/Nucleus accumbens (OCD)	24	Weaned
Germany, 2009 [355]	3	Tobacco/Nucleus accumbens (OCD, GTS)	30	Partially weaned
Germany, 2009 [359]	5	Alcohol/Nucleus accumbens	38	3/5 weaned
China, 2011 [364] China, 2012 [389]	1	Heroin/Nucleus accumbens	36	Weaned
	1	Heroin/Nucleus accumbens	?	partially weaned
Netherlands, 2012 [358]	1	Heroin/Nucleus accumbens	6	Weaned
Portugal, 2012 [390]	1	Cocaine/Nucleus accumbens	6	Partially weaned

result because he remains dependent on a methadone treatment [389]. In 2012, an Amsterdam team performed the same procedure but this time, with a portion of the electrode within the ALIC and end without the nucleus accumbens. For 4 months, the Dutch team correlated the consumption of heroin as the electrode pads stimulated (180 Hz, 3.5 V). They observed in this patient 47 heroin (0.5–0.6 g/j) for 22 years, until the middle part of the anterior limb of the internal capsule was stimulated, the average consumption increased at 0, 87 g per day while it dropped to 0.10 g when it came to the dorsal and 0.25 g for the nucleus accumbens. A complete withdrawal, but with an episode of relapse after 2 weeks, was finally obtained at 6 months [358]. In Lisbon, encouraging results, but with a shorter monitoring period, were reported in a patient dependent on cocaine since 14 years [390]. Upon stimulation by the electrodes implanted in the ALIC and the posterior part of the nucleus accumbens, the patient said, *the high caused by cocaine are much less intense and I take less pleasure from them, I am able to stop my intake even after the first dose* (Table 4.13).

Conclusion

Psychosurgical treatment, in particular lesional techniques, for addiction can lead to ethical problems regarding free and informed consent and conflicts of interest. We return to these points in the chapter on bioethics,[96] however we can already question the choice of offering patients lesional techniques. Whether in Russia or China policies regarding heroin are punitive [391] and drug trafficking is

---

[96] cf. p. 426.

punishable by death in China [392]. Moreover, these two countries offer little or no access to drug treatment programs such as methadone clinics [393, 394]. The absence of such therapy offers can not compare the efficacy of this surgery replacement therapy [395]. Aware of ethical issues, the majority of surgical teams working on these themes have oriented toward reversible deep brain stimulation techniques that appear promising and are more economical than replacement therapy with methadone [396]. However, financially attractive or reversible DBS of the nuclei accumbens may be, certain reservations must be made. Ethicists like Canadian Racine Canadian or Australian Hall are concerned about potential abuses of stimulation in addiction [397]. They believe today that clinical results remain fragile and it would be wise, at first, to wait until stimulation has proven less controversial in psychiatric disorders. Moreover, these neuroethicists recommend[97] that these therapeutic techniques be strictly regulated and remain exclusively used for refractory forms of addictions where the best treatment, including substitution, have failed. These authors emphasize the absolute necessity of obtaining consent by a fully independent authority and specify that this type of treatment cannot be administered within a context of coercion or injunctive care.

Eating Disorders

Abstract Morbid obesity is becoming a major public health problem; teams are looking at the neuromodulation of the hypothalamus, a center regulating hunger and satiety, in the treatment of this pathology. To date, very few interventions were performed, sometimes with unexpected results. As with anorexia nervosa, which shares some clinical features with OCD, and with some patients suffering from both disorders, deep brain stimulation of the anterior limb of the internal capsule has, in recent years, had a beneficial effect in a few patients.

Obesity

Obesity is defined as a *Body Mass Index* (BMI)[98] greater than 30 kg/m^2, and affects more than 500 million people on the planet. The cost to society would, by country, 2–7 % of health expenditure [398]. In the United States, for example, these costs would average a hundred billion dollars a year [399]. At this huge cost associated with the occurrence of diseases (diabetes, cardiovascular disease, sleep apnea, cancer, arthritis…) and to reduce the life expectancy of about 20 years, in addition an impaired quality of life for millions of individuals [400]. This public health problem worsens over time. In the United States, it is considered that the

---

[97] Cf. p. 443.
[98] BMI = (Weight in kg)/(size in cm)^2.

prevalence of obesity among adults over 20 years has doubled from 1980 to 2000 [401] while that of children and adolescents has tripled [402]. Two-thirds of Americans are overweight ($25 < BMI < 30$ kg/m^2) leading to 300,000 deaths each year. In morbid obesity ($BMI > 40$ kg/m^2), low calorie diets or pharmacological therapies [403] have a low efficacy because of the high rate of relapse. For 20 years, bariatric surgery has strengthened the therapeutic arsenal. These popular interventions [404], are meant to limit the absorption of nutrients by using a gastric band to restrict food intake, or in gastroplasty, by reducing the size of the stomach to lower the production of ghrelin [405], a hormone synthesized by the stomach which causes hunger. A second category of interventions, called mixed, associated gastric restriction with the creation of a branch of the digestive tract to reduce the absorption of nutrients from the gut, a "gastric bypass." These interventions reduce weight by 20–60 % [406, 407] resulting in a net decrease of comorbidities [406] and mortality [406] but in 10 % of cases a recurrence of obesity may be observed [408]. This percentage may exceed 40 % in extremely obese patients ($BMI > 50$ kg/m^2) [409]. Before bariatric surgery grows, psychosurgery lesional interventions have been proposed targeting the satiety centers in the thalamus. The disappointing results and frequent complications led to the abandonment of the practice. Today, with the new tools of deep brain stimulation, some teams have returned to this hypothalamic target. These clinical studies are reserved for extremely limited indications after failure of bariatric surgery. To understand these new developments, a reminder of the old hypothalamotomy intervention may be useful (Fig. 4.9).

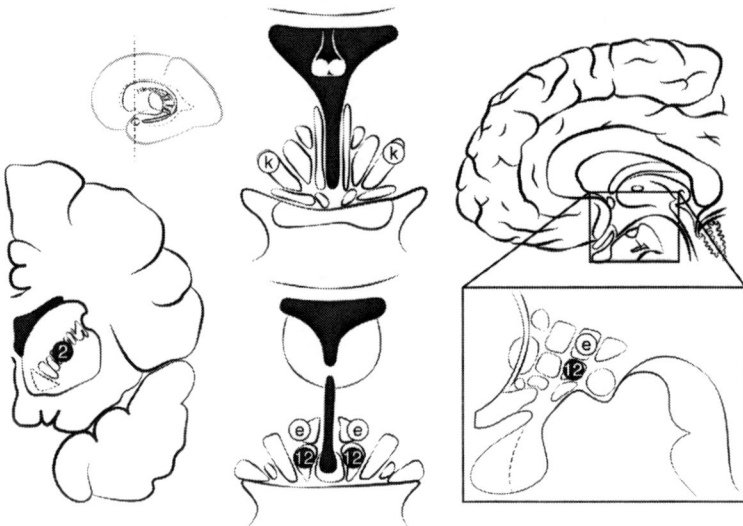

Fig. 4.9 Lesional or deep brain stimulation (*DBS*) targets in the treatment of eating disorders. (*e*) Dorsomedial hypothalamotomy: obesity, (*k*) lateral hypothalamotomy: obesity, (2) *DBS* of the anterior limb of the internal capsule: anorexia nervosa, (12) *DBS* of the ventromedial hypothalamus: obesity

Hypothalamotomy

The medial hypothalamus[99] houses the ventromedial and dorsomedial nuclei (Fig. 2.11, p. 68) responsible for hunger and thirst. The ventromedial nucleus, connected to the amygdala is involved in satiety[100] [410]. A lesion of this structure causes an exacerbation of appetite leading to obesity. Conversely, electrical stimulation of the nucleus reduces the active food intake, lipolysis, and reduces body mass [411]. Next to the medial hypothalamus are the lateral nuclei (Figs. 2. 12, 2.13, 2.14, p. 69, 70, 71) whose action differs from that of the ventromedial nucleus in that they promote consumption behavior the lesions of these lateral cores, under the control of the cortex and amygdala causes weight loss [412] or cachexia[101] [413–415]. In contrast, electrical stimulation of these segments increases food intake, body weight, and lipogenesis [416]. In 1974, the Danish F. Quaade performed in three obese patients electrostimulation of the lateral hypothalamus triggering feelings of hunger [417]. A unilateral thermocoagulation of this region was also practiced at the same time. In all, five patients, weighing between 118 and 180 kg, received a lateral hypothalamotomy. The endocrinologist reported decreased transient appetite and weight among this small cohort of patients [418]. Given these disappointing results and high risk of neurological complications, these interventions were quickly abandoned.

Deep Brain Stimulation

The Lateral Hypothalamus

Some authors [419] hypothesized that the weight gain, average 9 kg [420], which was frequently observed [420, 421] in patients treated by stimulation of subthalamic nuclei in the treatment of Parkinson's disease could be due to a chronic effect of stimulation of the lateral hypothalamus. A priori, the high frequency (130 Hz) should instead be an inhibitor effect similar to an injury, and therefore, conversely, cause weight loss. This bystander effect, in the hypothalamus, during stimulation of the thalamic nuclei is probably more complex, unless this weight gain is due to the improvement of power due to the reduction of abnormal movements even energy savings made possible by stopping dyskinesia [411]. Work done in obese rats showed that bilateral high frequency stimulation of the lateral hypothalamus resulted in a 16 % decrease 20 days after surgery despite a high calorie food. Following this work and observations made by Quaade, research

---

[99] Cf. p. 112.

[100] A hormone secreted by the white adipose tissue, leptin (from the Greek, λεπτός) sometimes also called the "hunger hormone," controls this at the level of the ventromedial nucleus.

[101] A state of weight loss and generalized fatigue caused by severe malnutrition or the terminal phase of a disease.

protocols are currently underway to assess the effectiveness of a high frequency stimulation of the lateral hypothalamus, similar to an injury but reversible and adaptable in patients suffering from a morbidly obesity (BMI > 40 kg/m^2) for which bariatric surgery has failed [422].

The Ventromedial Hypothalamus

The ventromedial nuclei are responsible for the feeling of satiety. Their damage causes an exacerbation of appetite and thus obesity [423]. Conversely, electrical stimulation, at a low frequency of this nucleus causes weight loss in rats. Recently, the work of N. Torres, S. Chabardes and A. Benobie, in Grenoble have shown that stimulation of thirty minutes at high frequency (130 Hz), of the ventromedial nucleus caused an increase in food intake in rats, while the low frequency (30 Hz) decreased intake [411]. Related results, with a decrease in adipose mass, were obtained in macaques by intraventricular stimulation of this area [424]. With 4 h a day, the high frequency stimulation leads, paradoxically, to a decrease in weight. Work nearby, led this time in pigs by De Sallesm team showed a decrease in weight of the animals after chronic low frequency stimulation (50 Hz) [425]. According to these researchers the weight reduction is not linked to a decrease in food intake but rather a change in metabolism. For now, this region was targeted only twice in humans. The first operation was conducted in 2008 by the Canadian team of C. Hamani and A. Lozano in a patient weighing 190 kg (IMC = 55 kg/m^2) [426]. A discreet, 6 % decrease in weight after 5 months was recorded at a low frequency stimulation (50 Hz, 3–4 V) without a change in diet or exercise. Stimulation at high frequency (130 Hz) for 6 months did not lead to weight reduction. At the end of the stimulation, the patient regained the lost weight, suggesting the reversibility of the effect of the stimulation. This intervention was remarkable not because of the modest weight loss, but because the 50-year-old patient, had a significant improvement in memory performance during high frequency stimulation. It was determined that the electrodes were more in contact with the fornix than the ventromedial nuclei. We know that the fornix are involved in the memory system, the Papez circuit, by connecting, in a reciprocal manner, the hippocampi to the mammillary bodies. This discovery led to the development of a research program in the treatment of Alzheimer's disease. Stimulation of the fornix in patients suffering from this neurodegenerative disease may be stopping the memory decline through a process of neurogenesis[102] [427]. The second action to stimulate the ventromedial hypothalamus was held in 2010 in an obese patient. Again, the gesture had unintended consequences: during stimulation (130 Hz, 1–7 V) the patient developed a severe panic attack. This effect, already seen in animals probably arises from the connections between this region of the hypothalamus and the amygdala. (Fig. 2.7, p. 59) [428, 429].

---

[102] Plasticity and neurogenesis in deep brain stimulation cf. p. 200.

The Nucleus Accumbens[103]

In 2010, the Amsterdam team, treating severe OCD by deep brain stimulation of the nucleus accumbens, implanted electrodes in a patient who, in addition to the obsessive-compulsive symptoms, was obese (BMI = 37) and a chronic smoker. Stimulation of this nucleus (185 Hz, 3,5 V) led to a decrease in the Y-BOCS score from 38 to 2 after 5 months, a loss of 44 kg (BMI = 25) and smoking cessation [356]. This result underlines the importance of the nucleus accumbens in compulsive, bulimic, and addictive behaviors. Closer examination of the links between the cortico-striato-thalamo-cortical circuits (CSTC), involved in OCD, and those of the reward involved in addictions is also necessary. Much clinical and laboratory evidence suggests that obesity is associated with dysregulation of the dopaminergic reward system [430–432]. Anatomically, moreover, there are reciprocal connections between the lateral hypothalamus, *hunger center*, and the nucleus accumbens, *pleasure center* [433, 434]. Abnormalities of this system would alter the functioning of the prefrontal and anterior cingulate cortex, itself the origin of inhibitory control to resist compulsive behaviors [334, 347, 388, 430]. Functional imaging studies have also shown an inverse correlation between the activity of these regions and BMI [435]. For now, the stimulation of the nucleus accumbens has not been the subject of research in the treatment of obesity [430].

Conclusion

Whether animal testing, old hypothalamotomy interventions or, today, deep brain stimulation, evidence is accumulating for the possible benefits of a neuromodulation treatment for refractory morbid obesity. Protocols for clinical research are underway to evaluate the efficacy and safety of such treatment [422]. These results, as well as the incidence and severity of complications which may arise during the neuromodulation should be compared with those of bariatric surgery. For the latter, a successful intervention is defined by a weight loss greater than 45 % in the year following the intervention. The success rate of these interventions amounted on average to 97 % for the bypass against 30 % for gastric banding and complications affected 33 % and 22 of subjects respectively. A team in Philadelphia compared the complications of bariatric surgery to those "of equivalent severity" from deep brain stimulation. From these different rates of success and complications, and some perplexing calculations, the authors conclude that deep brain stimulation must reach at least 83 % efficacy before becoming a valid alternative to bariatric surgery [436].

---

[103] Cf. p. 129.

Anorexia Nervosa

Abstract Anorexia nervosa, a condition that can be life-threatening, shares some clinical features with OCD. Based on this observation, teams have suggested using capsulotomy or deep brain stimulation techniques for patients in treatment failure. These results are preliminary and ethical hurdles remain: the sufferer is frequently in denial making it difficult to obtain consent.

Anorexia nervosa, with an insidious onset occurring typically excessive physical activity. The actual anorexia—i.e., loss of appetite—occurs only in a second phase, as a physiological consequence of prolonged fasting [437]. Weight loss is defined as a *Body Mass Index* (BMI)[104] less than 18.5 kg/m^2. Hospitalization usually occurs when the index falls below 14 kg/m^2, the prognosis being engaged below 13. Amenorrhea invariably has an early onset and late resolution. Associated with this triad, is the denial of the disease and thinness accompanied by an exaggerated interest in everything about food in a young patient who willingly over thinks. Psychiatric comorbidities are common whether anxiety disorder [438] or obsessive-compulsive disorders [438]. Biologically there is a dysregulation of the hypothalamic-pituitary axis, which amenorrhea demonstrates clinically, manifested by a decrease in thyroid and ovarian hormones.

The DSM-IV criteria for a diagnosis of anorexia nervosa are:

(a) refusal to maintain weight above the minimum normal weight (BMI < 18.5 kg/m^2);
(b) intense fear of gaining weight despite being underweight;
(c) altered perception of weight or shape of ones own body;
(d) undue influence of weight on self-esteem or denial of current thinness;
(e) amenorrhea for at least three consecutive cycles in menstruating women;

Nearly three-quarters of the patients were women [438], the prevalence of this disorder varies between 0.3 and 1 % [439] and concerns Western countries more [440]. Psychotherapy is the mainstay of treatment and also involves the parents of the adolescent whether by therapeutic alliance or family therapy. This therapeutic treatment sometimes requires hospitalization in cachectic states (BMI < 13 kg/m^2) in order to establish a *contract weight* which underpins future visits and the gradual weight gain. For 10 years, cognitive-behavioral therapy (CBT) have also demonstrated their effectiveness [441, 442], however psychotropic treatments are of little use. After a decade, healing is seen in a little less than half of the patients while a third has an *intermediate* cure [443]. In the remaining patients the disease becomes chronic or, in 5 % of cases, leads to death.

---

[104] BDI = Weight in kg/(Size in cm)^2.

Lesional Surgery During the Sixties

In North America, the craze that has taken over psychiatry in favor of surgical techniques has led some teams [444–447] to offer leucotomies to patients with advanced cachectic states. The effectiveness of these interventions, sometimes offered in life-threatening emergency situations [448, 449], remains difficult to assess. These interventions involved ten patients [450], and if weight gain was sometimes observed episodes of bulimia that followed and especially personality changes have seriously compromised the potential benefits of these generally coarse surgeries. In the late 1960s, A. Crisp at St George's Hospital à Londres London treated five patients with severe anorexia. By transorbitary leucotomies[105] for the first two, and stereotactic limbic leucotomies for the following three [450]. The justification for such psychiatrist actions was based on the similarities between this disease and obsessive-compulsive disorder. Four of these patients were followed by the British team for over 20 years. Three of them found a "reasonable quality of life" and an acceptable weight, while the first, operated by transorbital lobotomy, committed suicide. In 1993, a Chilean team performed a bilateral dorsomedial thalamotomy in two patients [451]. Monitoring, ranging from 2 to 4 years, seemed to show a significant weight gain and improved the quality of life with this man and this woman. The work by the Belgian team led by Nuttin on animal models for anorexia nervosa[106] has, indeed, shown an increased metabolism of the dorsal medial thalamus but also the cingulate cortex and ventral striatum [452]: three structures involved in the cortico-striato-thalamo-cortical loop.[107] Thalamotomies or even the high frequency stimulation in these rats, however, did not lead to weight gain [453]. Other functional imaging studies performed in patients with anorexia nervosa also point to abnormalities in the dorsolateral cortex, cingulate cortex, and striatum [454].

Therapeutic Prospects

According to studies, 10–40 % [438, 455] of anorexic patients present diagnostic criteria for obsessive personality or obsessive-compulsive disorder. The obsessive fear of gaining weight, recurrent and intrusive thoughts about body image, as well as the ritual meal planning and calorie counting are closer to obsessive-compulsive disorder. When authentic symptoms OCD are also present, they are often related to symmetry, order, accuracy, and cleanliness. Clinical similarities found in

---

[105] Cf. p. 42.

[106] This model involves restraining the animal's feeding to one and a half hours per day while giving the rat continuous access to a wheel. After a while, the animal develops hyperactive behavior and stops feeding spontaneously which leads to starvation and often death. (Routtenberg, A. 1968. "Self-starvation" of rats living in activity wheels: adaptation effects. J Comp Physiol Psychol 66:234–238).

[107] Cf. p. 139.

functional imaging results guide research in these two diseases toward a mal-function of the cortico-striato-thalamo-cortical circuit. In 2003, Nuttin with col-leagues at the University of Leuven reported on a 39-year-old woman with severe OCD and anorexia nervosa who had seen all her symptoms disappear after deep brain stimulation of the anterior limb of the internal capsule. Subsequently, she returned to a normal weight. The same progress has been made in 2005 in a 46-year-old patient suffering the same comorbidities. The team recently reported a third case, a 38-year-old woman with OCD since the age of 4 [456]. Symptoms began with fears of contamination by excrement and were accompanied by ritual washing. Later appeared the morbid fear of harming others and obsessive checking that she was being understood by her interlocutor by compulsively asking. For her anorexia nervosa, the patient was hospitalized a dozen times and the lowest weight was 27 kg (BMI = 9 kg/m^2). Given the severity of symptoms and repeated treatment failure, an anterior capsulotomy was performed. One year after surgery, the OCD had markedly decreased while the weight had increased from 40 (BMI = 13 kg/m^2) to 76 kg (BMI = 22 kg/m^2). From 2006 to 2011, a team led by B. Sun at Shanghai University operated on 104 patients with anorexia nervosa often asso-ciated with other psychiatric comorbidities. Among the 61 patients followed for more than a year, 56 were treated by anterior capsulotomy[108] and 12 by deep brain stimulation of the nucleus accumbens. These Chinese authors calculated that the mean BMI of 13.8 kg/m^2 had increased to 20.9 kg/m^2. With the exception of four subjects, menstrual cycles returned in all the patients. A majority of depressive symptoms, or obsessive fears also seemed to have disappeared [457].

In 2013, Lozano's team in Toronto published in the *Lancet* the results of a phase I study on six patients treated with the DBS of the subgenual area. By definition, this type of study aims primarily to determine the feasibility and the harmlessness of a therapy. This objective was achieved since the authors recorded the occurrence of only one epileptic episode 15 days after surgery. In terms of therapeutic efficacy, the mean BMI increased from 16.1 to 16.6 kg/m^2 9 months after surgery, only two patients were significantly improved (20 and 21 kg/m^2). Other avenues are being considered, including the hypothalamus. As we have seen, eating behaviors are under the control of two opposing structures: the lateral hypothalamus and the ventromedial hypothalamus. A lesion of the latter leads to overeating and obesity, while the low frequency electrical stimulation reduces food intake. The Grenoble team of A. Benabid, estimates that using opposite stimulation parameters it would be possible to treat severe forms of anorexia nervosa, but for now, no study has yet started [458]. Beyond questions about the optimal anatomical target, one of the main problems of the disease is probably the difficulty of obtaining informed consent from patients whose denial is a defense mechanism: denying their thinness, disputing the severity of their condition, dis-qualification of eating disorders, or any mental suffering.

---

[108] Eight of these anorexic patients had, at least 6 months prior, already received an operation for the placement of electrodes for stimulation of the nuclei accumbens.

Post-traumatic Stress Disorder

Abstract A state of post-traumatic stress, which follows a particularly traumatic event, is a mental disorder with potentially disastrous consequences. The amygdala, but also other structures of the limbic system, have abnormalities in people who suffer from this syndrome. Work targeting the amygdala is currently under investigation in the treatment of this pathology.

Post-traumatic stress disorder (PTSD) Post-traumatic stress disorder *combat fatigue, shell shocks*, or *war neurosis*. During their existence, 5–6 % of men and 10–14 % of women[109] will be affected by this syndrome which ranks fourth among psychiatric diseases [459]. The DSM-IV manual specifies that the subject must have witnessed an event in which individuals have been seriously injured or died, or his physical integrity was threatened. The diagnostic manual adds that *The reaction of the person to this event should include an intense fear, helplessness or horror* [153]. Thereafter the patient will persistently relive the traumatic event by repetitive memories, often actual "flashbacks," or intrusive nightmares and avoid anything that may be associated with the trauma. Besides emotional blunting, the patient has autonomic symptoms (restlessness, sleep disorder, anger, irritability, or disorder concentrating) and pain impacting their social and professional activities. Whether reliving the traumatic event, emotional numbing or autonomic activity, all of the symptoms must last more than a month before the diagnosis is retained. This psychic injury may be complicated in 60–75 % of cases by substance abuse, depression, and even suicide [459, 460]. The pathology remains under diagnosed because, as psychologist V. Dosseto notes, *the experience of shame, guilt and inhibition associated with these patients explains their reluctance to consult*. Usually, the treatment of this syndrome involves psychotherapy, including cognitive-behavioral therapy (CBT), antidepressants [459], the EMDR[110] [461, 462] and sometimes rTMS [463, 464]. Higher levels of noradrenaline[111] and thyroid hormones have been observed in these patients and may explain some of the symptoms such as panic attacks, insomnia, and hypervigilance and lowered blood cortisol levels[112] [465]. In these patients, recent studies point to functional neuroanatomical alterations in the amygdala, the cingulate cortex, and hippocampus [466, 467]. Functional imaging shows that amygdala activity is increased in patients with PTSD [466, 468]. A U.S. study of veterans who had received severe head injuries showed that soldiers with amygdala lesions developed little or no PTSD. In contrast, in patients being followed for this psychiatric condition,

---

[109] A total of 55 % of female victims of rape present PTSD, versus 7.5 % of subjects involved in traffic accidents or 14 % who have suffered the accidental death of a close friend or relative.

[110] Eye Movement Desensitization and Reprocessing is a neuro-emotional therapy based on eye movement. Results for PTSD are under evaluation.

[111] Noradrenergic circuit cf. p. 150.

[112] During the initial phase, a period of extreme stress, a sudden and significant increase in cortisol is observed (Fig. 2.15, p. 73), inhibition is secondary.

functional imaging did reveal hyperactivity in the amygdala [469]. The amygdala is involved in the processing of sensory information which may contain emotional content [470], storing memories with a strong emotional charge [312], as well as their recall [471]. Other studies, however, observe decreased activity in the anterior cingulate and orbitofrontal cortex [472]. It should be noted that in healthy subjects amygdala activity is curbed by the medial prefrontal cortex. The hippocampus, meanwhile, appears atrophied in patients with PTSD [473–475] and, in addition, a smaller hippocampus appears to be a risk factor for PTSD [476]. This latter observation would tend to show that the hippocampus could suppress the repetitive nature of traumatic recall. Recent work with animal models have shown that high frequency brain stimulation, notably of the amygdala, decreased PTSD symptoms [477, 478]. Despite the tentative nature of these first, encouraging results obtained in rodents, the authors suggest that some patients with severe and treatment-refractory PTSD could in the future benefit from a surgical therapy, either lesional or stimulation-based, targeting the amygdala or striato-prefrontal circuit [351, 479].

References

1. Denys D (2006) Pharmacotherapy of obsessive-compulsive disorder and obsessive-compulsive spectrum disorders. Psychiatr Clin North Am 29(2):553–584. doi:10.1016/j.psc.2006.02.013
2. Brody AL, Saxena S, Schwartz JM, Stoessel PW, Maidment K, Phelps ME et al (1998) FDG-PET predictors of response to behavioral therapy and pharmacotherapy in obsessive compulsive disorder. Psychiatry Res 84(1):1–6
3. Rauch SL, Shin LM, Dougherty DD, Alpert NM, Fischman AJ, Jenike MA (2007) Predictors of fluvoxamine response in contamination-related obsessive compulsive disorder: a PET symptom provocation study. Neuropsychopharmacology 27(5):782–791. doi:10.1016/S0893-133X(02)00351-2 S0893133X02003512 [pii]
4. Szeszko PR, Robinson D, Alvir JM, Bilder RM, Lencz T, Ashtari M et al (1999) Orbital frontal and amygdala volume reductions in obsessive-compulsive disorder. Arch Gen Psychiatry 56(10):913–919
5. Gilbert AR, Moore GJ, Keshavan MS, Paulson LA, Narula V, Mac Master FP et al (2000) Decrease in thalamic volumes of pediatric patients with obsessive-compulsive disorder who are taking paroxetine. Arch Gen Psychiatry 57(5):449–456
6. Scarone S, Colombo C, Livian S, Abbruzzese M, Ronchi P, Locatelli M et al (1992) Increased right caudate nucleus size in obsessive-compulsive disorder: detection with magnetic resonance imaging. Psychiatry Res 45(2):115–121
7. Robinson D, Wu H, Munne RA, Ashtari M, Alvir JM, Lerner G et al (1995) Reduced caudate nucleus volume in obsessive-compulsive disorder. Arch Gen Psychiatry 52(5):393–398
8. Jenike MA, Breiter HC, Baer L, Kennedy DN, Savage CR, Olivares MJ et al (1996) Cerebral structural abnormalities in obsessive-compulsive disorder. A quantitative morphometric magnetic resonance imaging study. Arch Gen Psychiatry 53(7):625–632
9. McGuire PK, Bench CJ, Frith CD, Marks IM, Frackowiak RS, Dolan RJ (1994) Functional anatomy of obsessive-compulsive phenomena. Br J Psychiatry 164(4):459–468

10. Rauch SL, Jenike MA, Alpert NM, Baer L, Breiter HC, Savage CR et al (1994) Regional cerebral blood flow measured during symptom provocation in obsessive-compulsive disorder using oxygen 15-labeled carbon dioxide and positron emission tomography. Arch Gen Psychiatry 51(1):62–70

11. Schwartz JM, Stoessel PW, Baxter LR Jr, Martin KM, Phelps ME (1996) Systematic changes in cerebral glucose metabolic rate after successful behavior modification treatment of obsessive-compulsive disorder. Arch Gen Psychiatry 53(2):109–113

12. Baxter LR Jr, Schwartz JM, Bergman KS, Szuba MP, Guze BH, Mazziotta JC et al (1992) Caudate glucose metabolic rate changes with both drug and behavior therapy for obsessive-compulsive disorder. Arch Gen Psychiatry 49(9):681–689

13. Swedo SE, Pietrini P, Leonard HL, Schapiro MB, Rettew DC, Goldberger EL et al (1992) Cerebral glucose metabolism in childhood-onset obsessive-compulsive disorder: revisualization during pharmacotherapy. Arch Gen Psychiatry 49(9):690–694

14. Saxena S, Brody AL, Maidment KM, Dunkin JJ, Colgan M, Alborzian S et al (1999) Localized orbitofrontal and subcortical metabolic changes and predictors of response to paroxetine treatment in obsessive-compulsive disorder. Neuropsychopharmacology 21(6):683–693. doi:10.1016/S0893-133X(99)00082-2 [pii] S0893133X99000822

15. Rauch SL, Dougherty DD, Malone D, Rezai A, Friehs G, Fischman AJ et al (2006) A functional neuroimaging investigation of deep brain stimulation in patients with obsessive-compulsive disorder. J Neurosurg 104(4):558–565. doi:10.3171/jns.2006.104.4.558

16. Haynes WI, Mallet L (2010) High-frequency stimulation of deep brain structures in obsessive-compulsive disorder: the search for a valid circuit. Eur J Neurosci 32(7):1118–1127. doi:10.1111/j.1460-9568.2010.07418.x

17. Carmin CN, Wiegartz PS, Yunus U, Gillock KL (2002) Treatment of late-onset OCD following basal ganglia infarct. Depress Anxiety 15(2):87–90 [pii] 10.1002/da.10024

18. Thobois S, Jouanneau E, Bouvard M, Sindou M (2004) Obsessive-compulsive disorder after unilateral caudate nucleus bleeding. Acta Neurochir (Wien) 146(9):1027–1031. doi:10.1007/s00701-004-0312-6 (discussion 31)

19. Baxter LC et al (2001) Cortical-subcortical systems in the mediation of OCD: modeling the brain's mediation of a classic "neurosis". In: Lichter DG, Cummings JL (eds) Frontal-subcortical circuits in psychiatric and neurological disorders. Guilford Press, New York, pp 207–230

20. Modell JG, Mountz JM, Curtis GC, Greden JF (1989) Neurophysiologic dysfunction in basal ganglia/limbic striatal and thalamocortical circuits as a pathogenetic mechanism of obsessive-compulsive disorder. J Neuropsychiatry Clin Neurosci 1(1):27–36

21. Lipsman N, Neimat JS, Lozano AM (2007) Deep brain stimulation for treatment-refractory obsessive-compulsive disorder: the search for a valid target. Neurosurgery 61(1):1–11. doi:10.1227/01.neu.0000279719.75403.f7 [pii] 00006123-200707000-00001 (discussion -3)

22. Merckelbach H, Wessel I (2000) Memory for actions and dissociation in obsessive-compulsive disorder. J Nerv Ment Dis 188(12):846–848

23. Sher KJ, Frost RO, Kushner M, Crews TM, Alexander JE (1989) Memory deficits in compulsive checkers: replication and extension in a clinical sample. Behav Res Ther 27(1):65–69 [pii] 0005-7967(89)90121-6

24. Gabriels L, Nuttin B (2012) Deep brain stimulation in the VC/VS for the treatment of OCD: role of the bed nucleus of the stria terminalis. In: Denys D, Feenstra M, Schuurman R (eds) Deep brain stimulation: a new frontier in psychiatry. Springer, Berlin, pp 35–41

25. Sauteraud A (2005) Le trouble obsessionnel-compulsif: Le manuel du thérapeute. Odile Jacob

26. Millet B, Jaafari N (2004) Approches thérapeutiques dans le trouble obsessionnel compulsif. Ann Med Psychol (Paris) 162:411–417

27. Polosan MM, B. Bougerol, T. Olié, J-P. Devaux, B (2003) Traitement psychochirurgical des TOC malins: à propos de trois cas. L'Encéphale XXIX(Cahier 1):514–552

28. France Comité consultatif national d'éthique pour les sciences de la vie et de la santé (2005) Avis sur la neurochirurgie fonctionnelle d'affections psychiatriques sévères. Ethique et recherche biomédicale Rapport 2002. la Documentation française, Paris

29. Lippitz BE, Mindus P, Meyerson BA, Kihlstrom L, Lindquist C (1999) Lesion topography and outcome after thermocapsulotomy or gamma knife capsulotomy for obsessive-compulsive disorder: relevance of the right hemisphere. Neurosurgery 44(3):452–458 (discussion 8-60)

30. Oliver B, Gascon J, Aparicio A, Ayats E, Rodriguez R, Maestro De Leon JL et al (2003) Bilateral anterior capsulotomy for refractory obsessive-compulsive disorders. Stereotact Funct Neurosurg 81(1–4):90–95. doi:10.1159/000075110 [pii] 75110

31. Ruck C, Karlsson A, Steele JD, Edman G, Meyerson BA, Ericson K et al (2008) Capsulotomy for obsessive-compulsive disorder: long-term follow-up of 25 patients. Arch Gen Psychiatry 65(8):914–921. doi:10.1001/archpsyc.65.8.914 [pii] 65/8/914

32. Baer L, Rauch SL, Ballantine HT Jr, Martuza R, Cosgrove R, Cassem E et al (1995) Cingulotomy for intractable obsessive-compulsive disorder. Prospective long-term follow-up of 18 patients. Arch Gen Psychiatry 52(5):384–392

33. Dougherty DD, Baer L, Cosgrove GR, Cassem EH, Price BH, Nierenberg AA et al (2002) Prospective long-term follow-up of 44 patients who received cingulotomy for treatment-refractory obsessive-compulsive disorder. Am J Psychiatry 159(2):269–275

34. Woerdeman PA, Willems PW, Noordmans HJ, Berkelbach van der Sprenkel JW, van Rijen PC (2006) Frameless stereotactic subcaudate tractotomy for intractable obsessive-compulsive disorder. Acta Neurochir (Wien) 148(6):633–637. doi:10.1007/s00701-006-0769-6 (discussion 7)

35. Kelly D, Richardson A, Mitchell-Heggs N (1973) Stereotactic limbic leucotomy: neurophysiological aspects and operative technique. Br J Psychiatry 123(573):133–140

36. Mallet L, Polosan M, Jaafari N, Baup N, Welter ML, Fontaine D et al (2008) Subthalamic nucleus stimulation in severe obsessive-compulsive disorder. N Engl J Med 359(20):2121–2134. doi:10.1056/NEJMoa0708514 [pii] 359/20/2121

37. Chabardes S, Polosan M, Krack P, Bastin J, Krainik A, David O et al (2012) Deep brain stimulation for obsessive-compulsive disorder: subthalamic nucleus target. World Neurosurg. doi:10.1016/j.wneu.2012.03.010 [pii]S1878-8750(12)00413-5

38. Nuttin B, Cosyns P, Demeulemeester H, Gybels J, Meyerson B (1999) Electrical stimulation in anterior limbs of internal capsules in patients with obsessive-compulsive disorder. Lancet 354(9189):1526. doi:10.1016/S0140-6736(99)02376-4 [pii] S0140-6736(99)02376-4

39. Nuttin BJ, Gabriels LA, Cosyns PR, Meyerson BA, Andreewitch S, Sunaert SG et al (2003) Long-term electrical capsular stimulation in patients with obsessive-compulsive disorder. Neurosurgery 52(6):1263–1272 (discussion 72-4)

40. Greenberg BD, Gabriels LA, Malone DA Jr, Rezai AR, Friehs GM, Okun MS et al (2010) Deep brain stimulation of the ventral internal capsule/ventral striatum for obsessive-compulsive disorder: worldwide experience. Mol Psychiatry 15(1):64–79. doi:10.1038/mp.2008.55 [pii] mp200855

41. Sturm V, Lenartz D, Koulousakis A, Treuer H, Herholz K, Klein JC et al (2003) The nucleus accumbens: a target for deep brain stimulation in obsessive-compulsive- and anxiety-disorders. J Chem Neuroanat 26(4):293–299 S0891061803001030 [pii]

42. Denys D, Mantione M, Figee M, van den Munckhof P, Koerselman F, Westenberg H et al (2010) Deep brain stimulation of the nucleus accumbens for treatment-refractory obsessive-compulsive disorder. Arch Gen Psychiatry 67(10):1061–1068. doi:10.1001/archgenpsychiatry.2010.122 [pii] 67/10/1061

43. Franzini A, Messina G, Gambini O, Muffatti R, Scarone S, Cordella R et al (2010) Deep-brain stimulation of the nucleus accumbens in obsessive compulsive disorder: clinical, surgical and electrophysiological considerations in two consecutive patients. Neurol Sci 31(3):353–359. doi:10.1007/s10072-009-0214-8

44. Jimenez-Ponce F, Velasco-Campos F, Castro-Farfan G, Nicolini H, Velasco AL, Salin-Pascual R et al (2009) Preliminary study in patients with obsessive-compulsive disorder

treated with electrical stimulation in the inferior thalamic peduncle. Neurosurgery 65(6 Suppl):203–209. doi:10.1227/01.NEU.0000345938.39199.90 [pii] 00006123-200912001-00026 (discussion 9)

45. Liu K, Zhang H, Liu C, Guan Y, Lang L, Cheng Y et al (2008) Stereotactic treatment of refractory obsessive compulsive disorder by bilateral capsulotomy with 3 years follow-up. J Clin Neurosci 15(6):622–629. doi:10.1016/j.jocn.2007.07.086 [pii] S0967-5868(07) 00497-3

46. Bingley TL, Leksell L, Meyerson BA, Rylander G (1977) Long-term results of stereotactic capsulotomy in chronic obsessive-compulsive neurosis. In: Sweet WOS, Martin Rodriguez JG (eds) Neurosurgical treatment in psychiatry, pain and epilepsy. University Park Press, Baltimore, pp 287–289

47. Herner T (1961) Treatment of mental disorders with frontal stereotaxic thermo-lesions. Acta Psychiatr Scand 36(158):1–140

48. Cosgrove GR (2009) Cingulotomy for depression and OCD. In: Lozano A (ed) Textbook of stereotactic and functional neurosurgery, vol 1, 2nd edn. Springer, NY, pp 2887–2896

49. Taub A, Lopes AC, Fuentes D, D'Alcante CC, de Mathis ME, Canteras MM et al (2009) Neuropsychological outcome of ventral capsular/ventral striatal gamma capsulotomy for refractory obsessive-compulsive disorder: a pilot study. J Neuropsychiatry Clin Neurosci 21(4):393–397. doi:10.1176/appi.neuropsych.21.4.393 [pii] 21/4/393

50. Lévêque MC, Régis J (2012) Radiosurgery for the treatment of psychiatric disorders: a review world neurosurgery

51. Ballantine HT Jr, Bouckoms AJ, Thomas EK, Giriunas IE (1987) Treatment of psychiatric illness by stereotactic cingulotomy. Biol Psychiatry 22(7):807–819 [pii] 0006-3223(87)90080-1

52. Foltz EL, White LE (1968) The role of rostral cingulumotomy in "pain" relief. Int J Neurol 6(3–4):353–373

53. Spangler WJ, Cosgrove GR, Ballantine HT, Jr, Cassem EH, Rauch SL, Nierenberg A et al (1996) Magnetic resonance image-guided stereotactic cingulotomy for intractable psychiatric disease. Neurosurgery 38(6):1071–1076 (discussion 6–8)

54. Rauch SL, Kim H, Makris N, Cosgrove GR, Cassem EH, Savage CR et al (2000) Volume reduction in the caudate nucleus following stereotactic placement of lesions in the anterior cingulate cortex in humans: a morphometric magnetic resonance imaging study. J Neurosurg 93(6):1019–1025. doi:10.3171/jns.2000.93.6.1019

55. Rauch SL, Makris N, Cosgrove GR, Kim H, Cassem EH, Price BH et al (2001) A magnetic resonance imaging study of regional cortical volumes following stereotactic anterior cingulotomy. CNS Spectr 6(3):214–222

56. Jung HH, Kim CH, Chang JH, Park YG, Chung SS, Chang JW (2006) Bilateral anterior cingulotomy for refractory obsessive-compulsive disorder: long-term follow-up results. Stereotact Funct Neurosurg 84(4):184–189. doi:10.1159/000095031 [pii] 95031

57. Kim CH, Chang JW, Koo MS, Kim JW, Suh HS, Park IH et al (2003) Anterior cingulotomy for refractory obsessive-compulsive disorder. Acta Psychiatr Scand 107(4):283–290 [pii] 087

58. Richter EO, Davis KD, Hamani C, Hutchison WD, Dostrovsky JO, Lozano AM (2004) Cingulotomy for psychiatric disease: microelectrode guidance, a callosal reference system for documenting lesion location, and clinical results. Neurosurgery 54(3):622–628 (discussion 8–30)

59. Jenike MA, Baer L, Ballantine T, Martuza RL, Tynes S, Giriunas I et al (1991) Cingulotomy for refractory obsessive-compulsive disorder. A long-term follow-up of 33 patients. Arch Gen Psychiatry 48(6):548–555

60. Goktepe EO, Young LB, Bridges PK (1975) A further review of the results of sterotactic subcaudate tractotomy. Br J Psychiatry 126:270–280

61. Hodgkiss AD, Malizia AL, Bartlett JR, Bridges PK (1995) Outcome after the psychosurgical operation of stereotactic subcaudate tractotomy, 1979–1991. J Neuropsychiatry Clin Neurosci 7(2):230–234

62. Kartsounis LD, Poynton A, Bridges PK, Bartlett JR (1991) Neuropsychological correlates of stereotactic subcaudate tractotomy: a prospective study. Brain 114(Pt 6):2657–2673
63. Kelly D, Richardson A, Mitchell-Heggs N, Greenup J, Chen C, Hafner RJ (1973) Stereotactic limbic leucotomy: a preliminary report on forty patients. Br J Psychiatry 123(573):141–148
64. Gabriels L (2009) DBS for OCD. In: Lozano A (ed) Textbook of stereotactic and functional neurosurgery, vol 1, 2nd edn. Springer, NY, pp 2887–2896
65. HAS (2005) Troubles obsessionnels compulsifs (TOC) résistants: prise en charge et place de la neurochirurgie fonctionnelle. In: professionnels HAdSH-Sevda (ed) Paris, p 80
66. de Koning PP, van den Munckhof P, Figee M, Schuurman PR, Denys D (2012) Deep brain stimulation in obsessive-compulsive disorder targeted at the nucleus accumbens. In: Denys D, Feenstra M, Schuurman R (eds) Deep brain stimulation: a new frontier in psychiatry. Springer, Berlin, pp 43–51
67. Mindus P, Rasmussen SA, Lindquist C (1994) Neurosurgical treatment for refractory obsessive-compulsive disorder: implications for understanding frontal lobe function. J Neuropsychiatry Clin Neurosci 6(4):467–477
68. Jenike MA (1998) Neurosurgical treatment of obsessive-compulsive disorder. Br J Psychiatry Suppl 35:79–90
69. Haynes WM (2012) Trouble obsessionnel compulsif, la place de la stimulation cérébrale profonde. Neurologies 15(144):37–40
70. Nau J (2008) Stimulation cérébrale profonde contre les TOC. Revue Médicale Suisse 181
71. Mallet L, Mesnage V, Houeto JL, Pelissolo A, Yelnik J, Behar C et al (2002) Compulsions, Parkinson's disease, and stimulation. Lancet 360(9342):1302–1304. doi:S0140-6736(02) 11339-0
72. Fontaine D, Mattei V, Borg M, von Langsdorff D, Magnie MN, Chanalet S et al (2004) Effect of subthalamic nucleus stimulation on obsessive-compulsive disorder in a patient with Parkinson disease Case report. J Neurosurg 100(6):1084–1086. doi:10.3171/jns.2004. 100.6.1084
73. Cosyns P, Gabriels L, Nuttin B (2003) Deep brain stimulation in treatment refractory obsessive compulsive disorder. Verh K Acad Geneeskd Belg 65(6):385–399 (discussion 99-400)
74. Gabriels L, Cosyns P, Nuttin B, Demeulemeester H, Gybels J (2003) Deep brain stimulation for treatment-refractory obsessive-compulsive disorder: psychopathological and neuropsychological outcome in three cases. Acta Psychiatr Scand 107(4):275–282. doi:10.1034/j.1600-0447.2003.00066.x
75. Nuttin B, Gybels J, Cosyns P, Gabriels L, Meyerson B, Andreewitch S et al (2003) Deep brain stimulation for psychiatric disorders. Neurosurg Clin N Am 14(2):xv–xvi
76. Goodman WK, Foote KD, Greenberg BD, Ricciuti N, Bauer R, Ward H et al (2010) Deep brain stimulation for intractable obsessive compulsive disorder: pilot study using a blinded, staggered-onset design. Biol Psychiatry 67(6):535–542. doi:10.1016/j.biopsych.2009.11.028 [pii] S0006-3223(09)01426-7
77. Huff W, Lenartz D, Schormann M, Lee SH, Kuhn J, Koulousakis A et al (2010) Unilateral deep brain stimulation of the nucleus accumbens in patients with treatment-resistant obsessive-compulsive disorder: Outcomes after one year. Clin Neurol Neurosurg. 112(2):137–143. doi:10.1016/j.clineuro.2009.11.006 [pii] S0303-8467(09)00303-5
78. Aouizerate B, Cuny E, Martin-Guehl C, Guehl D, Amieva H, Benazzouz A et al (2004) Deep brain stimulation of the ventral caudate nucleus in the treatment of obsessive-compulsive disorder and major depression Case report. J Neurosurg 101(4):682–686. doi:10.3171/jns.2004.101.4.0682
79. Haynes WI, Mallet L (2012) What is the role of the subthalamic nucleus in OCD. Elements and insights from DBS. In: Denys D, Feenstra M, Schuurman R (eds) Deep brain stimulation: a new frontier in psychiatry. Springer, Berlin, pp 53–60

80. Abelson JL, Curtis GC, Sagher O, Albucher RC, Harrigan M, Taylor SF et al (2005) Deep brain stimulation for refractory obsessive-compulsive disorder. Biol Psychiatry 57(5):510–516. doi:10.1016/j.biopsych.2004.11.042 [pii] S0006-3223(04)01285-5

81. Greenberg BD, Malone DA, Friehs GM, Rezai AR, Kubu CS, Malloy PF et al (2006) Three-year outcomes in deep brain stimulation for highly resistant obsessive-compulsive disorder. Neuropsychopharmacology 31(11):2384–2393. doi:10.1038/sj.npp.1301165 [pii] 1301165

82. Pepper J, Hariz M (2012) Anterior capsulotomy versus dbs for obsessive compulsive disorder: a review of the literature. In: XXth Congress of the European Society for stereotactic and functional neurosurgery; 27 Sep 2012, Cascais, Portugal

83. Gilles de la Tourette G (1885) Etude sur une affection nerveuse caracterisée par l'incoordination motrice accompagnée d'écholalie et de coprolalie. Arch Neurol 9(19):158–200

84. Berardelli A, Curra A, Fabbrini G, Gilio F, Manfredi M (2003) Pathophysiology of tics and Tourette syndrome. J Neurol 250(7):781–787. doi:10.1007/s00415-003-1102-4

85. Moutaud B (2009) «C'est un problème neurologique ou psychiatrique ?» Ethnologie de la stimulation cérébrale profonde appliquée au trouble obsessionnel compulsif. Université Paris Descartes, Paris

86. Lombroso PJ, Mack G, Scahill L, King RA, Leckman JF (1991) Exacerbation of Gilles de la Tourette's syndrome associated with thermal stress: a family study. Neurology 41(12):1984–1987

87. Leckman JF, Riddle MA, Hardin MT, Ort SI, Swartz KL, Stevenson J et al (1989) The yale global tic severity scale: initial testing of a clinician-rated scale of tic severity. J Am Acad Child Adolesc Psychiatry 28(4):566–573. doi:10.1097/00004583-198907000-00015 [pii] S0890-8567(09)65477-0

88. Goetz CG, Pappert EJ, Louis ED, Raman R, Leurgans S (1999) Advantages of a modified scoring method for the rush video-based tic rating scale. Mov Disord 14(3):502–506

89. Sassi M, Porta M, Servello D (2011) Deep brain stimulation therapy for treatment-refractory Tourette's syndrome: a review. Acta Neurochir (Wien) 153(3):639–645. doi:10.1007/s00701-010-0803-6

90. Robertson MM (1989) The Gilles de la Tourette syndrome: the current status. Br J Psychiatry 154:147–169

91. Visser-Vandewalle V (2009) Surgical procedure for Tourette's Syndrome. In: Lozano A (ed) Textbook of stereotactic and functional neurosurgery, 2nd edn. Springer, NY, pp 2963–2969

92. Jankovic J (2001) Tourette's syndrome. N Engl J Med 345(16):1184–1192. doi:10.1056/NEJMra010032

93. Kurlan R, Behr J, Medved L, Como P (1988) Transient tic disorder and the spectrum of Tourette's syndrome. Arch Neurol 45(11):1200–1201

94. Krack P, Hariz MI, Baunez C, Guridi J, Obeso JA (2010) Deep brain stimulation: from neurology to psychiatry? Trends Neurosci 33(10):474–484. doi:10.1016/j.tins.2010.07.002 [pii] S0166-2236(10)00105-0

95. Abramowitz JS, Taylor S, McKay D (2009) Obsessive-compulsive disorder. Lancet 374(9688):491–499. doi:10.1016/S0140-6736(09)60240-3 [pii] S0140-6736(09)60240-3

96. Leckman JF, Bloch MH, Scahill L, King RA (2006) Tourette syndrome: the self under siege. J Child Neurol 21(8):642–649

97. Jankovic J, Sekula S (1998) Dermatological manifestations of Tourette syndrome and obsessive-compulsive disorder. Arch Dermatol 134(1):113–114

98. Hyde TM, Aaronson BA, Randolph C, Rickler KC, Weinberger DR (1992) Relationship of birth weight to the phenotypic expression of Gilles de la Tourette's syndrome in monozygotic twins. Neurology 42(3 Pt 1):652–658

99. Leckman JF, Dolnansky ES, Hardin MT, Clubb M, Walkup JT, Stevenson J et al (1990) Perinatal factors in the expression of Tourette's syndrome: an exploratory study. J Am Acad Child Adolesc Psychiatry. 29(2):220–226. doi:10.1097/00004583-199003000-00010 [pii] S0890-8567(09)65511-8

100. Swerdlow NR, Young AB (2001) Neuropathology in Tourette syndrome: an update. Adv Neurol 85:151–161
101. Singer HS, Minzer K (2003) Neurobiology of Tourette's syndrome: concepts of neuroanatomic localization and neurochemical abnormalities. Brain Dev 25(Suppl 1):S70–S84. doi:S038776040390012X
102. Vesterhus P (1971) Tics in children. Differential diagnosis, etiology and therapy. Tidsskr Nor Laegeforen 91(4):285–288
103. Peterson BS, Skudlarski P, Anderson AW, Zhang H, Gatenby JC, Lacadie CM et al (1998) A functional magnetic resonance imaging study of tic suppression in Tourette syndrome. Arch Gen Psychiatry 55(4):326–333
104. Goldstein M, Anderson LT, Reuben R, Dancis J (1985) Self-mutilation in Lesch-Nyhan disease is caused by dopaminergic denervation. Lancet 1(8424):338–339. doi:S0140-6736(85)91107-9
105. Jinnah HA, Wojcik BE, Hunt M, Narang N, Lee KY, Goldstein M et al (1994) Dopamine deficiency in a genetic mouse model of Lesch-Nyhan disease. J Neurosci 14(3 Pt 1):1164–1175
106. Sallee FR, Nesbitt L, Jackson C, Sine L, Sethuraman G (1997) Relative efficacy of haloperidol and pimozide in children and adolescents with Tourette's disorder. Am J Psychiatry 154(8):1057–1062
107. Diallo R (2007) Prise en charge thérapeutique des tics dans la maladie de Gilles de la Tourette. Revue Neurologique 163(3):375–386
108. Lang A (2001) Update on the treatment of tics. In: Cohen DJ et al (eds) Advances in neurology. Tourette syndrome. Lippincott Williams and Wilkins, Philadelphia, pp 355–362
109. Temel Y, Visser-Vandewalle V (2004) Surgery in Tourette syndrome. Mov Disord. 19(1):3–14. doi:10.1002/mds.10649
110. Martinez-Fernandez R, Zrinzo L, Aviles-Olmos I, Hariz M, Martinez-Torres I, Joyce E et al (2011) Deep brain stimulation for Gilles de la Tourette syndrome: a case series targeting subregions of the globus pallidus internus. Mov Disord 26(10):1922–1930. doi:10.1002/mds.23734
111. Hariz MI, Robertson MM (2010) Gilles de la Tourette syndrome and deep brain stimulation. Eur J Neurosci 32(7):1128–1134. doi:10.1111/j.1460-9568.2010.07415.x
112. Servello D, Porta M, Sassi M, Brambilla A, Robertson MM (2008) Deep brain stimulation in 18 patients with severe Gilles de la Tourette syndrome refractory to treatment: the surgery and stimulation. J Neurol Neurosurg Psychiatry 79(2):136–142. doi:10.1136/jnnp.2006.104067
113. Servello D, Sassi M, Brambilla A, Defendi S, Porta M (2010) Long-term, post-deep brain stimulation management of a series of 36 patients affected with refractory gilles de la tourette syndrome. Neuromodulation 13(3):187–194. doi:10.1111/j.1525-1403.2009.00253.x
114. Viswanathan A, Jimenez-Shahed J, Baizabal Carvallo JF, Jankovic J (2012) Deep brain stimulation for Tourette syndrome: target selection. Stereotact Funct Neurosurg 90(4):213–224. doi:10.1159/000337776
115. Baer L, Rauch SL, Jenike MA, Cassem NH, Ballantine HT, Manzo PA et al (1994) Cingulotomy in a case of concomitant obsessive-compulsive disorder and Tourette's syndrome. Arch Gen Psychiatry 51(1):73–74
116. Visser-Vandewalle V, Ackermans L, van der Linden C, Temel Y, Tijssen MA, Schruers KR et al (2006) Deep brain stimulation in Gilles de la Tourette's syndrome. Neurosurgery 58(3):E590. doi:10.1227/01.NEU.0000207959.53198.D6 [piii] 00006123-200603000-00032
117. Idris Z, Ghani AR, Mar W, Bhaskar S, Wan Hassan WN, Tharakan J et al (2010) Intracerebral haematomas after deep brain stimulation surgery in a patient with Tourette syndrome and low factor XIIIA activity. J Clin Neurosci 17(10):1343–1344. doi:10.1016/j.jocn.2010.01.054 [pii] S0967-5868(10)00249-3

118. Martinez-Torres I, Hariz MI, Zrinzo L, Foltynie T, Limousin P (2009) Improvement of tics after subthalamic nucleus deep brain stimulation. Neurology 72(20):1787–1789. doi:10. 1212/WNL.0b013e3181a60a0c

119. Flaherty AW, Williams ZM, Amirnovin R, Kasper E, Rauch SL, Cosgrove GR et al (2005) Deep brain stimulation of the anterior internal capsule for the treatment of Tourette syndrome: technical case report. Neurosurgery 57(4 Suppl):E403. doi:00006123-200510004-00029 [pii] (discussion E)

120. Neuner I, Podoll K, Lenartz D, Sturm V, Schneider F (2009) Deep brain stimulation in the nucleus accumbens for intractable Tourette's syndrome: follow-up report of 36 months. Biol Psychiatry 65(4):e5–e6. doi:10.1016/j.biopsych.2008.09.030 [pii] S0006-3223(08)01170-0

121. Maciunas RJ, Maddux BN, Riley DE, Whitney CM, Schoenberg MR, Ogrocki PJ et al (2007) Prospective randomized double-blind trial of bilateral thalamic deep brain stimulation in adults with Tourette syndrome. J Neurosurg 107(5):1004–1014. doi:10. 3171/JNS-07/11/1004

122. Vandewalle V, van der Linden C, Groenewegen HJ, Caemaert J (1999) Stereotactic treatment of Gilles de la Tourette syndrome by high frequency stimulation of thalamus. Lancet 353(9154):724. doi:S0140673698059649

123. Dehning S, Mehrkens JH, Muller N, Botzel K (2008) Therapy-refractory Tourette syndrome: beneficial outcome with globus pallidus internus deep brain stimulation. Mov Disord 23(9):1300–1302. doi:10.1002/mds.21930

124. Vilela Filho O, Ragazzo PC, Silva DJ, Souza JT, Oliveira PM, Ribeiro TMC (2007) Bilateral globus pallidus externus deep brain stimulation (GPe-DBS) for the treatment of Tourette syndrome: an ongoing prospective controlled study. Stereotact Funct Neurosurg 85:42–43

125. Babel TB, Warnke PC, Ostertag CB (2001) Immediate and long term outcome after infrathalamic and thalamic lesioning for intractable Tourette's syndrome. J Neurol Neurosurg Psychiatry 70(5):666–671

126. Cappabianca P, Spaziante R, Carrabs G, de Divitiis E (1987) Surgical stereotactic treatment for Gilles de la Tourette's syndrome. Acta Neurol (Napoli) 9(4):273–280

127. Cooper IS (1962) Dystonia reversal by operation on basal ganglia. Arch Neurol 7:132–145

128. Hassler R (1982) Stereotaxic surgery for psychiatric disturbances. In: Schaltenbrand G et al (eds) Stereotaxy of the human brain. Thieme-Stratton Inc., New York, pp 570–590

129. Korzenev AV, Shoustin VA, Anichkov AD, Polonskiy JZ, Nizkovolos VB, Oblyapin AV (1997) Differential approach to psychosurgery of obsessive disorders. Stereotact Funct Neurosurg 68(1–4 Pt 1):226–230

130. Leckman JF, de Lotbiniere AJ, Marek K, Gracco C, Scahill L, Cohen DJ (1993) Severe disturbances in speech, swallowing, and gait following stereotactic infrathalamic lesions in Gilles de la Tourette's syndrome. Neurology 43(5):890–894

131. Rauch SL, Baer L, Cosgrove GR, Jenike MA (1995) Neurosurgical treatment of Tourette's syndrome: a critical review. Compr Psychiatry 36(2):141–156

132. Nadvornik P, Sramka M, Lisy L, Svicka I (1972) Experiences with dentatotomy. Confin Neurol 34(5):320–324

133. Visser-Vandewalle V, Temel Y, Boon P, Vreeling F, Colle H, Hoogland G et al (2003) Chronic bilateral thalamic stimulation: a new therapeutic approach in intractable Tourette syndrome: report of three cases. J Neurosurg 99(6):1094–1100. doi:10.3171/jns.2003.99.6. 1094

134. Bajwa RJ, de Lotbiniere AJ, King RA, Jabbari B, Quatrano S, Kunze K et al (2007) Deep brain stimulation in Tourette's syndrome. Mov Disord 22(9):1346–1350. doi:10.1002/mds. 21398

135. Egidi M et al (eds) (2005) Thalamic DBS in Tourette's syndrome: case report. In: 14th meeting of the WSSFN, Rome

136. Diederich NJ, Kalteis K, Stamenkovic M, Pieri V, Alesch F (2005) Efficient internal pallidal stimulation in Gilles de la Tourette syndrome: a case report. Mov Disord 20(11):1496–1499. doi:10.1002/mds.20551

137. Ackermans L, Temel Y, Cath D, van der Linden C, Bruggeman R, Kleijer M et al (2006) Deep brain stimulation in Tourette's syndrome: two targets? Mov Disord 21(5):709–713. doi:10.1002/mds.20816

138. Gallagher CL, Garell PC, Montgomery EB Jr (2006) Hemi tics and deep brain stimulation. Neurology 66(3):E12. doi:10.1212/01.wnl.0000190258.92496.a4 [pii] 66/3/E12

139. Shahed J, Poysky J, Kenney C, Simpson R, Jankovic J (2007) GPi deep brain stimulation for Tourette syndrome improves tics and psychiatric comorbidities. Neurology 68(2):159–160. doi:10.1212/01.wnl.0000250354.81556.90 [pii] 68/2/159

140. Dueck A, Wolters A, Wunsch K, Bohne-Suraj S, Mueller JU, Haessler F et al (2009) Deep brain stimulation of globus pallidus internus in a 16-year-old boy with severe tourette syndrome and mental retardation. Neuropediatrics 40(5):239–242. doi:10.1055/s-0030-1247519

141. Houeto JL, Karachi C, Mallet L, Pillon B, Yelnik J, Mesnage V et al (2005) Tourette's syndrome and deep brain stimulation. J Neurol Neurosurg Psychiatry 76(7):992–995. doi:10.1136/jnnp.2004.043273 [pii] 76/7/992

142. Kuhn J, Lenartz D, Mai JK, Huff W, Lee SH, Koulousakis A, Klosterkoetter J, Sturm V (2007) Deep brain stimulation of the nucleus accumbens and the internal capsule in therapeutically refractory Tourette-syndrome. J Neurol 254:963–965

143. Zabek M, Sobstyl M, Koziara H, Dzierzecki S (2008) Deep brain stimulation of the right nucleus accumbens in a patient with Tourette syndrome: case report. Neurol Neurochir Pol 42(6):554–559. doi:11799

144. Welter ML, Mallet L, Houeto JL, Karachi C, Czernecki V, Cornu P et al (2008) Internal pallidal and thalamic stimulation in patients with Tourette syndrome. Arch Neurol 65(7):952–957. doi:10.1001/archneur.65.7.952 [pii] 65/7/952

145. Ackermans L, Duits A, van der Linden C, Tijssen M, Schruers K, Temel Y et al (2011) Double-blind clinical trial of thalamic stimulation in pa- tients with Tourette syndrome. Brain 134:832–844

146. Como PG (2001) Neuropsychological function in Tourette syndrome. Adv Neurol 85:103–111

147. Mink JW, Walkup J, Frey KA, Como P, Cath D, Delong MR et al (2006) Patient selection and assessment recommendations for deep brain stimulation in Tourette syndrome. Mov Disord 21(11):1831–1838. doi:10.1002/mds.21039

148. Pansaon Piedad JC, Rickards HE, Cavanna AE (2012) What patients with gilles de la tourette syndrome should be treated with deep brain stimulation and what is the best target? Neurosurgery 71(1):173–192. doi:10.1227/NEU.0b013e3182535a00

149. Kessler RC, Chiu WT, Demler O, Merikangas KR, Walters EE (2005) Prevalence, severity, and comorbidity of 12-month DSM-IV disorders in the National Comorbidity Survey Replication. Arch Gen Psychiatry 62(6):617–627. doi:10.1001/archpsyc.62.6.617 [pii] 62/6/617

150. Lopez AD, Mathers CD, Ezzati M, Jamison DT, Murray CJ (2006) Global and regional burden of disease and risk factors, 2001: systematic analysis of population health data. Lancet 367(9524):1747–1757. doi:10.1016/S0140-6736(06)68770-9 [pii] S0140-6736(06)68770-9

151. Joukamaa M, Heliovaara M, Knekt P, Aromaa A, Raitasalo R, Lehtinen V (2001) Mental disorders and cause-specific mortality. Br J Psychiatry 179:498–502

152. Moussavi S, Chatterji S, Verdes E, Tandon A, Patel V, Ustun B (2007) Depression, chronic diseases, and decrements in health: results from the World Health Surveys. Lancet 370(9590):851–858. doi:10.1016/S0140-6736(07)61415-9

153. American Psychiatric Association (2000) American Psychiatric Association. Task Force on DSM-IV. Diagnostic and statistical manual of mental disorders: DSM-IV-TR, 4th ed. American Psychiatric Association, Washington, DC

154. Beck AT, Ward CH, Mendelson M, Mock J, Erbaugh J (1961) An inventory for measuring depression. Arch Gen Psychiatry 4:561–571

155. Hamilton M (1967) Development of a rating scale for primary depressive illness. Br J Soc Clin Psychol 6(4):278–296

156. Anderson RJ, Frye MA, Abulseoud OA, Lee KH, McGillivray JA, Berk M et al (2012) Deep brain stimulation for treatment-resistant depression: efficacy, safety and mechanisms of action. Neurosci Biobehav Rev 36(8):1920–1933. doi:10.1016/j.neubiorev.2012.06.001

157. Rauch SL (2003) Neuroimaging and neurocircuitry models pertaining to the neurosurgical treatment of psychiatric disorders. Neurosurg Clin N Am 14(2):213–223, vii–viii

158. Mayberg HS (2003) Modulating dysfunctional limbic-cortical circuits in depression: towards development of brain-based algorithms for diagnosis and optimised treatment. Br Med Bull 65:193–207

159. Drevets WC (1998) Functional neuroimaging studies of depression: the anatomy of melancholia. Annu Rev Med 49:341–361. doi:10.1146/annurev.med.49.1.341

160. George MS, Ketter TA, Parekh PI, Rosinsky N, Ring HA, Pazzaglia PJ et al (1997) Blunted left cingulate activation in mood disorder subjects during a response interference task (the Stroop). J Neuropsychiatry Clin Neurosci 9(1):55–63

161. Drevets WC, Bogers W, Raichle ME (2002) Functional anatomical correlates of antidepressant drug treatment assessed using PET measures of regional glucose metabolism. Eur Neuropsychopharmacol 12(6):527–544. doi:S0924977X02001025 [pii]

162. Drevets WC (2007) Orbitofrontal cortex function and structure in depression. Ann NY Acad Sci 1121:499–527. doi:10.1196/annals.1401.029 [pii] annals.1401.029

163. Drevets WC, Videen TO, Price JL, Preskorn SH, Carmichael ST, Raichle ME (1992) A functional anatomical study of unipolar depression. J Neurosci 12(9):3628–3641

164. Brody AL, Saxena S, Silverman DH, Alborzian S, Fairbanks LA, Phelps ME et al (1999) Brain metabolic changes in major depressive disorder from pre- to post-treatment with paroxetine. Psychiatry Res 91(3):127–139

165. Mayberg HS, Brannan SK, Mahurin RK, Jerabek PA, Brickman JS, Tekell JL et al (1997) Cingulate function in depression: a potential predictor of treatment response. Neuroreport 8(4):1057–1061

166. Pizzagalli D, Pascual-Marqui RD, Nitschke JB, Oakes TR, Larson CL, Abercrombie HC et al (2001) Anterior cingulate activity as a predictor of degree of treatment response in major depression: evidence from brain electrical tomography analysis. Am J Psychiatry 158(3):405–415

167. Mayberg HS (2003) Positron emission tomography imaging in depression: a neural systems perspective. Neuroimaging Clin N Am 13(4):805–815

168. Kennedy SH, Evans KR, Kruger S, Mayberg HS, Meyer JH, McCann S et al (2001) Changes in regional brain glucose metabolism measured with positron emission tomography after paroxetine treatment of major depression. Am J Psychiatry 158(6):899–905

169. Kennedy SH, Konarski JZ, Segal ZV, Lau MA, Bieling PJ, McIntyre RS et al (2007) Differences in brain glucose metabolism between responders to CBT and venlafaxine in a 16-week randomized controlled trial. Am J Psychiatry 164(5):778–788. doi:10.1176/appi.ajp.164.5.778 [pii] 164/5/778

170. Goldapple K, Segal Z, Garson C, Lau M, Bieling P, Kennedy S et al (2004) Modulation of cortical-limbic pathways in major depression: treatment-specific effects of cognitive behavior therapy. Arch Gen Psychiatry 61(1):34–41. doi:10.1001/archpsyc.61.1.3461/1/34 [pii] 61/1/34

171. Mayberg HS, Liotti M, Brannan SK, McGinnis S, Mahurin RK, Jerabek PA et al (1999) Reciprocal limbic-cortical function and negative mood: converging PET findings in depression and normal sadness. Am J Psychiatry 156(5):675–682

172. Johansen-Berg H, Gutman DA, Behrens TE, Matthews PM, Rushworth MF, Katz E et al (2008) Anatomical connectivity of the subgenual cingulate region targeted with deep brain stimulation for treatment-resistant depression. Cereb Cortex 18(6):1374–1383. doi:bhm167 10.1093/cercor/bhm167

173. Keller MB (2005) Issues in treatment-resistant depression. J Clin Psychiatry 66(Suppl 8):5–12

174. Nierenberg AA, Katz J, Fava M (2007) A critical overview of the pharmacologic management of treatment-resistant depression. Psychiatr Clin North Am 30(1):13–29. doi:10.1016/j.psc.2007.01.001 [pii] S0193-953X(07)00002-0
175. Fava M (2003) Diagnosis and definition of treatment-resistant depression. Biol Psychiatry 53(8):649–659. doi:S0006322303002312 [pii]
176. Rush AJ, Thase ME, Dube S (2003) Research issues in the study of difficult-to-treat depression. Biol Psychiatry 53(8):743–753. doi:S000632230300088X [pii]
177. Petersen T, Papakostas GI, Posternak MA, Kant A, Guyker WM, Iosifescu DV et al (2005) Empirical testing of two models for staging antidepressant treatment resistance. J Clin Psychopharmacol 25(4):336–341. doi:00004714-200508000-00008 [pii]
178. Souery D, Amsterdam J, de Montigny C, Lecrubier Y, Montgomery S, Lipp O et al (1999) Treatment resistant depression: methodological overview and operational criteria. Eur Neuropsychopharmacol 9(1–2):83–91. doi:S0924-977X(98)00004-2 [pii]
179. Parker GB, Malhi GS, Crawford JG, Thase ME (2005) Identifying "paradigm failures" contributing to treatment-resistant depression. J Affect Disord 87(2–3):185–191. doi:10.1016/j.jad.2005.02.015 [pii] S0165-0327(05)00072-8
180. Hauptman JS, DeSalles AA, Espinoza R, Sedrak M, Ishida W (2008) Potential surgical targets for deep brain stimulation in treatment-resistant depression. Neurosurg Focus 25(1):E3. doi:10.3171/FOC/2008/25/7/E3
181. Rasmussen K (2002) The practice of electroconvulsive therapy: recommendations for treatment, training, and privileging, 2nd edn. J ECT 18(1):58–59
182. Cabut S (2012) Neurologie : volte-face sur l'électrochoc. Le Monde
183. Szekely DP (2010) Les thérapeutiques non médicamenteuses en psychiatrie. Ann Med Psychol (Paris) 168:546–551
184. Grunhaus L, Schreiber S, Dolberg OT, Polak D, Dannon PN (2003) A randomized controlled comparison of electroconvulsive therapy and repetitive transcranial magnetic stimulation in severe and resistant nonpsychotic major depression. Biol Psychiatry 53(4):324–331. doi:S0006322302014993 [pii]
185. Dannon PN, Grunhaus L (2003) Repetitive transcranial magnetic stimulation is effective following repeated courses in the treatment of major depressive disorder—a case report. Hum Psychopharmacol 18(4):313–315. doi:10.1002/hup.478
186. Janicak PG, Dowd SM, Martis B, Alam D, Beedle D, Krasuski J et al (2002) Repetitive transcranial magnetic stimulation versus electroconvulsive therapy for major depression: preliminary results of a randomized trial. Biol Psychiatry 51(8):659–667. doi:S0006322301013543
187. Pridmore S, Bruno R, Turnier-Shea Y, Reid P, Rybak M (2000) Comparison of unlimited numbers of rapid transcranial magnetic stimulation (rTMS) and ECT treatment sessions in major depressive episode. Int J Neuropsychopharmacol 3(2):129–134. doi:10.1017/S1461145700001784 [pii] S1461145700001784
188. Richieri R, Adida M, Dumas R, Fakra E, Azorin JM, Pringuey D et al (2010) Affective disorders and repetitive transcranial magnetic stimulation: therapeutic innovations. Encephale 36(Suppl 6):S197–S201. doi:10.1016/S0013-7006(10)70057-9 [pii] S0013-7006(10)70057-9
189. Kopell BH, Halverson J, Butson CR, Dickinson M, Bobholz J, Harsch H et al (2011) Epidural cortical stimulation of the left dorsolateral prefrontal cortex for refractory major depressive disorder. Neurosurgery 69(5):1015–1029. doi:10.1227/NEU.0b013e318229cfcd (discussion 29)
190. Nahas Z, Anderson BS, Borckardt J, Arana AB, George MS, Reeves ST et al (2010) Bilateral epidural prefrontal cortical stimulation for treatment-resistant depression. Biol Psychiatry 67(2):101–109. doi:10.1016/j.biopsych.2009.08.021 [pii] S0006-3223(09)01020-8
191. Lisanby SH, Schlaepfer TE, Fisch HU, Sackeim HA (2001) Magnetic seizure therapy of major depression. Arch Gen Psychiatry 58(3):303–305

192. Lisanby SH, Luber B, Finck AD, Schroeder C, Sackeim HA (2001) Deliberate seizure induction with repetitive transcranial magnetic stimulation in nonhuman primates. Arch Gen Psychiatry 58(2):199–200

193. Kayser S, Bewernick BH, Grubert C, Hadrysiewicz BL, Axmacher N, Schlaepfer TE (2011) Antidepressant effects, of magnetic seizure therapy and electroconvulsive therapy, in treatment-resistant depression. J Psychiatr Res 45(5):569–576. doi:10.1016/j.jpsychires.2010.09.008

194. Kosel M, Frick C, Lisanby SH, Fisch HU, Schlaepfer TE (2003) Magnetic seizure therapy improves mood in refractory major depression. Neuropsychopharmacology 28(11):2045–2048. doi:10.1038/sj.npp.1300293

195. White PF, Amos Q, Zhang Y, Stool L, Husain MM, Thornton L et al (2006) Anesthetic considerations for magnetic seizure therapy: a novel therapy for severe depression. Anesth Analg 103(1):76–80. doi:10.1213/01.ane.0000221182.71648.a3 (table of contents)

196. Rowny SB, Benzl K, Lisanby SH (2009) Translational development strategy for magnetic seizure therapy. Exp Neurol 219(1):27–35. doi:10.1016/j.expneurol.2009.03.029

197. Christmas D, Eljamel MS, Butler S, Hazari H, MacVicar R, Steele JD et al (2011) Long term outcome of thermal anterior capsulotomy for chronic, treatment refractory depression. J Neurol Neurosurg Psychiatry 82(6):594–600. doi:10.1136/jnnp.2010.217901 [pii] jnnp.2010.217901

198. Dougherty DD, Weiss AP, Cosgrove GR, Alpert NM, Cassem EH, Nierenberg AA et al (2003) Cerebral metabolic correlates as potential predictors of response to anterior cingulotomy for treatment of major depression. J Neurosurg 99(6):1010–1017. doi:10.3171/jns.2003.99.6.1010

199. Steele JD, Christmas D, Eljamel MS, Matthews K (2008) Anterior cingulotomy for major depression: clinical outcome and relationship to lesion characteristics. Biol Psychiatry 63(7):670–677. doi:10.1016/j.biopsych.2007.07.019 [pii] S0006-3223(07)00731-7

200. Dalgleish T, Yiend J, Bramham J, Teasdale JD, Ogilvie AD, Malhi G et al (2004) Neuropsychological processing associated with recovery from depression after stereotactic subcaudate tractotomy. Am J Psychiatry 161(10):1913–1916. doi:10.1176/appi.ajp.161.10.1913 [pii] 161/10/1913

201. Montoya A, Weiss AP, Price BH, Cassem EH, Dougherty DD, Nierenberg AA et al (2002) Magnetic resonance imaging-guided stereotactic limbic leukotomy for treatment of intractable psychiatric disease. Neurosurgery 50(5):1043–1049 (discussion 9–52)

202. Malone DA Jr (2010) Use of deep brain stimulation in treatment-resistant depression. Cleve Clin J Med 77(Suppl 3):S77–S80. doi:10.3949/ccjm.77.s3.14 [pii] 77/Suppl_3/S77

203. Malone DA Jr, Dougherty DD, Rezai AR, Carpenter LL, Friehs GM, Eskandar EN et al (2009) Deep brain stimulation of the ventral capsule/ventral striatum for treatment-resistant depression. Biol Psychiatry 65(4):267–275. doi:10.1016/j.biopsych.2008.08.029 [pii] S0006-3223(08)01083-4

204. Bewernick BH, Hurlemann R, Matusch A, Kayser S, Grubert C, Hadrysiewicz B et al (2010) Nucleus accumbens deep brain stimulation decreases ratings of depression and anxiety in treatment-resistant depression. Biol Psychiatry 67(2):110–116. doi:10.1016/j.biopsych.2009.09.013 [pii] S0006-3223(09)01094-4

205. Bewernick BH, Kayser S, Sturm V, Schlaepfer TE (2012) Long-term effects of nucleus accumbens deep brain stimulation in treatment-resistant depression: evidence for sustained efficacy. Neuropsychopharmacology 37(9):1975–1985. doi:10.1038/npp.2012.44

206. Schlaepfer TE, Cohen MX, Frick C, Kosel M, Brodesser D, Axmacher N et al (2008) Deep brain stimulation to reward circuitry alleviates anhedonia in refractory major depression. Neuropsychopharmacology 33(2):368–377. doi:1301408 [pii] 10.1038/sj.npp.1301408

207. Jimenez F, Velasco F, Salin-Pascual R, Hernandez JA, Velasco M, Criales JL et al (2005) A patient with a resistant major depression disorder treated with deep brain stimulation in the inferior thalamic peduncle. Neurosurgery 57(3):585–593. doi:00006123-200509000-00027 [pii] (discussion 93)

208. Mayberg HS, Lozano AM, Voon V, McNeely HE, Seminowicz D, Hamani C et al (2005) Deep brain stimulation for treatment-resistant depression. Neuron 45(5):651–660. doi:10. 1016/j.neuron.2005.02.014 [pii] S0896-6273(05)00156-X

209. Puigdemont D, Perez-Egea R, Portella MJ, Molet J, de Diego-Adelino J, Gironell A et al (2011) Deep brain stimulation of the subcallosal cingulate gyrus: further evidence in treatment-resistant major depression. Int J Neuropsychopharmacol 1–13. doi:10.1017/ S1461145711001088 [pii] S1461145711001088

210. Lozano AM, Mayberg HS, Giacobbe P, Hamani C, Craddock RC, Kennedy SH (2008) Subcallosal cingulate gyrus deep brain stimulation for treatment-resistant depression. Biol Psychiatry 64(6):461–467. doi:10.1016/j.biopsych.2008.05.034 [pii] S0006-3223(08) 00703-8

211. Neimat JS, Hamani C, Giacobbe P, Merskey H, Kennedy SH, Mayberg HS et al (2008) Neural stimulation successfully treats depression in patients with prior ablative cingulotomy. Am J Psychiatry 165(6):687–693. doi:10.1176/appi.ajp.2008.07081298 [pii] 165/6/687

212. Kennedy SH, Giacobbe P, Rizvi SJ, Placenza FM, Nishikawa Y, Mayberg HS et al (2011) Deep brain stimulation for treatment-resistant depression: follow-up after 3 to 6 years. Am J Psychiatry 168(5):502–510. doi:10.1176/appi.ajp.2010.10081187 [pii] appi.ajp.2010. 10081187

213. Holtzheimer PE, Kelley ME, Gross RE, Filkowski MM, Garlow SJ, Barrocas A et al (2012) Subcallosal cingulate deep brain stimulation for treatment-resistant unipolar and bipolar depression. Arch Gen Psychiatry 69(2):150–158. doi:10.1001/archgenpsychiatry.2011.1456 [pii] archgenpsychiatry.2011.1456

214. Sartorius A, Kiening KL, Kirsch P, von Gall CC, Haberkorn U, Unterberg AW et al (2010) Remission of major depression under deep brain stimulation of the lateral habenula in a therapy-refractory patient. Biol Psychiatry 67(2):e9–e11. doi:10.1016/j.biopsych.2009.08. 027 [pii] S0006-3223(09)01047-6

215. Coenen VA, Bewernick B, Kayser S, Maedler B, Schlaepfer TE (2012) Deep brain stimulation of the human medial forebrain bundle (slmfb-dbs) for refractory depression— results from the foresee study. In: XXth Congress of the European Society for stereotactic and functional neurosurgery; 27 Sep 2012, Cascais, Portugal

216. Lozano AM, Giacobbe P, Hamani C, Rizvi SJ, Kennedy SH, Kolivakis TT et al (2012) A multicenter pilot study of subcallosal cingulate area deep brain stimulation for treatment-resistant depression. J Neurosurg 116(2):315–322. doi:10.3171/2011.10.JNS102122

217. Schlaepfer TE, Frick C, Zobel A, Maier W, Heuser I, Bajbouj M et al (2008) Vagus nerve stimulation for depression: efficacy and safety in a European study. Psychol Med 38(5):651–661. doi:10.1017/S0033291707001924 [pii] S0033291707001924

218. Rush AJ, George MS, Sackeim HA, Marangell LB, Husain MM, Giller C et al (2000) Vagus nerve stimulation (VNS) for treatment-resistant depressions: a multicenter study. Biol Psychiatry 47(4):276–286. doi:S0006-3223(99)00304-2

219. George MS, Rush AJ, Marangell LB, Sackeim HA, Brannan SK, Davis SM et al (2005) A one-year comparison of vagus nerve stimulation with treatment as usual for treatment-resistant depression. Biol Psychiatry 58(5):364–373. doi:10.1016/j.biopsych.2005.07.028 [pii] S0006-3223(05)00917-0

220. Kosel M, Brockmann H, Frick C, Zobel A, Schlaepfer TE (2011) Chronic vagus nerve stimulation for treatment-resistant depression increases regional cerebral blood flow in the dorsolateral prefrontal cortex. Psychiatry Res 191(3):153–159. doi:10.1016/j.pscychresns. 2010.11.004 [pii] S0925-4927(10)00385-9

221. Abosch A, Cosgrove GR (2008) Biological basis for the surgical treatment of depression. Neurosurg Focus 25(1):E2. doi:10.3171/FOC/2008/25/7/E2

222. Mashour GA, Walker EE, Martuza RL (2005) Psychosurgery: past, present, and future. Brain Res Brain Res Rev 48(3):409–419. doi:10.1016/j.brainresrev.2004.09.002 [pii] S0165-0173(04)00129-8

223. Leiphart JW, Valone FH 3rd (2010) Stereotactic lesions for the treatment of psychiatric disorders. J Neurosurg 113(6):1204–1211. doi:10.3171/2010.5.JNS091277

224. Shields DC, Asaad W, Eskandar EN, Jain FA, Cosgrove GR, Flaherty AW et al (2008) Prospective assessment of stereotactic ablative surgery for intractable major depression. Biol Psychiatry 64(6):449–454. doi:10.1016/j.biopsych.2008.04.009 [pii] S0006-3223(08)00431-9

225. Andrade P, Noblesse LH, Temel Y, Ackermans L, Lim LW, Steinbusch HW et al (2010) Neurostimulatory and ablative treatment options in major depressive disorder: a systematic review. Acta Neurochir (Wien) 152(4):565–577. doi:10.1007/s00701-009-0589-6

226. Sachdev PS, Sachdev J (2005) Long-term outcome of neurosurgery for the treatment of resistant depression. J Neuropsychiatry Clin Neurosci 17(4):478–485. doi:10.1176/appi. neuropsych.17.4.478 [pii] 17/4/478

227. Schoene-Bake JC, Parpaley Y, Weber B, Panksepp J, Hurwitz TA, Coenen VA (2010) Tractographic analysis of historical lesion surgery for depression. Neuropsychopharmacology 35(13):2553–2563. doi:10.1038/npp.2010.132 [pii] npp2010132

228. Delgado JMR, Graulich M (1972) Le conditionnement du cerveau et la liberté de l'esprit. Ch. Dessart

229. Romito LM, Raja M, Daniele A, Contarino MF, Bentivoglio AR, Barbier A et al (2002) Transient mania with hypersexuality after surgery for high frequency stimulation of the subthalamic nucleus in Parkinson's disease. Mov Disord 17(6):1371–1374. doi:10.1002/mds.10265

230. Kulisevsky J, Berthier ML, Gironell A, Pascual-Sedano B, Molet J, Pares P (2002) Mania following deep brain stimulation for Parkinson's disease. Neurology 59(9):1421–1424

231. Herzog J, Reiff J, Krack P, Witt K, Schrader B, Muller D et al (2003) Manic episode with psychotic symptoms induced by subthalamic nucleus stimulation in a patient with Parkinson's disease. Mov Disord 18(11):1382–1384. doi:10.1002/mds.10530

232. Houeto JL, Mesnage V, Mallet L, Pillon B, Gargiulo M, du Moncel ST et al (2002) Behavioural disorders, Parkinson's disease and subthalamic stimulation. J Neurol Neurosurg Psychiatry 72(6):701–707

233. Witt K, Krack P, Deuschl G (2006) Change in artistic expression related to subthalamic stimulation. J Neurol 253(7):955–956. doi:10.1007/s00415-006-0127-x

234. Schneider F, Habel U, Volkmann J, Regel S, Kornischka J, Sturm V et al (2003) Deep brain stimulation of the subthalamic nucleus enhances emotional processing in Parkinson disease. Arch Gen Psychiatry 60(3):296–302. doi:yoa10144

235. Witt K, Daniels C, Herzog J, Lorenz D, Volkmann J, Reiff J et al (2006) Differential effects of L-dopa and subthalamic stimulation on depressive symptoms and hedonic tone in Parkinson's disease. J Neuropsychiatry Clin Neurosci 18(3):397–401. doi:10.1176/appi. neuropsych.18.3.397 [pii] 18/3/397

236. Houeto JL, Mallet L, Mesnage V, Tezenas du Montcel S, Behar C, Gargiulo M et al (2006) Subthalamic stimulation in Parkinson disease: behavior and social adaptation. Arch Neurol 63(8):1090–1095. doi:10.1001/archneur.63.8.1090 [pii] 63/8/1090

237. Berney A, Vingerhoets F, Perrin A, Guex P, Villemure JG, Burkhard PR et al (2002) Effect on mood of subthalamic DBS for Parkinson's disease: a consecutive series of 24 patients. Neurology 59(9):1427–1429

238. Funkiewiez A, Ardouin C, Caputo E, Krack P, Fraix V, Klinger H et al (2004) Long term effects of bilateral subthalamic nucleus stimulation on cognitive function, mood, and behaviour in Parkinson's disease. J Neurol Neurosurg Psychiatry 75(6):834–839

239. Temel Y, Blokland A, Ackermans L, Boon P, van Kranen-Mastenbroek VH, Beuls EA et al (2006) Differential effects of subthalamic nucleus stimulation in advanced Parkinson disease on reaction time performance. Exp Brain Res 169(3):389–399. doi:10.1007/s00221-005-0151-6

240. Burkhard PR, Vingerhoets FJ, Berney A, Bogousslavsky J, Villemure JG, Ghika J (2004) Suicide after successful deep brain stimulation for movement disorders. Neurology 63(11):2170–2172. doi:63/11/2170

241. Soulas T, Gurruchaga JM, Palfi S, Cesaro P, Nguyen JP, Fenelon G (2008) Attempted and completed suicides after subthalamic nucleus stimulation for Parkinson's disease. J Neurol Neurosurg Psychiatry 79(8):952–954. doi:10.1136/jnnp.2007.130583 [pii] jnnp.2007. 130583

242. Witt K, Daniels C, Reiff J, Krack P, Volkmann J, Pinsker MO et al (2008) Neuropsychological and psychiatric changes after deep brain stimulation for Parkinson's disease: a randomised, multicentre study. Lancet Neurol 7(7):605–614. doi:10.1016/S1474-4422(08)70114-5 [pii] S1474-4422(08)70114-5

243. Smeding HM, Speelman JD, Koning-Haanstra M, Schuurman PR, Nijssen P, van Laar T et al (2006) Neuropsychological effects of bilateral STN stimulation in Parkinson disease: a controlled study. Neurology 66(12):1830–1836. doi:10.1212/01.wnl.0000234881.77830.66 [pii] 66/12/1830

244. Bejjani BP, Damier P, Arnulf I, Thivard L, Bonnet AM, Dor- mont D, Cornu P, Pidoux B, Samson Y, Agid Y (1999) Transient acute depression induced by high-frequency deep-brain stimulation. N Engl J Med 340:1476–1480

245. Temel Y, Kessels A, Tan S, Topdag A, Boon P, Visser-Vandewalle V (2006) Behavioural changes after bilateral subthalamic stimulation in advanced Parkinson disease: a systematic review. Parkinsonism Relat Disord 12(5):265–272. doi:10.1016/j.parkreldis.2006.01.004 [pii] S1353-8020(06)00026-5

246. Wichmann TD, DeLong MR (2006) Deep brain stimulation for neurologic and neuropsychiatric disorders. Neuron 52:197–204

247. Velasco F, Velasco M, Jimenez F, Velasco AL, Salin-Pascual R. Neurobiological background for performing surgical intervention in the inferior thalamic peduncle for treatment of major depression disorders. Neurosurgery 57(3):439–448. doi:00006123-200509000-00001 [pii] (discussion 48)

248. Brody AL, Barsom MW, Bota RG, Saxena S (2001) Prefrontal-subcortical and limbic circuit mediation of major depressive disorder. Semin Clin Neuropsychiatry 6(2):102–112. doi:S1084361201000119

249. Drevets WC, Ongur D, Price JL (1998) Neuroimaging abnormalities in the subgenual prefrontal cortex: implications for the pathophysiology of familial mood disorders. Mol Psychiatry 3(3):220–226, 190–191

250. Drevets WC, Price JL, Simpson JR Jr, Todd RD, Reich T, Vannier M et al (1997) Subgenual prefrontal cortex abnormalities in mood disorders. Nature 386(6627):824–827. doi:10.1038/386824a0

251. Mayberg HS (1994) Frontal lobe dysfunction in secondary depression. J Neuropsychiatry Clin Neurosci 6(4):428–442

252. Mayberg HS, Brannan SK, Tekell JL, Silva JA, Mahurin RK, McGinnis S et al (2000) Regional metabolic effects of fluoxetine in major depression: serial changes and relationship to clinical response. Biol Psychiatry 48(8):830–843. doi:S0006-3223(00)01036-2

253. Mottaghy FM, Keller CE, Gangitano M, Ly J, Thall M, Parker JA et al (2002) Correlation of cerebral blood flow and treatment effects of repetitive transcranial magnetic stimulation in depressed patients. Psychiatry Res 115(1–2):1–14. doi:S092549270200032X

254. Nobler MS, Oquendo MA, Kegeles LS, Malone KM, Campbell CC, Sackeim HA et al (2001) Decreased regional brain metabolism after ect. Am J Psychiatry 158(2):305–308

255. Malizia AL (1997) The frontal lobes and neurosurgery for psychiatric disorders. J Psychopharmacol 11(2):179–187

256. Sedrak M, Gorgulho A, De Salles AF, Frew A, Behnke E, Ishida W et al (2008) The role of modern imaging modalities on deep brain stimulation targeting for mental illness. Acta Neurochir Suppl 101:3–7

257. Winter C, Vollmayr B, Djodari-Irani A, Klein J, Sartorius A (2011) Pharmacological inhibition of the lateral habenula improves depressive-like behavior in an animal model of treatment resistant depression. Behav Brain Res 216(1):463–465. doi:10.1016/j.bbr.2010. 07.034 [pii] S0166-4328(10)00535-8

258. Sartorius A, Henn FA (2007) Deep brain stimulation of the lateral habenula in treatment resistant major depression. Med Hypotheses 69(6):1305–1308. doi:10.1016/j.mehy.2007.03. 021 [pii] S0306-9877(07)00247-2

259. McNeely HE, Mayberg HS, Lozano AM, Kennedy SH (2008) Neuropsychological impact of Cg25 deep brain stimulation for treatment-resistant depression: preliminary results over 12 months. J Nerv Ment Dis 196(5):405–410. doi:10.1097/NMD.0b013e3181710927 [pii] 0005053-200805000-00007

260. Pizzagalli DA, Holmes AJ, Dillon DG, Goetz EL, Birk JL, Bogdan R et al (2009) Reduced caudate and nucleus accumbens response to rewards in unmedicated individuals with major depressive disorder. Am J Psychiatry 166(6):702–710. doi:10.1176/appi.ajp.2008.08081201

261. Luigjes J, van den Brink W, Feenstra M, van den Munckhof P, Schuurman PR, Schippers R et al (2012) Deep brain stimulation in addiction: a review of potential brain targets. Mol Psychiatry 17(6):572–583. doi:10.1038/mp.2011.114

262. Rolls ET (2004) The functions of the orbitofrontal cortex. Brain Cogn 55(1):11–29. doi:10. 1016/S0278-2626(03)00277-X S027826260300277X

263. Drevets WC (2000) Neuroimaging studies of mood disorders. Biol Psychiatry 48(8):813–829. doi:S0006-3223(00)01020-9

264. Ferraro G, Montalbano ME, Sardo P, La Grutta V (1996) Lateral habenular influence on dorsal raphe neurons. Brain Res Bull 41(1):47–52. doi:S0361923096001700

265. Coenen VA, Schlaepfer TE, Maedler B, Panksepp J (2011) Cross-species affective functions of the medial forebrain bundle-implications for the treatment of affective pain and depression in humans. Neurosci Biobehav Rev 35(9):1971–1981. doi:10.1016/j.neubiorev. 2010.12.009

266. Dougherty DT, Thase ME, Howland RH, Evans KC, Harsch H, Kondziolka D (eds) (2008) Feasibility study of an implantable cortical stimulation system for patients with major depressive disorder. In: Society of Biological Psychiatry 63rd Annual Meeting, Washington, DC

267. Spielmans GI (2012) Unimpressive efficacy and unclear safety assessment of epidural cortical stimulation for refractory major depressive disorder. Neurosurgery 70(1):E268-E269. doi:10.1227/NEU.0b013e31823a3206 (author reply E9)

268. George MS, Sackeim HA, Rush AJ, Marangell LB, Nahas Z, Husain MM et al (2000) Vagus nerve stimulation: a new tool for brain research and therapy. Biol Psychiatry 47(4):287–295. doi:S0006-3223(99)00308-X

269. Sackeim HA, Rush AJ, George MS, Marangell LB, Husain MM, Nahas Z et al (2001) Vagus nerve stimulation (VNS) for treatment-resistant depression: efficacy, side effects, and predictors of outcome. Neuropsychopharmacology 25(5):713–728. doi:10.1016/ S0893-133X(01)00271-8 [pii] S0893133X01002718

270. Shuchman M (2007) Approving the vagus-nerve stimulator for depression. N Engl J Med 356(16):1604–1607. doi:10.1056/NEJMp078035 [pii] 356/16/1604

271. Rush AJ, Marangell LB, Sackeim HA, George MS, Brannan SK, Davis SM et al (2005) Vagus nerve stimulation for treatment-resistant depression: a randomized, controlled acute phase trial. Biol Psychiatry 58(5):347–354. doi:10.1016/j.biopsych.2005.05.025 [pii] S0006-3223(05)00620-7

272. Nahas Z, Marangell LB, Husain MM, Rush AJ, Sackeim HA, Lisanby SH et al (2005) Two-year outcome of vagus nerve stimulation (VNS) for treatment of major depressive episodes. J Clin Psychiatry 66(9):1097–1104

273. Martin JL, Martin-Sanchez E (2012) Systematic review and meta-analysis of vagus nerve stimulation in the treatment of depression: variable results based on study designs. Eur Psychiatry 27(3):147–155. doi:10.1016/j.eurpsy.2011.07.006 [pii] S0924-9338(11)00125-8

274. Corfmat J, Januel D, Braha S, Moulier V (2012) The placebo effect: general information and specificities in psychiatry (depression and schizophrenia). Encephale 38(1):50–57. doi:10. 1016/j.encep.2011.01.010 [pii] S0013-7006(11)00011-X

275. Schatzberg AF, Kraemer HC (2000) Use of placebo control groups in evaluating efficacy of treatment of unipolar major depression. Biol Psychiatry 47(8):736–744. doi:S0006-3223(00)00846-5

276. Rush AJ, Sackeim HA, Marangell LB, George MS, Brannan SK, Davis SM et al (2005) Effects of 12 months of vagus nerve stimulation in treatment-resistant depression: a naturalistic study. Biol Psychiatry 58(5):355–363. doi:10.1016/j.biopsych.2005.05.024 [pii] S0006-3223(05)00619-0

277. Corcoran CD, Thomas P, Phillips J, O'Keane V (2006) Vagus nerve stimulation in chronic treatment-resistant depression: preliminary findings of an open-label study. Br J Psychiatry 189:282–283. doi:10.1192/bjp.bp.105.018689 [pii] 189/3/282

278. Yudofsky SC, Silver JM, Jackson W, Endicott J, Williams D (1986) The overt aggression scale for the objective rating of verbal and physical aggression. Am J Psychiatry 143(1):35–39

279. Valle D (2005) Estado actual de la radiocirugía psiquiátrica con gamma Knife en México. Medical Sur

280. del Valle RdA, Garnica SR, Aguilar E, Pérez-Pastenes M (2006) Radiocirurgia psiquiatrica con gammaknife. Salud Mental 29(1):18–27

281. Jimenez-Ponce F, Soto-Abraham JE, Ramirez-Tapia Y, Velasco-Campos F, Carrillo-Ruiz JD, Gomez-Zenteno P (2011) Evaluation of bilateral cingulotomy and anterior capsulotomy for the treatment of aggressive behavior. Cir Cir 79(2):107–113

282. Jimenez F, Soto JE, Velasco F, Andrade P, Bustamante JJ, Gomez P et al (2012) Bilateral cingulotomy and anterior capsulotomy applied to patients with aggressiveness. Stereotact Funct Neurosurg 90(3):151–160. doi:10.1159/000336746 [pii] 000336746

283. Sano K, Mayanagi Y (1988) Posteromedial hypothalamotomy in the treatment of violent, aggressive behaviour. Acta Neurochir Suppl (Wien) 44:145–151

284. Ramamurthi B (1988) Stereotactic operation in behaviour disorders. Amygdalotomy and hypothalamotomy. Acta Neurochir Suppl (Wien) 44:152–157

285. Cif L, Biolsi B, Gavarini S, Saux A, Robles SG, Tancu C et al (2007) Antero-ventral internal pallidum stimulation improves behavioral disorders in Lesch-Nyhan disease. Mov Disord 22(14):2126–2129. doi:10.1002/mds.21723

286. Taira T, Kobayashi T, Hori T (2003) Disappearance of self-mutilating behavior in a patient with lesch-nyhan syndrome after bilateral chronic stimulation of the globus pallidus internus: case report. J Neurosurg 98(2):414–416. doi:10.3171/jns.2003.98.2.0414

287. Broggi G, Franzini A (2009) Treatment of aggressive behavior. In: Lozano A (ed) Textbook of stereotactic and functional neurosurgery, 2nd edn. Springer, NY, pp 2963–2969

288. Kluver H, Bucy PC (1997) Preliminary analysis of functions of the temporal lobes in monkeys. J Neuropsychiatry Clin Neurosci 9(4):606–620

289. Thomson AF, Walker AE (1950) Behavioral alterations following lesions of the medial surface of the temporal lobe. Folia Psychiatr Neurol Neurochir Neerl 53(2):444–452

290. Terzian H, Ore GD (1955) Syndrome of Kluver and Bucy; reproduced in man by bilateral removal of the temporal lobes. Neurology 5(6):373–380

291. Ursin H (1960) The temporal lobe substrate of fear and anger. A review of recent stimulation and ablation studies in animals and humans. Acta Psychiatr Scand 35:378–396

292. Narabayashi H, Nagao T, Saito Y, Yoshida M, Nagahata M (1963) Stereotaxic amygdalotomy for behavior disorders. Arch Neurol 9:1–16

293. Balasubramaniam V, Ramamurthi B (1968) Stereotaxic amygdalotomy. Proc Aust Assoc Neurol 5(2):277–278

294. Hitchcock E, Cairns V (1973) Amygdalotomy. Postgrad Med J 49(578):894–904

295. Chitanondh H (1966) Stereotaxic amygdalotomy in the treatment of olfactory seizures and psychiatric disorders with olfactory hallucination. Confin Neurol 27(1):181–196

296. Heimburger RF, Whitlock CC, Kalsbeck JE (1966) Stereotaxic amygdalotomy for epilepsy with aggressive behavior. JAMA 198(7):741–745

297. Narabayashi H, Uno M (1966) Long range results of stereotaxic amygdalotomy for behavior disorders. Confin Neurol 27(1):168–171

298. Hitchcock ER, Laitinen L, Vaernet K (eds) (1970) Psychosurgery. In: Proceedings. International Conference on Psychosurgery, Copenhagen, Springfield, Ill, Denmark
299. Small IF, Heimburger RF, Small JG, Milstein V, Moore DF (1977) Follow-up of stereotaxic amygdalotomy for seizure and behavior disorders. Biol Psychiatry 12(3):401–411
300. Mempel E, Witkiewicz B, Stadnicki R, Luczywek E, Kucinski L, Pawlowski G et al (1980) The effect of medial amygdalotomy and anterior hippocampotomy on behavior and seizures in epileptic patients. Acta Neurochir Suppl (Wien) 30:161–167
301. Fountas KN, Smith JR, Lee GP (2007) Bilateral stereotactic amygdalotomy for self-mutilation disorder. Case report and review of the literature. Stereotact Funct Neurosurg 85(2–3):121–128. doi:10.1159/000098527 [pii] 000098527
302. Mark VHE, Frank R (1970) Violence and the brain, 1st edn, Medical Dept, New York
303. Missa J-N (2001) Psychochirurgie. In: Hautois GM, Missa J-N (eds) Nouvelle encyclopédie de bioéthique médecine, environnement, biotechnologie avec la collab. de Marie-Geneviève Pinsart et Pascal Chabot. Bruxelles [Paris]: De Boeck université, p 922
304. Osmundsen J (1965 May) Matador with a radio stops bull. New York Times 17(1965):1
305. United State Senate (1977) Project MKULTRA, the CIA's program of research into behavioral modification. In: Ninety-Fifth Congress FS (ed) U.S. Government Printing Office, Washington
306. David MP, Lepoire J, Dilenge D (1961) Chapitre IV - Troubles mentaux (Psycho-chirurgie). Neurochirurgie, Collection médico-chirurgicale à révision annuelle. Flammarion édit, Paris, pp 927–963
307. Schergna EMS (1969) Treatment of character disorders with stereotaxic anterior cingulotomy. Riv Sper Freniatr Med Leg Alien Ment 93(3):795–802
308. Mingrino SS et al (eds) (1970) Stereotaxic anterior cingulotomy in the treatment of sever behavior disorders. In: International conference on psychosurgery, copenhagen, Springfield, Ill, Denmark
309. Sano K, Mayanagi Y, Sekino H, Ogashiwa M, Ishijima B (1970) Results of timulation and destruction of the posterior hypothalamus in man. J Neurosurg 33(6):689–707. doi:10.3171/jns.1970.33.6.0689
310. Arjona VE (1974) Sterotactic hypothalamotomy in erethic children. Acta Neurochir Suppl (Wien) 21:185–191
311. Schvarcz JR, Driollet R, Rios E, Betti O (1972) Stereotactic hypothalamotomy for behaviour disorders. J Neurol Neurosurg Psychiatry 35(3):356–359
312. Franzini A, Ferroli P, Leone M, Broggi G (2003) Stimulation of the posterior hypothalamus for treatment of chronic intractable cluster headaches: first reported series. Neurosurgery 52(5):1095–1099 (discussion 9–101)
313. Hernando V, Pastor J, Pedrosa M, Pena E, Sola RG (2008) Low-frequency bilateral hypothalamic stimulation for treatment of drug-resistant aggressiveness in a young man with mental retardation. Stereotact Funct Neurosurg 86(4):219–223. doi:10.1159/000131659 [pii] 000131659
314. Benazzouz A, Hallett M (2000) Mechanism of action of deep brain stimulation. Neurology 55(12 Suppl 6):S13–S16
315. Bejjani BP, Houeto JL, Hariz M, Yelnik J, Mesnage V, Bonnet AM et al (2002) Aggressive behavior induced by intraoperative stimulation in the triangle of Sano. Neurology 59(9):1425–1427
316. Goetz CG (2007) Textbook of clinical neurology, vol 355, Elsevier, The Netherlands
317. Nyhan WL, Wong DF (1996) New approaches to understanding Lesch-Nyhan disease. N Engl J Med 334(24):1602–1604. doi:10.1056/NEJM199606133342411
318. Lesch M, Nyhan WL (1964) A familial disorder of uric acid metabolism and central nervous system function. Am J Med 36:561–570
319. Norstrand IF (1982) Lesch-Nyhan syndrome. N Engl J Med 306(22):1368
320. Mizuno TI, Yugari Y (1974) Letter: self mutilation in Lesch-Nyhan syndrome. Lancet 1(7860):761

321. Nyhan WL (1968) Clinical features of the Lesch-Nyhan syndrome. Introduction—clinical and genetic features. Fed Proc 27(4):1027–1033

322. Ernst M, Zametkin AJ, Matochik JA, Pascualvaca D, Jons PH, Hardy K et al (1996) Presynaptic dopaminergic deficits in Lesch-Nyhan disease. N Engl J Med 334(24):1568–1572. doi:10.1056/NEJM199606133342403

323. Casas-Bruge M, Almenar C, Grau IM, Jane J, Herrera-Marschitz M, Ungerstedt U (1985) Dopaminergic receptor supersensitivity in self-mutilatory behaviour of Lesch-Nyhan disease. Lancet 1(8435):991–992. doi:S0140-6736(85)91773-8

324. Coubes P, Roubertie A, Vayssiere N, Hemm S, Echenne B (2000) Treatment of DYT1-generalised dystonia by stimulation of the internal globus pallidus. Lancet 355(9222):2220–2221. doi:10.1016/S0140-6736(00)02410-7 [pii] S0140-6736(00)02410-7

325. Andaluz N, Taha JM, Dalvi A (2001) Bilateral pallidal deep brain stimulation for cervical and truncal dystonia. Neurology 57(3):557–558

326. Trottenberg T, Volkmann J, Deuschl G, Kuhn AA, Schneider GH, Muller J et al (2005) Treatment of severe tardive dystonia with pallidal deep brain stimulation. Neurology 64(2):344–346. doi:10.1212/01.WNL.0000149762.80932.55 [pii] 64/2/344

327. Vercueil L, Pollak P, Fraix V, Caputo E, Moro E, Benazzouz A et al (2001) Deep brain stimulation in the treatment of severe dystonia. J Neurol 248(8):695–700

328. Pralong E, Pollo C, Coubes P, Bloch J, Roulet E, Tetreault MH et al (2005) Electrophysiological characteristics of limbic and motor globus pallidus internus (GPI) neurons in two cases of Lesch-Nyhan syndrome. Neurophysiol Clin 35(5–6):168–173. doi:10.1016/j.neucli.2005.12.004 [pii] S0987-7053(05)00081-X

329. Deon LL, Kalichman MA, Booth CL, Slavin KV, Gaebler-Spira DJ (2012) Pallidal deep-brain stimulation associated with complete remission of self-injurious behaviors in a patient with Lesch-Nyhan syndrome: a case report. J Child Neurol 27(1):117–120. doi:10.1177/0883073811415853 [pii] 0883073811415853

330. Programme UNIDC (2007) World drug report. Oxford University Press, Northamptonshire

331. Ferri MA, Amato L, Davoli M (2006) Alcoholics anonymous and other 12-step programmes for alcohol dependence. Cochrane Data-base Syst Rev 3:CD005032

332. Heinze HJ, Heldmann M, Voges J, Hinrichs H, Marco-Pallares J, Hopf JM, Münte TF (2009) Counteracting incentive sensitization in severe alcohol dependence using deep brain stimulation of the nucleus accumbens: clinical and basic science aspects. Front Hum Neurosci 3:22. doi:10.3389/neuro.09.022.2009

333. Di Chiara G, Imperato A (1988) Drugs abused by humans preferentially increase synaptic dopamine concentrations in the mesolimbic system of freely moving rats. Proc Natl Acad Sci USA 85(14):5274–5278

334. Kalivas PW, Volkow ND (2005) The neural basis of addiction: a pathology of motivation and choice. Am J Psychiatry 162(8):1403–1413. doi:10.1176/appi.ajp.162.8.1403 [pii] 162/8/1403

335. Stewart J, de Wit H, Eikelboom R (1984) Role of unconditioned and conditioned drug effects in the self-administration of opiates and stimulants. Psychol Rev 91(2):251–268

336. Robbins TW, Everitt BJ (1999) Drug addiction: bad habits add up. Nature 398(6728):567–570. doi:10.1038/19208

337. Wise RA, Bozarth MA (1987) A psychomotor stimulant theory of addiction. Psychol Rev 94(4):469–492

338. Hoebel BG, Monaco AP, Hernandez L, Aulisi EF, Stanley BG, Lenard L (1983) Self-injection of amphetamine directly into the brain. Psychopharmacology (Berl) 81(2):158–163

339. Alexander GE, DeLong MR, Strick PL (1986) Parallel organization of functionally segregated circuits linking basal ganglia and cortex. Annu Rev Neurosci 9:357–381. doi:10.1146/annurev.ne.09.030186.002041

340. Wise RA (1996) Addictive drugs and brain stimulation reward. Annu Rev Neurosci 19:319–340. doi:10.1146/annurev.ne.19.030196.001535

341. Wikler A (1948) Recent progress in research on the neurophysiologic basis of morphine addiction. Am J Psychiatry 105(5):329–338
342. Koob GF, Bloom FE (1988) Cellular and molecular mechanisms of drug dependence. Science 242(4879):715–723
343. Koob GF (2006) The neurobiology of addiction: a neuroadaptational view relevant for diagnosis. Addiction 101(Suppl 1):23–30. doi:10.1111/j.1360-0443.2006.01586.x [pii] ADD1586
344. Jentsch JD, Taylor JR (1999) Impulsivity resulting from frontostriatal dysfunction in drug abuse: implications for the control of behavior by reward-related stimuli. Psychopharmacology (Berl) 146(4):373–390. doi:91460373.213
345. Koob GF, Moal ML (2005) Neurobiology of addiction. Elsevier, The Netherlands
346. Tassin J-P (1998) Drogues, dépendance et dopamine. La recherche 2(306)
347. Lubman DI, Yucel M, Pantelis C (2004) Addiction, a condition of compulsive behaviour? Neuroimaging and neuropsychological evidence of inhibitory dysregulation. Addiction 99(12):1491–1502. doi:10.1111/j.1360-0443.2004.00808.x [pii] ADD808
348. Goldstein RZ, Volkow ND (2002) Drug addiction and its underlying neurobiological basis: neuroimaging evidence for the involvement of the frontal cortex. Am J Psychiatry 159(10):1642–1652
349. Ambroggi F, Ishikawa A, Fields HL, Nicola SM (2008) Basolateral amygdala neurons facilitate reward-seeking behavior by exciting nucleus accumbens neurons. Neuron 59(4):648–661. doi:10.1016/j.neuron.2008.07.004
350. Frenois F, Stinus L, Di Blasi F, Cador M, Le Moine C (2005) A specific limbic circuit underlies opiate withdrawal memories. J Neurosci 25(6):1366–1374. doi:10.1523/JNEUROSCI.3090-04.2005
351. Langevin JP (2012) The amygdala as a target for behavior surgery. Surg Neurol Int 3(Suppl 1):S40–S46. doi:10.4103/2152-7806.91609
352. Fang J, Gu JW, Yang WT, Qin XY, Hu YH (2012) Clinical observation of physiological and psychological reactions to electric stimulation of the amygdaloid nucleus and the nucleus accumbens in heroin addicts after detoxification. Chin Med J (Engl) 125(1):63–66
353. Medvedev SV, Anichkov AD, PoliakovIu I (2003) Physiological mechanisms of the effectiveness of bilateral stereotactic cingulotomy in treatment of strong psychological dependence in drug addiction. Fiziol Cheloveka 29(4):117–123
354. Li N, Wang J, Wang XL, Chang CW, Ge SN, Gao L et al (2012) Nucleus accumbens surgery for addiction. World Neurosurg. doi:10.1016/j.wneu.2012.10.007
355. Kuhn J, Bauer R, Pohl S, Lenartz D, Huff W, Kim EH et al (2009) Observations on unaided smoking cessation after deep brain stimulation of the nucleus accumbens. Eur Addict Res 15(4):196–201. doi:10.1159/000228930 [pii] 000228930
356. Mantione M, van de Brink W, Schuurman PR, Denys D (2010) Smoking cessation and weight loss after chronic deep brain stimulation of the nucleus accumbens: therapeutic and research implications: case report. Neurosurgery 66(1):E218. doi:10.1227/01.NEU.0000360570.40339.64 [pii] 00006123-201001000-00024 (discussion E)
357. Luigjes J, van den Brink W, Feenstra M, van den Munckhof P, Schuurman PR, Schippers R et al (2011) Deep brain stimulation in addiction: a review of potential brain targets. Mol Psychiatry. doi:10.1038/mp.2011.114 [pii] mp2011114
358. Valencia-Alfonso CE, Luigjes J, Smolders R, Cohen MX, Levar N, Mazaheri A et al (2012) Effective deep brain stimulation in heroin addiction: a case report with complementary intracranial electroencephalogram. Biol Psychiatry 71(8):e35–e37. doi:10.1016/j.biopsych.2011.12.013
359. Voges J, Muller U, Bogerts B, Munte T, Heinze HJ (2012) DBS surgery for alcohol addiction. World Neurosurg. doi:10.1016/j.wneu.2012.07.011
360. Kanaka TS, Balasubramaniam V (1978) Stereotactic cingulumotomy for drug addiction. Appl Neurophysiol 41(1–4):86–92
361. Brotis AG, Kapsalaki EZ, Paterakis K, Smith JR, Fountas KN (2009) Historic evolution of open cingulectomy and stereotactic cingulotomy in the management of medically

intractable psychiatric disorders, pain and drug addiction. Stereotact Funct Neurosurg 87(5):271–291. doi:10.1159/000226669 [pii] 000226669

362. Dieckmann G, Schneider H (1978) Influence of stereotactic hypothalamotomy on alcohol and drug addiction. Appl Neurophysiol 41(1–4):93–98

363. Witjas T, Baunez C, Henry JM, Delfini M, Regis J, Cherif AA et al (2005) Addiction in Parkinson's disease: impact of subthalamic nucleus deep brain stimulation. Mov Disord 20(8):1052–1055. doi:10.1002/mds.20501

364. Zhou H, Xu J, Jiang J (2011) Deep brain stimulation of nucleus accumbens on heroin-seeking behaviors: a case report. Biol Psychiatry 69(11):e41–e42. doi:10.1016/j.biopsych. 2011.02.012 [pii] S0006-3223(11)00147-8

365. Balasubramaniam V, Kanaka TS, Ramanujam PB (1973) Stereotaxic cingulumotomy for drug addiction. Neurol India 21(2):63–66

366. Foltz EL, White LE Jr (1962) Pain "relief" by frontal cingulumotomy. J Neurosurg 19:89–100. doi:10.3171/jns.1962.19.2.0089

367. Lenhard T, Brassen S, Tost H, Braus DF (2005) Long-term behavioural changes after unilateral stereotactic cingulotomy in a case of therapy-resistant alcohol dependence. World J Biol Psychiatry 6(4):264–266. doi:10.1080/15622970510029984 [pii] M6048386L6037760

368. Cohen RA, Kaplan RF, Moser DJ, Jenkins MA, Wilkinson H (1999) Impairments of attention after cingulotomy. Neurology 53(4):819–824

369. Jarraya B, Brugieres P, Tani N, Hodel J, Grandjacques B, Fenelon G et al (2010) Disruption of cigarette smoking addiction after posterior cingulate damage. J Neurosurg 113(6):1219–1221. doi:10.3171/2010.6.JNS10346

370. Muller D, Roeder F, Orthner H (1973) Further results of stereotaxis in the human hypothalamus in sexual deviations. First use of this operation in addiction to drugs. Neurochirurgia (Stuttg) 16(4):113–126. doi:10.1055/s-0028-1090504

371. Rieber I, Sigusch V (1979) Psychosurgery on sex offenders and sexual "deviants" in West Germany. Arch Sex Behav 8(6):523–527

372. Anonymous (1969) Brain surgery for sexual disorders. Br Med J 4(5678):250–251

373. Schmidt G, Schorsch E (1981) Psychosurgery of sexually deviant patients: review and analysis of new empirical findings. Arch Sex Behav 10(3):301–323

374. He S, Gao GD, Wang XL (2001)Effect of ventral pallidum lesions on drug seeking behavior in rats. Chin J Drug Depend (3):182–184

375. Gao G, Wang X, He S, Li W, Wang Q, Liang Q et al (2003) Clinical study for alleviating opiate drug psychological dependence by a method of ablating the nucleus accumbens with stereotactic surgery. Stereotact Funct Neurosurg 81(1–4):96–104. doi:10.1159/00007511175111

376. Xu JW, G. Zhou, H. Neurosurgical treatment on alleviating heroin psychological dependence. Chin J Neurosurg 21:590–593

377. Wang XL, He SM, Heng LJ (2005) Analysis of 1 year follow up results in patients who underwent bilateral nucleus accumbens ablation with stereotactic surgery for the treatment of drug dependence encephalopathy. Chin J Neurosurg 21(579–584)

378. Chen L, Li D, Xia X (2005) A clinical analysis on stereotactic surgery of multi-targets lesion for heroin dependence. Chin J Neurosurg 21:594–599

379. Zhao HK, Chang CW, Geng N, Gao L, Wang J, Wang X et al (2012) Associations between personality changes and nucleus accumbens ablation in opioid addicts. Acta Pharmacol Sin 33(5):588–593. doi:10.1038/aps.2012.10aps201210

380. Wu HM, Wang XL, Chang CW, Li N, Gao L, Geng N et al (2010) Preliminary findings in ablating the nucleus accumbens using stereotactic surgery for alleviating psychological dependence on alcohol. Neurosci Lett 473(2):77–81. doi:10.1016/j.neulet.2010.02.019 [pii] S0304-3940(10)00177-1

381. Kuhn J, Lenartz D, Huff W, Lee S, Koulousakis A, Klosterkoetter J et al (2007) Remission of alcohol dependency following deep brain stimulation of the nucleus accumbens: valuable therapeutic implications? J Neurol Neurosurg Psychiatry 78(10):1152–1153. doi:10.1136/jnnp.2006.113092 [pii] 78/10/1152

382. Vassoler FM, Schmidt HD, Gerard ME, Famous KR, Ciraulo DA, Kornetsky C et al (2008) Deep brain stimulation of the nucleus accumbens shell attenuates cocaine priming-induced reinstatement of drug seeking in rats. J Neurosci 28(35):8735–8739. doi:10.1523/JNEUROSCI.5277-07.2008 28/35/8735 [pii]

383. Knapp CM, Tozier L, Pak A, Ciraulo DA, Kornetsky C (2009) Deep brain stimulation of the nucleus accumbens reduces ethanol consumption in rats. Pharmacol Biochem Behav 92(3):474–479. doi:10.1016/j.pbb.2009.01.017 S0091-3057(09)00046-X [pii]

384. Henderson MB, Green AI, Bradford PS, Chau DT, Roberts DW, Leiter JC (2010) Deep brain stimulation of the nucleus accumbens reduces alcohol intake in alcohol-preferring rats. Neurosurg Focus 29(2):E12. doi:10.3171/2010.4.FOCUS10105

385. Heinze HJ HM, Voges J, Hinrichs H, Marco-Pallares J, Hopf JM, Müller UJ, Galazky I, Sturm V, Bogerts B, Münte TF (2009) Counteracting incentive sensitization in severe alcohol dependence using deep brain stimulation of the nucleus accumbens: clinical and basic science aspects. Front Human Neurosci 3(22)

386. Muller UJ, Sturm V, Voges J, Heinze HJ, Galazky I, Heldmann M et al (2009) Successful treatment of chronic resistant alcoholism by deep brain stimulation of nucleus accumbens: first experience with three cases. Pharmacopsychiatry 42(6):288–291. doi:10.1055/s-0029-1233489

387. Kuhn J, Grundler TO, Bauer R, Huff W, Fischer AG, Lenartz D et al (2011) Successful deep brain stimulation of the nucleus accumbens in severe alcohol dependence is associated with changed performance monitoring. Addict Biol 16(4):620–623. doi:10.1111/j.1369-1600.2011.00337.x

388. Stelten BM, Noblesse LH, Ackermans L, Temel Y, Visser-Vandewalle V (2008) The neurosurgical treatment of addiction. Neurosurg Focus 25(1):E5. doi:10.3171/FOC/2008/25/7/E5

389. Sun B, Liu W (2012) Surgical treatments for drug addictons in humans. In: Denys D, Feenstra M, Schuurman R (eds) Deep brain stimulation: a new frontier in psychiatry. Springer, Berlin, pp 131–140

390. Gonçalves-Ferreira A, Simões Do Couto F, Rainha Campos A, Lucas Neto L, Salgado L, Lauterbach M et al (2012) Deep brain stimulation for the treatment of refractory cocaine dependence. XXth Congress of the European Society for Stereotactic and Functional Neurosurgery; 27 Sep 2012, Cascais, Karger, Portugal

391. Goff P (2005) I was conscious as they pushed the needle deep into my brain. The Telegraph 2005:22

392. Philip BR (2009) Pour la première fois depuis 1951, la Chine exécute un Occidental. Le Monde. 2009 30 Décembre 2009

393. Cohen J (2004) HIV/AIDS in China. Changing course to break the HIV–heroin connection. Science 304(5676):1434–1435. doi:10.1126/science.304.5676.1434 [pii] 304/5676/1434

394. Krupitsky EM, Zvartau EE, Masalov DV, Tsoi MV, Burakov AM, Egorova VY et al (2004) Naltrexone for heroin dependence treatment in St. Petersburg, Russia. J Subst Abuse Treat 26(4):285–294. doi:10.1016/j.jsat.2004.02.002 [pii] S0740547204000078

395. Byrne G (1988) From Metrecal to methadone. Science 242(4884):1383

396. Stephen JH, Halpern CH, Barrios CJ, Balmuri U, Pisapia JM, Wolf JA et al (2011) Deep brain stimulation compared with methadone maintenance for the treatment of heroin dependence: a threshold and cost-effectiveness analysis. Addiction. doi:10.1111/j.1360-0443.2011.03656.x

397. Hall W, Carter A (2011) Is deep brain stimulation a prospective "cure" for addiction? F1000 Med Rep 3:4. doi:10.3410/M3-4

398. Deitel M (2002) The international obesity task force and "globesity". Obes Surg 12(5):613–614

399. Allison DB, Fontaine KR, Manson JE, Stevens J, VanItallie TB (1999) Annual deaths attributable to obesity in the United States. JAMA 282(16):1530–1538. doi:joc90587

400. Fontaine KR, Redden DT, Wang C, Westfall AO, Allison DB (2003) Years of life lost due to obesity. JAMA 289(2):187–193. doi:joc20945

401. Flegal KM, Carroll MD, Ogden CL, Johnson CL (2002) Prevalence and trends in obesity among US adults, 1999–2000. JAMA 288(14):1723–1727. doi:joc21463
402. Ogden CL, Flegal KM, Carroll MD, Johnson CL (2002) Prevalence and trends in overweight among US children and adolescents, 1999–2000. JAMA 288(14):1728–1732. doi:joc21462
403. Li Z, Maglione M, Tu W, Mojica W, Arterburn D, Shugarman LR et al (2005) Meta-analysis: pharmacologic treatment of obesity. Ann Intern Med 142(7):532–546. doi:142/7/532
404. Santry HP, Gillen DL, Lauderdale DS (2005) Trends in bariatric surgical procedures. JAMA 294(15):1909–1917. doi:10.1001/jama.294.15.1909 [pii] 294/15/1909
405. Zhang JV, Ren PG, Avsian-Kretchmer O, Luo CW, Rauch R, Klein C et al (2005) Obestatin, a peptide encoded by the ghrelin gene, opposes ghrelin's effects on food intake. Science 310(5750):996–999. doi:10.1126/science.1117255 [pii] 310/5750/996
406. Beedupalli J (2007) Bariatric surgery and mortality. N Engl J Med 357(25):2633 (author reply 4)
407. Chen R, Takahashi T, Kanda T (2007) Bariatric surgery for morbid obesity. N Engl J Med 357(11):1159 (author reply 60)
408. Sjostrom L, Lindroos AK, Peltonen M, Torgerson J, Bouchard C, Carlsson B et al (2004) Lifestyle, diabetes, and cardiovascular risk factors 10 years after bariatric surgery. N Engl J Med 351(26):2683–2693. doi:10.1056/NEJMoa035622 [pii] 351/26/2683
409. Christou NV, Look D, Maclean LD (2006) Weight gain after short- and long-limb gastric bypass in patients followed for longer than 10 years. Ann Surg. 244(5):734–740. doi:10.1097/01.sla.0000217592.04061.d5 [pii] 00000658-200611000-00018
410. Grundmann SJ, Pankey EA, Cook MM, Wood AL, Rollins BL, King BM (2005) Combination unilateral amygdaloid and ventromedial hypothalamic lesions: evidence for a feeding pathway. Am J Phys Regul Integr Comp Physiol 288(3):R702–R707. doi:10.1152/ajpregu.00460.2004
411. Torres N, Chabardes S, Benabid AL (2011) Rationale for hypothalamus-deep brain stimulation in food intake disorders and obesity. Adv Tech Stand Neurosurg 36:17–30. doi:10.1007/978-3-7091-0179-7_2
412. Anand BK, Brobeck JR (1951) Localization of a "feeding center" in the hypothalamus of the rat. Proc Soc Exp Biol Med 77(2):323–324
413. Goldney RD (1978) Craniopharyngioma simulating anorexia nervosa. J Nerv Ment Dis 166(2):135–138
414. Heron GB, Johnston DA (1976) Hypothalamic tumor presenting as anorexia nervosa. Am J Psychiatry 133(5):580–582
415. Weller RA, Weller EB (1982) Anorexia nervosa in a patient with an infiltrating tumor of the hypothalamus. Am J Psychiatry 139(6):824–825
416. Anand BK, Dua S, Shoenberg K (1955) Hypothalamic control of food intake in cats and monkeys. J Physiol 127(1):143–152
417. Quaade F, Vaernet K, Larsson S (1974) Stereotaxic stimulation and electrocoagulation of the lateral hypothalamus in obese humans. Acta Neurochir (Wien) 30(1–2):111–117
418. Quaade F (1974) Letter: stereotaxy for obesity. Lancet 1(7851):267
419. Bannier S, Montaurier C, Derost PP, Ulla M, Lemaire JJ, Boirie Y et al (2009) Overweight after deep brain stimulation of the subthalamic nucleus in Parkinson disease: long term follow-up. J Neurol Neurosurg Psychiatry 80(5):484–488. doi:10.1136/jnnp.2008.158576 jnnp.2008.158576
420. Novakova L, Ruzicka E, Jech R, Serranova T, Dusek P, Urgosik D (2007) Increase in body weight is a non-motor side effect of deep brain stimulation of the subthalamic nucleus in Parkinson's disease. Neuro Endocrinol Lett 28(1):21–25. doi:NEL280107A05
421. Tuite PJ, Maxwell RE, Ikramuddin S, Kotz CM, Billington CJ, Laseski MA et al (2005) Weight and body mass index in Parkinson's disease patients after deep brain stimulation surgery. Parkinsonism Relat Disord 11(4):247–252. doi:10.1016/j.parkreldis.2005.01.006 [pii] S1353-8020(05)00023-4

422. Tomycz ND, Whiting DM, Oh MY (2012) Deep brain stimulation for obesity–from theoretical foundations to designing the first human pilot study. Neurosurg Rev 35(1):37–42. doi:10.1007/s10143-011-0359-9 (discussion 3)
423. Brobeck JR (1963) Hypothalamus, appetite, and obesity. Physiol Pharmacol Physicians 18:1–6
424. Torres N, Chabardes S, Piallat B, Devergnas A, Benabid AL (2012) Body fat and body weight reduction following hypothalamic deep brain stimulation in monkeys: an intraventricular approach. Int J Obes 1–8
425. Melega WP, Lacan G, Gorgulho AA, Behnke EJ, De Salles AA (2012) Hypothalamic deep brain stimulation reduces weight gain in an obesity-animal model. PLoS One 7(1):e30672. doi:10.1371/journal.pone.0030672 [pii] PONE-D-11-17312
426. Hamani C, McAndrews MP, Cohn M, Oh M, Zumsteg D, Shapiro CM et al (2008) Memory enhancement induced by hypothalamic/fornix deep brain stimulation. Ann Neurol 63(1):119–123. doi:10.1002/ana.21295
427. Laxton AW, Tang-Wai DF, McAndrews MP, Zumsteg D, Wennberg R, Keren R et al (2010) A phase I trial of deep brain stimulation of memory circuits in Alzheimer's disease. Ann Neurol 68(4):521–534. doi:10.1002/ana.22089
428. Maeda H, Maki S (1989) A mapping study of hypothalamic defensive attack and related responses in cats. Neurosci Res 6(5):438–445. doi:0168-0102(89)90005-9
429. Mori Y, Ma J, Tanaka S, Kojima K, Mizobe K, Kubo C et al (2001) Hypothalamically induced emotional behavior and immunological changes in the cat. Psychiatry Clin Neurosci 55(4):325–332. doi:10.1046/j.1440-1819.2001.00871.x [pii] pcn871
430. Taghva A, Corrigan JD, Rezai AR (2012) Obesity and brain addiction circuitry: implications for deep brain stimulation. Neurosurgery. doi:10.1227/NEU. 0b013e31825972ab
431. Halpern CH, Wolf JA, Bale TL, Stunkard AJ, Danish SF, Grossman M et al (2008) Deep brain stimulation in the treatment of obesity. J Neurosurg 109(4):625–634. doi:10.3171/JNS/2008/109/10/0625
432. Halpern CH, Torres N, Hurtig HI, Wolf JA, Stephen J, Oh MY et al (2011) Expanding applications of deep brain stimulation: a potential therapeutic role in obesity and addiction management. Acta Neurochir (Wien). doi:10.1007/s00701-011-1166-3
433. Peyron C, Tighe DK, van den Pol AN, de Lecea L, Heller HC, Sutcliffe JG et al (1998) Neurons containing hypocretin (orexin) project to multiple neuronal systems. J Neurosci 18(23):9996–10015
434. Zahm DS (2000) An integrative neuroanatomical perspective on some subcortical substrates of adaptive responding with emphasis on the nucleus accumbens. Neurosci Biobehav Rev 24(1):85–105. doi:S0149-7634(99)00065-2
435. Killgore WD, Yurgelun-Todd DA (2005) Body mass predicts orbitofrontal activity during visual presentations of high-calorie foods. Neuroreport 16(8):859–863. doi:00001756-200505310-00016
436. Pisapia JM, Halpern CH, Williams NN, Wadden TA, Baltuch GH, Stein SC (2010) Deep brain stimulation compared with bariatric surgery for the treatment of morbid obesity: a decision analysis study. Neurosurg Focus 29(2):E15. doi:10.3171/2010.5.FOCUS10109
437. Lempérière T, Féline A (2006) Psychiatrie de l'adulte. Masson
438. Halmi KA, Tozzi F, Thornton LM, Crow S, Fichter MM, Kaplan AS et al (2005) The relation among perfectionism, obsessive-compulsive personality disorder and obsessive-compulsive disorder in individuals with eating disorders. Int J Eat Disord 38(4):371–374. doi:10.1002/eat.20190
439. Treasure J, Claudino AM, Zucker N (2010) Eating disorders. Lancet 375(9714):583–593. doi:10.1016/S0140-6736(09)61748-7 [pii] S0140-6736(09)61748-7
440. Gowers S, Bryant-Waugh R (2004) Management of child and adolescent eating disorders: the current evidence base and future directions. J Child Psychol Psychiatry 45(1):63–83
441. Pike KM, Walsh BT, Vitousek K, Wilson GT, Bauer J (2003) Cognitive behavior therapy in the posthospitalization treatment of anorexia nervosa. Am J Psychiatry 160(11):2046–2049

442. Ball J, Mitchell P (2004) A randomized controlled study of cognitive behavior therapy and behavioral family therapy for anorexia nervosa patients. Eat Disord 12(4):303–314. doi:10. 1080/10640260490521389 [pii] N6EW4WJ9BX8BJ09W
443. Steinhausen HC (2002) The outcome of anorexia nervosa in the 20th century. Am J Psychiatry 159(8):1284–1293
444. Carmody JT, Vibber FL (1952) Anorexia nervosa treated by prefrontal lobotomy. Ann Intern Med 36(2:2):647–652
445. Glazebrook AJ, Prosen H (1956) Compulsive neurosis with cachexia. Can Med Assoc J 75(1):40–42
446. Sargant W (1951) Leucotomy in psychosomatic disorders. Lancet 2(6673):87–91
447. Sifneos PE (1952) A case of anorexia nervosa treated successfully by leucotomy. Am J Psychiatry 109(5):356–360
448. Drury MO (1950) An emergency leucotomy. Br Med J 2(4679):609
449. Gayral L (1950) Emergency frontal leucotomy. Toulouse Med 51(8):502–506
450. Crisp AH, Kalucy RS (1973) The effect of leucotomy in intractable adolescent weight phobia (primary anorexia nervosa). Postgrad Med J 49(578):883–893
451. Zamboni R, Larach V, Poblete M, Mancini R, Mancini H, Charlin V et al (1993) Dorsomedial thalamotomy as a treatment for terminal anorexia: a report of two cases. Acta Neurochir Suppl (Wien) 58:34–35
452. van Kuyck K, Casteels C, Vermaelen P, Bormans G, Nuttin B, Van Laere K (2007) Motor- and food-related metabolic cerebral changes in the activity-based rat model for anorexia nervosa: a voxel-based microPET study. Neuroimage 35(1):214–221. doi:10.1016/j. neuroimage.2006.12.009 [pii] S1053-8119(06)01187-6
453. Luyten L, Welkenhuysen M, van Kuyck K, Fieuws S, Das J, Sciot R et al (2009) The effects of electrical stimulation or an electrolytic lesion in the mediodorsal thalamus of the rat on survival, body weight, food intake and running activity in the activity-based anorexia model. Brain Res Bull 79(2):116–122. doi:10.1016/j.brainresbull.2009.01.001 [pii] S0361-9230(09)00017-3
454. Pietrini F, Castellini G, Ricca V, Polito C, Pupi A, Faravelli C (2011) Functional neuroimaging in anorexia nervosa: a clinical approach. Eur Psychiatry 26(3):176–182. doi:10.1016/j.eurpsy.2010.07.011 [pii] S0924-9338(10)00155-0
455. Sherman BJ, Savage CR, Eddy KT, Blais MA, Deckersbach T, Jackson SC et al (2006) Strategic memory in adults with anorexia nervosa: are there similarities to obsessive compulsive spectrum disorders? Int J Eat Disord 39(6):468–476. doi:10.1002/eat.20300
456. Barbier J, Gabriels L, van Laere K, Nuttin B (2011) Successful anterior capsulotomy in comorbid anorexia nervosa and obsessive-compulsive disorder: case report. Neurosurgery 69(3):E745–E751. doi:10.1227/NEU.0b013e31821964d2 (discussion E51)
457. Sun B, Lin G, Zhan S, Zhang X (eds) (2012) Grading refractory anorexia nervosa for surgical treatment. In: XXth congress of the European society for stereotactic and functional neurosurgery; 26–29 Sep 2012, Cascais, Portugal
458. Benabid AL, Torres N (2012) New targets for DBS. Parkinsonism Relat Disord 18(Suppl 1):S21–S23. doi:10.1016/S1353-8020(11)70009-8 [pii] S1353-8020(11)70009-8
459. Yehuda R (2002) Post-traumatic stress disorder. N Engl J Med 346(2):108–114. doi:10. 1056/NEJMra012941
460. Guay S (2006) Les troubles liés aux événements traumatiques: Dépistage, évaluation et traitements. Presses de l'Université de Montréal
461. Cloitre M (2009) Effective psychotherapies for posttraumatic stress disorder: a review and critique. CNS Spectr 14(1 Suppl 1):32–43
462. Bisson JI, Ehlers A, Matthews R, Pilling S, Richards D, Turner S (2007) Psychological treatments for chronic post-traumatic stress disorder. Systematic review and meta-analysis. Br J Psychiatry 190:97–104. doi:10.1192/bjp.bp.106.021402
463. Watts BV, Landon B, Groft A, Young-Xu Y (2012) A sham controlled study of repetitive transcranial magnetic stimulation for posttraumatic stress disorder. Brain Stimul 5(1):38–43. doi:10.1016/j.brs.2011.02.002

464. Osuch EA, Benson BE, Luckenbaugh DA, Geraci M, Post RM, McCann U (2009) Repetitive TMS combined with exposure therapy for PTSD: a preliminary study. J Anxiety Disord 23(1):54–59. doi:10.1016/j.janxdis.2008.03.015

465. Morgan S (2012) L'Etat de stress post-traumatique : diagnostic, prise en charge et réflexions: sur les facteurs prédi. Publibook/Société des écrivains

466. Rauch SL, Whalen PJ, Shin LM, McInerney SC, Macklin ML, Lasko NB et al (2000) Exaggerated amygdala response to masked facial stimuli in posttraumatic stress disorder: a functional MRI study. Biol Psychiatry 47(9):769–776

467. Shin LM, Orr SP, Carson MA, Rauch SL, Macklin ML, Lasko NB et al (2004) Regional cerebral blood flow in the amygdala and medial prefrontal cortex during traumatic imagery in male and female Vietnam veterans with PTSD. Arch Gen Psychiatry 61(2):168–176. doi:10.1001/archpsyc.61.2.168

468. Liberzon I, Taylor SF, Amdur R, Jung TD, Chamberlain KR, Minoshima S et al (1999) Brain activation in PTSD in response to trauma-related stimuli. Biol Psychiatry 45(7):817–826

469. Koenigs M, Huey ED, Raymont V, Cheon B, Solomon J, Wassermann EM et al (2008) Focal brain damage protects against post-traumatic stress disorder in combat veterans. Nat Neurosci 11(2):232–237. doi:10.1038/nn2032

470. Anderson AK, Phelps EA (2001) Lesions of the human amygdala impair enhanced perception of emotionally salient events. Nature 411(6835):305–309. doi:10.1038/3507708335077083

471. Cahill L, Babinsky R, Markowitsch HJ, McGaugh JL (1995) The amygdala and emotional memory. Nature 377(6547):295–296. doi:10.1038/377295a0

472. Shin LM, McNally RJ, Kosslyn SM, Thompson WL, Rauch SL, Alpert NM et al (1999) Regional cerebral blood flow during script-driven imagery in childhood sexual abuse-related PTSD: a PET investigation. Am J Psychiatry 156(4):575–584

473. Gurvits TV, Shenton ME, Hokama H, Ohta H, Lasko NB, Gilbertson MW et al (1996) Magnetic resonance imaging study of hippocampal volume in chronic, combat-related posttraumatic stress disorder. Biol Psychiatry 40(11):1091–1099. doi:10.1016/S0006-3223(96)00229-6

474. Bremner JD, Randall P, Vermetten E, Staib L, Bronen RA, Mazure C et al (1997) Magnetic resonance imaging-based measurement of hippocampal volume in posttraumatic stress disorder related to childhood physical and sexual abuse—a preliminary report. Biol Psychiatry 41(1):23–32

475. Stein MB, Koverola C, Hanna C, Torchia MG, McClarty B (1997) Hippocampal volume in women victimized by childhood sexual abuse. Psychol Med 27(4):951–959

476. Gilbertson MW, Shenton ME, Ciszewski A, Kasai K, Lasko NB, Orr SP et al (2002) Smaller hippocampal volume predicts pathologic vulnerability to psychological trauma. Nat Neurosci 5(11):1242–1247. doi:10.1038/nn958

477. Langevin JP, De Salles AA, Kosoyan HP, Krahl SE (2010) Deep brain stimulation of the amygdala alleviates post-traumatic stress disorder symptoms in a rat model. J Psychiatr Res 44(16):1241–1245. doi:10.1016/j.jpsychires.2010.04.022

478. Stehberg J, Levy D, Zangen A (2009) Impairment of aversive memory reconsolidation by localized intracranial electrical stimulation. Eur J Neurosci 29(5):964–969. doi:10.1111/j.1460-9568.2009.06634.x

479. Robison RA, Taghva A, Liu CY, Apuzzo ML (2012) Surgery of the mind, mood, and conscious state: an idea in evolution. World Neurosurg. doi:10.1016/j.wneu.2012.03.005 [pii] S1878-8750(12)00345-2

Chapter 5
Some Legitimate Ethical Questions

Abstract The recent success of deep brain stimulation has led to a resurgence of psychosurgery. Deep brain stimulation further lowers the risks of effecting the personality and dignity of a person who may have been mistreated in the last century. This speciality which targets a small fringe number of psychiatric disorders, treats vulnerable patients. Thus, the fundamental principles of modern bioethics: autonomy, beneficence, nonmaleficence, and justice must be respected. Even stricter vigilance is necessary in the field of clinical research, where a multitude of dangers remain: the difficulty of gaining consent in certain patient populations, conflicts of interest within society, the appropriateness of treatment for addictions and aggressive disorders, the plights of children and prisoners.... In order to avoid past abuses and prevent future missteps, ethics committees have enacted protocols promoting transparency, multidisciplinarity, monitoring, and the best practices to ensure respect for the fundamental principles of bioethics. It is by adhering to these principles that psychosurgery may earn the trust of patients, doctors, and society as a whole.

Psychosurgery is a recent and controversial practice. With the advent of frontal lobotomies, which were tirelessly promoted by the American W. Freeman, high hopes surrounded the field of psychosurgery. From the late 1940s to the early 1950s, driven by the overcrowding of asylums and the absence of alternative treatments, this procedure experienced excessive development and use. These years were marked by the broadening of indications for the use of frontal lobotomies, many instances of mutilated personalities, lack of rigorous monitoring, and the violation of the principles of ethics [1]. Invoking ethics did not necessarily signify compliance with its principles, and the author of the first article on the subject, *Ethics of psychosurgery* [2], which was published in the *New England Journal of Medicine* in 1953, was Freeman himself! The advent of neuropharmacology, a more wary public and increasingly selective surgical techniques used by a limited number of teams contributed to improving this field. Despite this stricter framework, concerns remained. In 1970, the neurosurgeon M. David insisted that: *in psychosurgery, the question of ethics has always remained, it is about this field that the moral questions were asked most acutely, leading to heated, sometimes empassioned debates* [3]. It is, in fact, following the publication in 1975 of the *Belmont Report*, one of the founding texts of bioethics by the National Commission for the Protection of Human Subjects of Biomedical and Behavioral Research that the future of psychosurgery was determined [4]. This document established respect of the person, beneficence, and justice as fundamental principles of medical research [5]. The following year, in *Principles of Biomedical Ethics* [6]. T. Beauchamp and J. Childress integrated these principles into treatment practices, creating the four fundamental principles which are the pillars of bioethics today: the principles of *autonomy, beneficence, nonmaleficence,* and *justice.*

Autonomy

In bioethics, the principle of autonomy states that each patient is an autonomous individual. In other words, a patient is capable of making choices and decisions. This principle presents difficulties for psychosurgery when obtaining consent from patients whose judgment may be impaired. This challenge becomes acutely relevant when seeking informed consent for a treatment which may severely impact the individual. It is true that the effects of deep brain stimulation are reversible, which limits some of the neuropathological alterations seen in the past. However, complications do exist and the long-term effects remain poorly understood [7, 8].

A Lack of Discernment

Several of the diseases now treated by psychosurgery cause the patient to be incapable of understanding treatments and giving consent for them. Consent requires comprehension of the intervention and its implications in order to decide and commit to a choice in the long-term. The difficulty with consent is even starker in psychosurgery because it is precisely due to the disease's severity and pervasive impact on the life of the patient that surgical intervention becomes necessary. J.J. Kress points out that a severely obsessive patient can be *paralyzed by indecision because of endless hesitation*, while the morbid thoughts of a melancholic patient *create a terrible distortion of the concept of health* [9]. The psychiatrist adds, citing Ricoeur, that *all suffering is a loss of power over life*. However, in patients suffering from obsessive compulsive disorder who are cognizant of their disorder, the French National Consultative Ethics Committee states that *the issue of consent is no different from other medical specialties in which patients do not suffer from an illness which annihilates their judgment and they fully grasp reality* [1]. The problem is significantly different in patients suffering from severe depression, who may present a certain degree of cognitive impairment [10] or in patients treated with aggressive psychoactive drugs. If doubts regarding the patient's cognitive and decision-making abilities arise, the physician may resort to objective methods to evaluate the patient's mental capacity for sensible decision making. One such evaluation tool is the *MacArthur Competence Assessment Tool-Treatment (MacCAT-T)* [11]. However, reliable evaluation methods may be, they do not account for some of the emotional and autobiographical aspects that can inform a patient's decision making [7]. A patient's imagination regarding psychosurgery and its effects can also influence the patient's choices. It is sometimes necessary for the physician to provide a balance for certain nihilistic representations of psychosurgery portrayed by films such as *One Flew Over the Cuckoo's Nest* and *Shutter Island*. It may also be necessary for a physician to provide a balance for the unrealistic expectations the media can present for treatments such as deep brain stimulation [12].

The Struggle to Inform Correctly

Psychosurgery, and deep brain stimulation treatments specifically, still require at least another 5 years of additional research. The experimental nature of these procedures raises the question of how to provide *fair, clear and appropriate* information to patients [13]. The small number of patients involved, the remaining uncertainties of some of the results, the numerous side effects, and the problems with short and long-term treatment tolerance make the necessary information difficult to establish. While some risks can be identified—such as the probability of a brain hemorrhage or an infection—there is an inherent difference that comes with the stimulation of a new anatomical target, which leads to greater difficulty in calculating the risk of neuropsychological complications. We will return to this issue when discussing the principle of nonmaleficence. While a number of the neuropsychological modifications appear reversible by simply adjusting the parameters of stimulation, the behavioral consequences can be irreversible. One sees here the difficulty the physician can experience in providing "clear" information. The question of long-term effects poses an equal number of problems since information on many of these therapies rarely date back further than 15 years: will the effects be permanent? What are the risks of electrode displacement during aging? Will there be compatible stimulation control units in 20 years? Will the company reimburse patients for subsequent pacemakers until the patient's death?

The Issue of Nonautonomous Patients

In the United States, the *National Commission for the Protection of Human Subjects of Biomedical and Behavioral Research* in its 1977 recommendations specified that psychosurgical treatments could not be offered to prisoners or children. The decision regarding prisoners arose, in part, following disclosures by the Washington Post in 1972 of the use of interventions on three repeat offenders in a California prison. The judgment in the Kaimowitz case, in which it was revealed that the State of Michigan had funded research in psychosurgical treatment of sex offenders, also influenced the Commission's recommendations [14]. It is estimated that in West Germany, 72 sex offenders, more than half of whom were in prison, were "treated" by stereotactic hypothalamotomies between the years 1962 and 1979 [15] (Fig. 5.1, p. 287). In 1981, the sexologists G. Schmidt and E. Schorsch from the University of Hamburg critically reevaluated this series of procedures. Besides the fact that many of the clinical findings were difficult to interpret and that many of the patients were never followed post-procedure, they found that although the prisoners may have volunteered, they were most likely influenced by the hope of freedom that this treatment provided. These findings, the media coverage they garnered, and the conclusions of a report by the Federal Bureau of Health from that same year, led to the definitive end of these practices in Germany [16]. Hypothalamotomies as well as amygdalactomies have been performed on both children and adults presenting with "pathological aggressivity." The Belgium philosopher J.-N. Missa, points out that it was probably the Madras physicians *who practiced the destruction of the hypothalamus and the amygdala with the greatest fervor. Following in the footsteps of the Japanese K. Sano et al. [17] and H. Narabayashi, and the Indian V. Balasubramaniam, B. Ramamurthi [18] administered a high number of these procedures to children deemed aggressive or 'hyperkinetic.' Ramamurthi presented the results of his interventions and out of 1774 stereotactic operations over 28 years, 603 were aimed at treating children under 15 years of age whose behavior was judged to be aggressive [...] the results were considered to be good in 39 % of the cases and moderate in 37 % of the cases. [...]. For Ramamurthi, the results were considered to be good if the child became 'calm and quiet despite provocations' or if the child's family found the results satisfactory: 'the immeasurable value of the procedure for the family is indicated by the response of parents and relatives, whose quality of life has suddenly improved, as well as the increased demand for such operations* [19]. This dramatic experience provides insight into two ethical issues psychosurgery raises. That is, the problem of consent of a minor in this case, and the issue of conflicts of interest. According to B. Ramamurthi, this technique is not evaluated with the interests of the young patient in mind, but based on the satisfaction of his relatives. Rare pathologies for which this may be relevant are Tourettes syndrome and Lesch-Nyhan[1] disease. For Tourettes syndrome, indications for the appropriate use of deep brain stimulation in children occurs very rarely, due to the fact that we know that a large proportion of children see their condition improve or disappear in adulthood. However, the question of stimulation may still be posed when the manifestation of the syndrome can cause myelopathy or spinal cord injury [12, 21, 22]. Prudence is still required, however, as the side effects of stimulation on brain development [22] remain unknown.

---

[1]   Cf. p. 354.

Table III. Sexual Deviation of Patients Who Underwent
Stereotactic Hypothalamotomy ($N = 59$)[a,b]

Heterosexual ($N = 28$)	
Rape, adult women	11
Sexual contacts, girls (up to 14 years)	5
Exhibitionism, adult women	4
Exhibitionism, girls (up to 14 years)	4
Sadomasochistic contacts, girls (up to 14 years)	1
"hypersexual"[a]	3
Homosexual ($N = 28$)	
Sexual contacts, adult men[d]	2
Sexual contacts, boys (up to 14 years)	7
Sexual contacts, boys and adolescents (10-16 years)	9
Sexual contacts, adolescents (14-16 years)	8
Exhibitionism, boys (up to 14 years)	1
Sadomasochistic contacts, boys (up to 14 years)	1
Others ($N = 3$)	
Polymorphous pervert	1
Transvestitism and alcoholism	1
Sexually motivated incendiarism	1

Missing data: 13 cases, Göttingen
1 case, Homburg/Saar
2 cases, others

[a]From Müller et al., 1974; Horn, 1978; Supprian, 1979.
[b]According to diagnoses of surgeons or indicating psychiatrists.
[c]The only female patient is included in this category.
[d]One neurotic patient diagnosed erroneously as latent homosexual (see Müller et al., 1974, p. 102).

Fig. 5.1 Patients presenting sexual deviations who underwent hypothalamotomy procedures in the RFA from 1962 to 1979. According to [16]

Conflicts of Interest

It is not only the family, as in the preceding example, that can have conflicts of interest. The same can be true for physicians, the pharmaceutical industry, and society as a whole.

Society

Considering the opportunities for behavioral interventions leads one to consider the potential conflict between patients and society that may arise. In a report in *Functional Neurosurgery for Severe psychiatric Disorders*, the sages of the National Ethics Advisory Committee explained that in the early 1950s in the United States, *the desire to alleviate the issue of overcrowding and sub-medicalization of many asylums and hospitals was strong, and the lobotomy was seen as a way to calm and return a significant portion of the population to their homes. Considerations of 'economic efficiency' were no strangers to this growth, without great attention to selection criteria or patient consent*[2] [20–22]. Finally, it is especially with the advent of psychopharmacological interventions that asylums truly emptied and, as the psychiatrist and historian J. Hochmann emphasizes, these new medications allowed for *the disappearance of or rapid control over the loudest manifestations of insanity, leading to a shorter hospitalization, an increase in available space, and monitored outpatient treatment periods* [23]. At a time when talks of austerity run rampant, it is important to remain vigilant lest economic concerns lead to conflicts of interest. To this concern, one must add the issue of clinical management for a population which often disturbs the public, namely those with drug addictions, violent individuals, and those whose sexual orientations or practices have been, or remain in certain societies, stigmatized as deviant.

Sexuality

It was only 50 years ago that our Western society considered homosexuality, and even masturbation, deviant sexual behaviors requiring medical treatment. It was not until 1973 that homosexuality ceased to be classified as a mental disorder and was removed from the DSM. Until then, sexual orientation, or morality as it was called at certain times, sometimes necessitated psychosurgical treatment: In 1953, a social worker at Saint-Jean-de-Dieu Hospital in Montreal observed that: "Of the ten patients identified as chronic masturbators or homosexuals prior to the lobotomy, six seem to control their evil tendencies following the operation. They were no longer caught in the act following the procedure. [...]. Work was provided for these patients in order to keep them constantly occupied and to monitor their behavior with others" [27, 28]. In 1972, the psychiatrist Heath of Tulane University in New Orleans attempted to "initiate heterosexual behavior in a homosexual man" through stimulation of the septal area [24]. Although traces of such interventions in the literature are rare, they serve to remind us that the barrier between normality and pathology fluctuates depending on the epoch and the country. Doctors are not alone in defining what is or is not a psychiatric pathology; society and religion also influence this process, and sometimes do so negatively.

Addictions

Drug use, notably heroin and cocaine, affects 0.1–3 % of the world population according to the World Health Organization [25]. In 1973, in Madras, India, V. Balasubramaniam et al. [26] performed bilateral stereotactic cingulotomies in 28 patients. T. Kanaka and V. Balasubramaniam [27] and B. Ramamurthi et al. [28] followed suit in 1978, and used recruitment practices which remain questionable.

---

[2] Cf. p. **Erreur! Signet non défini.** Popularity of psychosurgery in the 1950s.

Their program was discontinued in the 1980s.[3] In Russia, between 1998 and 2002, a similar program led by the neurosurgeon S. Medvedev was established at the Brain Institute of St. Petersburg. Three hundred and forty eight heroin addicted patients were "treated" by stereotactic cryocingulotomy.[4] Medvedev reported that "30 % of the patients were cured of their addictions, while another 30 % suffered from one or two relapses in the first 2 months before being fully weaned." This practice was prohibited following a patient's complaints of headaches to the authorities. "Motivated by economic reasons, these interventions were practiced without an experimental model or controlled study, and without the approval of an ethics committee." The Russian academic B. Lichterman, whose comments were reported in the *Lancet*, stated that "as far as I know none of the results were reviewed by a committee of peers" [29]. Medvedev defended his "work" and stated that it had been approved by the Council for Addictions of the Russian Ministry of Health. In 2003, physicians at the Chinese military hospital in Xi'an, led by G. Gao, published results of bilateral stereotactic thermocoagulation interventions on the nucleus accumbens. The clinical results of this procedure on 28 heroin addicts were similar to those of Medvedev [30]. There was no mention of an ethics committee in these results either, and the authors did not elaborate on the selection criteria other than to state the patients were "free and without contra-indications." It is also unclear, in both the Russian and Chinese studies, whether or not neuropsychological assessments were conducted to determine if there were any cognitive or personality changes from the procedures. In 2009, German teams from Cologne and Magdeburg decided to resume study of the nucleus accumbens but, this time, using deep brain stimulation [31]. The program took place under much stricter ethical constraints and with a more limited number of patients. A successful weaning was achieved in all three patients with severe chronic alcoholism, but only a limited amount of time has elapsed since the interventions. For, although the technique is reversible, and despite the promising results, ethicists consider it premature [37]. Critics of brain stimulation for this indication take issue with the weak scientific evidence concerning the appropriateness of this target, the cost, and the risks of surgical procedure [38]. In addition, they recommend that, if new implants are made, they be registered in an international registry in order to avoid the publication of biased material focused primarily on positive results [32]. On this point, they are supported by the French teams who insist that it is necessary

---

[3] In 2000 when referring to the end of this program, B. Ramamurthi curiously declared that "After paranoia surrounding psychosurgery swept first through the US and then Japan and several European countries, the use of cingulotomies in the treatment of addiction, Author's Note was discredited. It was argued that putting the power to alter mental states in the hands of surgeons was too dangerous. If encouraged to do so, neurosurgeons might use it to change good natured Americans into evil communists" in [99].

[4] This stereotactic procedure, which relies on a dental mold rather than a stereotactic frame, uses a "cryoprobe" chilled to -70 °C to bilaterally destroy the anterior part of the cingulate gyrus, Brodmann area 24.

for double-blind studies[5] to be undertaken following the implant procedure [40]. Everyone agrees and recognizes, however, that this treatment must only be undertaken for those patients in which several weaning attempts, undertaken in optimal conditions, have failed [37, 38, 40]. Finally, for certain addictions, such as to heroin, the existence of alternative medication deemed effective discredits, a priori, surgical solutions, unlike for cases with no pharmacological alternatives such as amphetamines and cocaine addiction [33].

Hetero-aggressive Behavior

Hetero-aggressive behavior, like addiction to drugs, can lead to criminalization. In such instances, society can find itself in a conflict of interest. We addressed this issue in terms of freedom of consent when referring to the plight of incarcerated sex offenders and hypothalamotomy treatment. In 2007, the American K. Fountas suggested that lesion psychosurgery treatments for aggressive behavior had disappeared with the advent of psychopharmacological options and the stigma using surgery in such situations [34]. Three recent publications, however, cast doubt on this optimistic claim. The first two reports concern Mexican teams who have performed cingulotomies, capsulotomies and limbic leucotomies in individuals with aggressive behavior [35, 36]. Gamma-Knife radiosurgery was used and conditions of consent were not addressed in the 2011 publication. Three of the patients had previously been "treated" with a bilateral frontal leucotomy or cingulotomy. The story of the youngest patient, a 16-year old, is sobering: "The sixth patient, a teenager, is the son of a neurosurgeon and colleague who presented with symptoms of self- and hetero-aggressive behavior associated with a mental retardation. First, this patient underwent a bilateral capsulotomy under general anesthesia. The protocol stipulated that this procedure be combined at a later date with a bilateral limbic leucotomy as well as a hypothalatomy in order to control the auto-aggressive behavior. The impulsivity of the patient was significantly reduced in the first 2 months, however, the patient developed cerebral radiation necrosis before the end of the 6–8 months. An open cingulotomy was performed in another hospital. His current clinical state is unknown" [36]. This tragic story makes one wonder about the degree of consent obtained from this young patient suffering from mental retardation. Without looking at the questions the surgeries themselves raise, and in addition to the fact that the patient was a minor, one is entitled to question the fact that he was the son of a colleague. This recent but thankfully exceptional case underlines the necessity for strict guidelines regulating these interventions. The second publication concerns 12 individuals, 9 of which suffered from mental retardation, and 3 from schizophrenia, who were "treated" with capsulotomies and bilateral cingulotomies. The average age of the patients was 28-

---

[5] Neither the patient nor the psychiatrists following her know whether the stimulation is functioning or not.

years old, and two were minors. The authors reported that 3 months after surgery, the frequency of verbal and physical aggression had decreased by 60 %. In 42 % of patients, transitory complications were observed: binging (4), drowsiness (3), disinhibition (2), hypersexuality (2), infection (1), paraparesis (1). A majority of patients were unable to be located 6 months after the intervention [36]. If the authors do cite that "an ethics committee has reviewed each case according to the Declaration of Helsinki," and that this study financed by the General Hospital of Mexico was conducted "in accordance with the laws and best practices monitored by the research committee of the General Hospital," the question can still be asked whether the behavioral problems of these patients constituted more of a problem for their family and society than for themselves. In addition, the fact that they all suffered from a diminished mental capacity due to mental retardation or a dissociative disorder, brings to question the validity of their free and informed consent to participate in the clinical research. At this point, it is useful to recall an extract from the Nuremberg Code, enacted in 1947 following the trial of Nazi doctors, that B. Baertschi explains in an excellent book on neuroethics: "The voluntary consent of the human subject is absolutely essential. This means that the person involved should have the legally defined capacity to give consent; the person must be in a position to choose freely, without the intervention of any elements of force, of fraud, duress, or coercion. [...]. The experience must have practical results that benefit society in a way which cannot be achieved by any other means; the intervention must not be performed at random and unnecessarily. [...]. The experience must be undertaken in a way which avoids any suffering and unnecessary physical or mental harm" [37]. In 2004, the Italians A. Franzini and G. Broggi reported on the case of two patients suffering from violent and impulsive behavior which could not be controlled by medication who underwent surgery to have electrodes implanted for deep stimulation of the posterior hypothalamus [38]. Both patients, who were in their mid-thirties, suffered from mental retardation linked to prenatal cerebral anoxia and congenital toxoplasmosis. The Milan team specified that one patient experienced complications due to severe liver complications following his medication, while the second needed to be kept in isolation due to his destructive behavior. After one year of observation, the authors found a clear clinical amelioration in the first patient, who is now no longer committed, and the second no longer presents aggressive behavior and has thus been able to join an occupational therapy center. In the case of both of these patients monitored long term, it is important to note the conclusions of the authors: "The reversibility of this action and the absence of adverse effects during chronic bilateral stimulation of the posterior part of the hypothalamus suggests that this technique is ethically acceptable. Deep brain stimulation helped improve the quality of life of two patients for which previous treatment had failed." In 2008, J. Kuhn and V. Sturm's German team reported an encouraging new case [39] as well as V. Hernando and R. Sola with, in this last case, low frequency stimulation [40].

Medical Practitioners and Researchers

Apart from society, which may exert pressure if the patient disrupts standard functioning or creates costs which are too high, physicians in charge of obtaining consent for the psychosurgery can also face a conflict of interest. C. Jeanrenaud, in his book on law, states this notion: "there is a conflict of interest when the choices of the physician, the researcher, or the expert regarding an essential domain such as the patient's well-being, the integrity of the research, or the merits of a recommendation, are at risk of compromising other concurrent objectives such as economic gain, notoriety, or the ability to raise funds for the research." Two biographers of Freeman, Valenstein and El-Hai, recall how important the search for notoriety and prestige was to the psychiatrist from Washington in motivating his tireless promotion of the transorbital lobotomy. Characterized as "arrogant, confident and proselytizing," he contrasted the "sweet and humble" attitude of Moniz [22]. However, neither held disdain for honors and decorations (Fig. 5.2).

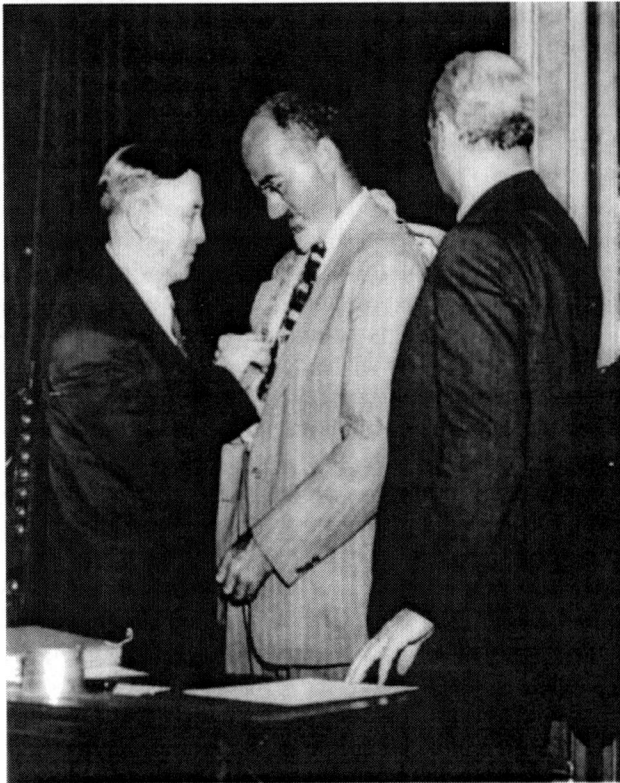

Fig. 5.2 Moniz honors Freeman. In 1948, he was made a foreign member of the Academy of Sciences of Portugal during a ceremony on the margins of the first International Congress of Psychosurgery in Lisbon

In *Great and Desperates Cures* [22], Valenstein describes Moniz's attitude in his quest for the 1949 Nobel Prize and his lobbying of the committee after the prize had escaped him twice in 1928 and 1933 for his work on cerebral angiography. More recently, the French psychiatrist A. Bottero, a fierce critic of psychosurgery [41], has warned us about physicians and researchers: *the problem that arises from experimental treatments is the impartial, passionless examination of its efficacy. It is their responsibility to prove the efficacy of an activity upon which their reputation rests; they are both judge and jury. One needs an enormous amount of enthusiasm and audacity to even engage in the study of a treatment which the majority do not approve of. We aim high in such an endeavor, and the risk of failure is always present. Driven by the conviction that they must do well, researchers frequently confound their hypotheses with reality, and neglect contradictory information* [42].

The financial savings that physicians hoped to gain from these new techniques are low: the need for monitoring and selection of patients requires a large number of employees and the intervention themselves demand a significant technical setup. In France for example, where deep brain stimulation is a part of the treatment for Parkinson's disease, the treatment is almost exclusively provided in public hospitals, due to the fact that the intervention brings little to no profit to a private practice. Whereas these practices have not let to a windfall for practitioners, the same cannot be true for the pharmaceutical industry.

The Ambivalence of the Pharmaceutical Industry

The pharmaceutical industry is not interested in ablative psychosurgery, which consists of creating lesions by thermocoagulation or Gamma-Knife, because the equipment necessary for these procedures is mostly reusable, and if it is not reusable, it is inexpensive. The situation is quite different for deep brain stimulation, and if the industry of implantable devices truly has the best interests of patients at heart, it is equally driven by the interest to make profit. These two objectives do not systematically coincide and commercial motivation sometimes impedes free and innovative research [43]. In 2006, it was estimated that the cost of the intervention was 37,000 euros, nearly 15,000 of which paid for the electrodes and the stimulator [44]. In addition to this, it is necessary to replace the neurostimulator every 5–6 years, due to its limited battery life, at a cost of about 10,000 euros. These numbers demonstrate the financial challenge these implantable devices represent; the worldwide market, all medical devices included, is estimated to represent close to 150 billion euros [45]. It is estimated that companies spend on average 7 % of this amount on research and development. For a number of ethicists, this participation in clinical research is ethically questionable. Of course, the involvement of companies provides the financial means to undertake clinical research to ensure the efficacy and safety of deep brain stimulation in psychiatric pathologies. Companies provide needed resources without which many treatments would never have come to fruition. However, researchers who are able to work due to these funds can develop conflicts of interest [43, 46, 47]. Erickson-Davis, an ethicist from Columbia University, is extremely critical of research done on deep brain stimulation in the treatment of obsessive compulsive disorders [46]. Most notably, she points to *Food and Drug Administration* (FDA) certification procedures which can be influenced by the lobbying of the implant device industry. This New York School of Public Health researcher, identified a company which bypassed the more rigorous and slow *Premarket Approval Application* (PMA) by using the *Humanitarian Device Exemption* (HDE) procedure instead (usually used for Class III devices). In fact, the HDE is generally used for medical devices targeting illnesses that touch fewer than four million Americans per year. The implant company argued that there is only a limited number of patients suffering with obsessive compulsive disorders who do not benefit from other medical treatments and who are sufficiently handicapped to justify recourse to this *compassionate* procedure which is generally reserved for so-called *orphan diseases*. Erickson-Davis sees this, instead, as a way to avoid a long and uncertain process for a treatment whose efficacy has yet to be proven. A similar article was published in 2007 in the *New England Journal of Medicine*. The author, Mr. Shuchman, remarked on the FDA approval of *vagus nerve stimulation in the treatment of drug-resistant depression*, 2 years before. He focused on the efforts of a competing implant device company to obtain this precious approval. He cites C. Grassley, an American senator and member of the Finance Committee, who was surprised to learn in 2006 that *the FDA could approve the vagus nerve stimulation for treatment-resistant depression even though FDA scientists were unable to establish its efficacy. Rather than allowing the scientific process to continue, a senior FDA member overturned the work of more then 20 FDA scientist who wished to rule against its approval* [48]. The high-standing FDA member, however, approved this treatment in order to enable randomized, double-blind studies using differing stimulation parameters. In the meantime, two large insurance companies supported senator Grassley and refused to reimburse the device in the absence of sufficient proof of its efficacy. The *New England Journal of Medicine* correspondent stated that, without the reimbursement from the insurance company, the researching company would have difficulty obtaining patients to execute the necessary clinical studies. The preceding examples illustrate the close ties between clinical research and industry Lobbying that can lead to conflicts of interest. It is for this reason that in 2002, influential practitioners of psychosurgery, most notably the Belgium Nuttin and the American Greenberg, demanded that clinical research in this domain adhere to stringent ethical rules and have a level of transparency, a topic which will be explored below in the section entitled "Safeguards" [49].

Should the Patient Be "in Control?"

Press that button again, please! wrote a recent North-American medical journal
[50] pointing to the wish of certain patients to be able to modify the parameters of
the devices providing their deep brain stimulation. We know that the modification
of intensity, frequency, and configuration of the studs being used can have more-
or-less immediate effects depending on the region in which the electrodes reside.
The clinical effect can be practically immediate in the subthalamic nucleus, for
instance, or lagging by several weeks, such as is the case in the ventral striatum.
Deep brain simulation, when used for Parkinson's disease or psychiatric pathologies, can lead to a feel of euphoria, well-being [51–53], and manic periods [54–
56]. Periods of hypersexuality [57–59] have been reported with equal frequency,
as well as the sensation of an approaching orgasm or even of a *high* similar to that
felt when taking opiates [60]. One can understand, therefore, the wish of some
patients to maintain stimulation parameters that cause these feelings. This com-
plicates the situation since this no longer constitutes an attempt to return *to the
normal state*, but rather, is an attempt to experience a better state. We thus leave
the domain of healing for that of doping.[6] It is therefore understandable that
physicians may refuse to allow patients to control their own "stimulation parameters." We could reply that this is a loss of autonomy compared to drug treatments
which patients administer themselves. One of the objectives of brain stimulation,
which we will develop in a later chapter, is to help the patient regain autonomy and
reduce the debilitating psychiatric symptoms experienced. The physician's control
over the stimulation parameters can interfere with the regaining of autonomy. The
anthropologist B. Moutaud's analysis helps clarify this subject. Having spent many
months with patients suffering from obsessive compulsive disorders and being
treated by deep brain stimulation, the anthropologist observed that the patient *no
longer has control of his treatment (he can no longer adapt his treatment along the
lines of normal living and his needs). He is a new patient being monitored with
consultations. If this technique I meant to return his autonomy, he finds himself
dependant on a neurologist and deep brain stimulation, with or without the
slightest control over the illness. He must readapt to his relationship with his
treatment. In the instance that there is a problem, or a perceived problem (the
sensations of the deep brain stimulation have become reduced, the stimulation
parameters were not well calculated during the last visit, etc.) the patient's only
recourse is to make an appointment, come back for a consultation, and explain
what he is feeling. The consequences of this can be that the patient views himself as
dependant on the technique, negating the notions of returning autonomy which are
integral to the treatment project. This loss of autonomy over his treatment due to a
constant need for the physician can lead the patient to try and re-appropriate the*

---

[6] Cf. p. 464, Towards an Augmented Human.

treatment, his illness, and his experience to himself (in the same way that he controlled these things during chemotherapy). Certain patients even ask if, perhaps, they can purchase their on parameter controller [61]. This possibility for the patient to "regulate himself," raises the question of how much patient discretion the stimulation parameters can allow. Is it just a binary choice of turning on or off the stimulation, this is currently the case, or can she be given access to the more complex regulations such as intensity, frequency, or even over the configuration of the stimulation implants?[7] The risks of complication are large, even when the treatment is administered by a physician with the necessary expertise to control the delicate regulations. However, as the anthropologist above mentions, patients may argue that he should have control over the stimulation parameters in the same way that she has control over adapting his psychotropic medications depending on his clinical state. The scientific literature has reported several incidents in which the changing of the parameters of cerebral stimulation have led to feelings of peace, euphoria, hypersexuality or "sensations resembling those caused by opium" [52, 57, 60, 62, 63]. Faced with a patient who is satisfied with these physical states, what should the physician's attitude be? Of course, these cases are exceptional, however, we can imagine that the increased investigation of psychiatric patholo-gies will lead to an increased number of these observations. Indeed, the anatomical structures targeted by *psychomodulation* have a more marked emotional valence (nucleus accumbens, ventral striatum, the limbic portion of the subthalamic nucleus) than those dealing with neuromodulation for abnormal movements. In his remarkable anthropological work, Moutaud identifies, through the experience of the two patients, another point: *when the technique causes instances of hypomania in Yvan and Melville, they describe a destabilizing experience in which they had no control but had, in hindsight, a clear understanding: the understanding that they had no control over the effects of the deep brain stimulation and its consequences, which could be a brutal experience. The treated are pulled into two modalities of sickness, at once the object of fundamental understanding, an organism repre-senting an experimental model of symptoms, and the subject of a treatment.*

Beneficence

It is only with regards to efficacy that we can discuss the moral issues of psycho-surgery: it can only be judged on facts, on results, paired with long-term statistical data across many years. As always, the real question is must we refuse a patient with a severe mental pathology for which all other treatments have failed the chance to escape a miserable condition or life-long hospitalization though surgical intervention?

David M., Guilly P. La neurochirurgie. "Que sais-je?", Paris: PUF; 1970.

---

[7] Cf. p. 205 Technique and parameters for DBS.

Marcel David, a well-known French neurosurgeon and one of its pioneers, focuses on the importance for psychiatrists and neurosurgeons of keeping a patient's best interests at the forefront of one's mind. Today, thanks to advances in psychopharmacology, life-long hospitalization is uncommon. Unfortunately however, this practice does persist on the margins of the psychiatric patient population for whom the pharmaceutical advances have not materialized. "The suffering that accompanies psychiatric illness inspires the search for new treatments that are concerned with the dignified and humane management of patients, and are not indifferent to the solitude, constraints, and forfeiture of the ill" [1]. It is thanks to this principle of striving to do good for a patient (beneficence) that the National Ethics Advisory Board gave its approval to *Functional Neurosurgery for Severe Psychiatric Afflictions* in 2005. Deep brain stimulation, and its reversible nature, is what gave psychosurgery its "second chance." We have already outlined, in the chapter devoted to psychosurgical lesioning techniques, that the results from capsulotomies and cingulotomies are satisfying: more than half of patients suffering from depression or severe obsessive pathologies see a significant diminishment of symptoms. We know that despite these encouraging findings ethics committees remain concerned about the risk of neuropsychological complications. Because, although these risks have diminished thanks to advances in stereotactic techniques, the consequences are more likely to be permanent due to the fact that lesions are, by nature, irreversible. Brain stimulation arose in large part to avoid this shortfall while still achieving similar clinical results. Although many patients see an improvement in their social lives, the issue of determining the factors which predict this outcome persists [64]. At this point, it is important to underline the concepts put forth by M. Schermer from Erasmus University in the Netherlands: the concept of "proportionality and subsidiarity" [65]. *Subsidiarity*, more a political than ethical concept, refers to the principle "by which a central authority can only carry out the tasks which lower ranking bodies cannot" [66]. Referencing this principle, the Rotterdam ethicist insists that psychosurgical treatments can only be used as a last recourse after the failure of pharmacological and psychotherapeutic interventions. Herein lies a problem frequently encountered when outlining the inclusion protocols for psychosurgical research: what are the criteria for pharmacological failure? To include a patient in a clinical study, the physicians must adhere to strict guidelines: what different pharmacological or psychotherapeutic treatments must follow or have been tried prior to the study? What group of molecules must have been tested? With what dosage? For how long? These strict criteria require that all possible treatment combinations have bee tried and failed. These multiple treatment combinations, often over a long period of time, can sometimes make it unethical for physicians to impose yet more pharmacological treatments on a patient. M. David had already begun to ask himself in 1970 whether "we have the right to impose numerous interventions on a melancholic patient who, after all the other treatments, has tried to commit suicide and who we know will, sooner or later, succeed in this enterprise?" [3] The second principle, *proportionality*, introduces the concept of nonmaleficence (do-no-harm) that we will develop later on. *Proportionality* entails that the clinical symptoms of the patient are severe enough to justify the possible negative risks of a new treatment, in this case psychosurgery. This concept forces psychiatrist and neurosurgeons to carefully consider the risk–benefit calculation which is inherent in all medical practice before any psychosurgical treatment. The concepts of *subsidiarity* and *proportionality* can be in conflict with the concept of *autonomy*. Here we can imagine a patient who considers himself sufficiently handicapped by his illness— or the secondary effects of his pharmacological treatment—and who therefore wants a psychosurgical treatment while her physician does not feel that the handicap is severe enough. In the same way, the concepts of *beneficence* (do good) and *nonmaleficence* (do-no-harm) for a patient can also come into opposition.

Nonmaleficence

The concept of do-no-harm recalls Hippocrates' maxim: *Primum non noncere.*[8] It also draws upon the notion of a risk–benefit calculation, mentioned above. Risks include the complications from the treatment, the implanted devices, and the undesirable effects of the stimulation. Concerning the surgical treatment, the risk of an intracerebral hematoma, which can provoke neurological symptoms, is about 4 %, while the probability of one or more epileptic episodes is 1.5 %. Transitory episodes of confusion occur in 15 % of post-op patients [67]. For implantable devices, the incidence of infections and dysfunction is around 3 %. These results taken from a meta-analysis of close to 1,000 Parkinson's patients with subthalamic implants can be extrapolated to deep brain stimulation treatments for psychiatric pathologies. When considering the undesirable effects of this stimulation, the situation is more complex. In Parkinson's patients treated with subthalamic stimulation the neuropsychological effects can be diffuse. The medical literature also mentions cases of impulsive behavior [68], aggression [69], hypersexuality and mania [54, 58, 70–72], apathy or depression [73–78], and suicidal thoughts [71, 76–82]. A very small number of patients describe feelings of strangeness [83], loss of meaning, alteration of their identity [84], and behavioral changes which could affect their family or professional relations. M. Schupback, of the Parisian team led by Y. Agid at the Salpêtrière Hospital, estimates that close to two-thirds of patients experience conjugal difficulties following the operation with more than 10 % divorcing in the 2 years following the intervention [83, 85]. According to the researchers, this finding can be explained by the regaining of autonomy, which changes the balance in the couple's relationship, as well as by the difficulty a patient might experience in abandoning his status as patient, followed by resentment from the spouse for not regaining the "normal life" hoped for. The

---

[8] In Epidemics (I, 5), dated around 410 BCE, Hippocrates defines the purpose of medicine thus: ἀσκέειν, περὶ τὰ νουσήματα, δύο, ὠφελέειν, ἢ μὴ βλάπτειν (to have with regards to disease two objectives in sight: to be useful or at least do-no-harm).

Salpêtrière team also found negative behavioral changes in the professional activity of patients. In short, although the motor improvements provided by this therapy are undeniable, the neuropsychological effects are more nuanced. Titles of articles published in this field support this: *The doctor is happy, the patient less so?* [86] or *A distressed spirit in a body that has been fixed* [83]. A patient's statement also illustrates this problem: *Before I wanted to but I could not. Now, I can, but I do not want to.* However, the neuropsychological effects of subthalamic stimulation are a secondary result of stimulation of an anatomical target primarily responsible for motor function. Neurosurgeons attempt, in theory, to target only the motor behavior of this structure. What will be the neuropsychological effects of stimulation once anatomical structures with much greater control over emotional behavior (such as the nucleus accumbens, the ventral striatum, the limbic portion of the subthalamic nucleus) are targeted? It is still too early to know since, as with Parkinson disease, a sufficient number of patients with long-term follow-up is necessary. The probability of these undesirable effects must be balanced with the benefits of the treatment. We, thus, return to the probabilistic nature of medicine, the *stochastic art,* as the ancients liked to say. The concept of *risk–benefit* calculations introduces yet another concept, that of the *cost–benefit* calculation.

Justice

Deep brain stimulation is one of the most expensive treatments. As we saw, a procedure can cost approximately 40,000 euros, plus the cost of changing the neurostimulator every 5 years [44]. If these costs, or a portion of them, can be reimbursed through the ability to return to work, savings from reduced use of medication, and the end of long hospital stays, the cost still remains high for society. The severe clinical state of patients being treated using these procedures, however, clearly inspires solidarity. The increased resource constraints that the future will bring will necessitate financial-medical studies to evaluate the cost–benefit relation of these interventions. Unlike Parkinson's disease, which affects older individuals, we can legitimately hope that therapeutic success in depression, which affects younger patients, will result in increased productivity, and therefore reduced cost to society [87].

Safeguards

Many authors have explored what structures and protocols should be established to ensure that clinical research in psychosurgery respects the principles of autonomy, beneficence, nonmaleficence, and justice [1, 49, 65, 87–89]. These guidelines are summarized in Table 5.1. There is unanimous agreement that all research programs must be approved by *ethics committees.* This recommendation assumes that

Table 5.1 Ethical principles and guidelines

Principles	Guidelines
Autonomy	Research programs should be **approved by an independent ethics committee** [1, 49, 65, 87–89]
	The patient's **informed consent** [1, 49, 65, 87, 88, 97], including on the need for postsurgical care and long-term follow-up must be obtained [13, 89]
	Transparency: the team must **reveal potential conflicts of interest** to guardians, ethical committees, and patients when informed consent is being sought [1, 49, 87, 88, 97]
	The practice must be **limited to adults, excluding inmates,** and all others unable to give free and informed consent [1, 65, 89]
	A **multidisciplinary** team should evaluate the patient's judgement [65, 87, 97]
	A patient may withdraw at any time [49, 88]
	An **independent psychiatrist** should confirm the indication in the absence of a selection committee
Beneficence	Strict inclusion and exclusion criteria considering disease severity, prior treatment failure, and impact on the subject's quality of life [1, 49, 65, 87–89, 97]
	The sole objective being to heal the patient or relieve his suffering to the exclusion of all other aims judicial, political, or improving mental abilities in the absence of a pathology [49, 65, 87, 88, 98]
	Multidisciplinary evaluation of the patient before inclusion [49, 87, 97]
	Results should be evaluated by a **second team** independently from the team leading the research [65]
	Standardized scales, evaluations, and nomenclature should be used to facilitate comparison of results [97]
Nonmaleficence	**Need for long-term follow-up** [65, 97, 98]
	Systematic post-surgical **neuropsychological evaluations** [65, 87] and evaluations of the quality of life [97]
	Creation of an international registry compiling results as well as complications and failures in order to offset the bias for positive results in publications [65, 87, 89]
	Psychosurgical **stimulation must be preferred to lesioning,** which is irreversible [1, 87, 89]
	Longitudinal studies examining the neuropsychological complications from deep brain stimulation in the treatment of abnormal movements [89]
	Radiosurgery can be called upon but should be evaluated using the results of deep brain stimulation as a control [1]
Justice	Patients should not **bear the financial burden of treatments and complications** [87, 89]
	The purpose should not be financial nor should the aim be to reduce healthcare costs [1, 87]
	Given the lack of access to stimulation-based treatments in developing countries, **results of lesioning and stimulation techniques should be compared** whenever possible [89]
Various	Procedures, follow-up, and adjustments of stimulation devices should only be performed in **approved clinical research centers** [49, 65, 87, 88]
	The research team should include at least: one **team of neurosurgeons with experience** in deep brain stimulation, one **team of psychiatrists with expertise in the relevant pathology.** If either of these two teams lacks prior experience in this field, they must call upon a reference center [49, 88, 89, 98]
	Psychosurgery is still in the **clinical research phase** [87, 89] and whenever possible studies should be prospective, double-blind, randomized and, for radiosurgery, compared to placebo [89]
	Clear information about the results and limitations of these techniques should be provided to the media to combat excessive expectations [87]
	Results of future studies may reveal the necessity for additional ethics guidelines [89]

at this point all work in psychosurgery must be viewed exclusively as research and not standard practice. The *transparency* of a research project's financing and its ties to the implantable device industry is imperative for evaluation of the potential conflicts of interest. Inclusion of patients must depend on meeting strict criteria regarding the *severity* of the psychiatric illness, the negative impact on the subject's life, and *failure* of standard well-carried out psychotherapeutic and pharmacological treatments. Minors, prisoners, and all other vulnerable population cannot be included in the clinical research. Certain psychiatric pathologies, such as hetero-aggressive behavioral problems, tend to be excluded by these guidelines due to the risk for abuse. For these patients, free consent can be problematic due to the pressure society places on them. It is essential that the selection of patients, the surgical procedure, and the follow-up monitoring be undertaken by a *multidisciplinary* team composed of psychiatrists, experts on the pathology in question, as well as neurosurgeons knowledgeable in stereotactic techniques. The emphasis should be placed on the novel deep brain stimulation techniques, whose effects are reversible, and which must be used preferentially over older lesioning techniques. However, we must not forget that these stimulation techniques, whether superficial or deep, may cause still unknown irreversible complications. From the beginning of the 1980s, even before the official advent of deep brain stimulation [90], the French neurosurgeons G. Lazorthes and R. Sedan, as well as the Swiss J. Siegfried already began questioning what the long-term consequences of these techniques might be, and, for this reason, whether this type of treatment is ethical or not [8]. For this and other reasons, the monitoring of these post-operation patients must include regular neuropsychological evaluations. The methodology of this prospective research must be rigorous and, whenever possible, entail a randomized, double-blind study. Thus, we see that the 2009 FDA decision to approve deep brain stimulation treatment for TOC under the *humanitarian device exemption* is a double-edged sword. Although it does give patients access to a technological development much more quickly since the exemption removes the long process that usually accompanies the authorization of an implantable device, many influential names in the specialty were in fact against the certification [91]. Regarding the clinical results, many authors claim that it is necessary to establish an international *registry* compiling information about each anatomical structure and each pathology in order to compare all of the available data and to identify undesirable outcomes. This is an attempt to avoid the bias in scientific publications where "positive results" are more likely to be published. In order to ensure social justice, research protocols must allow for the inclusion of all adults, regardless of origin, and ensure that their illness will be managed and monitored for complications. All authors agree that this new stimulation technique cannot be used for political reasons, social reasons, or to augment the capacities of normal individuals.

Although in the 1950s lax ethical rules and the absence of strict oversight prematurely halted the development of psychosurgery, the situation has since changed. The desire to guard against past mistakes has led supporters of psychosurgery to be particularly critical and to enact strict safeguards to limit future mistakes. Reflection on the practice of deep brain stimulation for both neurological and psychiatric indications has in fact been spurred on by psychosurgery. As M. Hariz highlights [90], it was not until 1999 and the first two deep brain stimulation therapies for mental illness [92, 93] that the issue of ethics rose to the forefront [49, 94, 95] despite the fact that this surgical technique had been used since 1987 [96] in treating Parkinson's disease and dystonia.

References

1. France Comité consultatif national d'éthique pour les sciences de la vie et de la santé. Avis sur la neurochirurgie fonctionnelle d'affections psychiatriques sévères. Ethique et recherche biomédicale Rapport 2002. Paris: la Documentation française; 2005
2. Freeman W (1953) Ethics of psychosurgery. N Engl J Med 249(20):798–801. doi:10.1056/NEJM195311122492003
3. David M, Guilly P (1970) La Neurochirurgie. Que sais-je? vol 1369. Presses universitaires de France, Paris
4. United States. National Commission for the Protection of Human Subjects of Biomedical and Behavioral Research (1977) Psychosurgery: report and recommendations, vol xviii. DHEW publication no (OS)77-0001, p 76
5. Marzano MM (2008) L' éthique appliquée. Que sais-je?, vol 3823. Presses universitaires de France, Paris
6. Beauchamp TL, Childress JF (1979) Principles of biomedical ethics. Oxford University Press, Oxford
7. Skuban TH, Woopen C, Kuhn J (2011) Informed consent in deep brain stimulation—ethical considerations in a stress field of pride and prejudice. Front Integr Neurosci 5(7):1–2
8. Siegfried J, Lazorthes Y, Sedan R (1980) Indications and ethical considerations of deep brain stimulation. Acta Neurochir Suppl (Wien) 30:269–274
9. Kress J-J (1994) Quelle est la place du consentement éclairé du patient dans le traitement neuroleptique? Conférence de consensus: texte des experts. Frisson-Roche, Paris
10. Appelbaum PS, Grisso T, Frank E, O'Donnell S, Kupfer DJ (1999) Competence of depressed patients for consent to research. Am J Psychiatry 156(9):1380–1384
11. Breden TM, Vollmann J (2004) The cognitive based approach of capacity assessment in psychiatry: a philosophical critique of the MacCAT-T. Health Care Anal 12(4):273–283. doi:10.1007/s10728-004-6635-x (discussion 65–72)
12. Bell E, Maxwell B, McAndrews MP, Sadikot A, Racine E (2010) Hope and patients' expectations in deep brain stimulation: healthcare providers' perspectives and approaches. J Clin Ethics 21(2):112–124
13. Glannon W (2010) Consent to deep brain stimulation for neurological and psychiatric disorders. J Clin Ethics 21(2):104–111
14. Shuman SI (1977) Psychosurgery and the medical control of violence: autonomy and deviance. Wayne State University Press, Detroit
15. Roeder F, Orthuer H, Mtiller D (1972) The stereotaxis treatment of pedophilic homosexuality and other sexual deviations. In: Hitchcock E, Laitinen L, Vaernet K (eds) Psychosurgery. Charles Thomas, Springfield, Ill, pp 87–111
16. Schmidt G, Schorsch E (1981) Psychosurgery of sexually deviant patients: review and analysis of new empirical findings. Arch Sex Behav 10(3):301–323
17. Sano K, Mayanagi Y, Sekino H, Ogashiwa M, Ishijima B (1970) Results of stimulation and destruction of the posterior hypothalamus in man. J Neurosurg 33(6):689–707. doi:10.3171/jns.1970.33.6.0689

18. Ramamurthi B (1988) Stereotactic operation in behaviour disorders. Amygdalotomy and hypothalamotomy. Acta Neurochir Suppl (Wien) 44:152–157
19. Missa J-N (2001) Psychochirurgie. In: Hautois GM (ed) Nouvelle encyclopédie de bioéthique médecine, environnement, biotechnologie avec la collab. de Marie-Geneviève Pinsart et Pascal Chabot. de Boeck université, Bruxelles, p 922
20. Mashour GA, Walker EE, Martuza RL (2005) Psychosurgery: past, present, and future. Brain Res Brain Res Rev 48(3):409–419. doi:10.1016/j.brainresrev.2004.09.002. S0165-0173(04) 00129-8 [pii]
21. Feldman RP, Goodrich JT (2001) Psychosurgery: a historical overview. Neurosurgery 48 (3):647–657 (discussion 57–59)
22. Valenstein ES (1986) Great and desperate cures: the rise and decline of psychosurgery and other radical treatments for mental illness. Basic Books, New York
23. Hochmann J (2004) Histoire de la psychiatrie. Que sais-je? vol 1428. Presses universitaires de France, Paris
24. Moan CH, Heath RG (1972) Septal stimulation for the initiation of heterosexual behavior in a homosexual male. Exp Psychiatry 3(1):23–26
25. WHO (2007) United Nations international drug control programme: World drug report. Oxford University Press, Northamptonshire
26. Balasubramaniam V, Kanaka TS, Ramanujam PB (1973) Stereotaxic cingulumotomy for drug addiction. Neurol India 21(2):63–66
27. Kanaka TS, Balasubramaniam V (1978) Stereotactic cingulotomy for drug addiction. Appl Neurophysiol 41(1–4):86–92
28. Ramamurthi B, Ravi R, Narayanan R (1980) Functional neurosurgery in psychiatric illnesses. Indian J Psychiatry 22(3):261–264
29. Orellana C (2002) Controversy over brain surgery for heroin addiction in Russia. Lancet Neurol 1(6):333. S1474442202001758 [pii]
30. Gao G, Wang X, He S, Li W, Wang Q, Liang Q et al (2003) Clinical study for alleviating opiate drug psychological dependence by a method of ablating the nucleus accumbens with stereotactic surgery. Stereotact Funct Neurosurg 81(1–4):96–104. doi:10.1159/000075111 [pii]
31. Muller UJ, Sturm V, Voges J, Heinze HJ, Galazky I, Heldmann M et al (2009) Successful treatment of chronic resistant alcoholism by deep brain stimulation of nucleus accumbens: first experience with three cases. Pharmacopsychiatry 42(6):288–291. doi:10.1055/s-0029-1233489
32. Carter AB, Racine E, Hall W (2011) Ethical issues raised by proposals to treat addiction using deep brain stimulation. Neuroethics 4:129–142
33. Vorspan F, Mallet L, Corvol JC, Pelissolo A, Lepine JP (2011) Treating addictions with deep brain stimulation is premature but well-controlled clinical trials should be performed. Addiction 106(8):1535–1536. doi:10.1111/j.1360-0443.2011.03450.x (author reply 7–8)
34. Fountas KN, Smith JR (2007) Historical evolution of stereotactic amygdalotomy for the management of severe aggression. J Neurosurg 106(4):710–713. doi:10.3171/jns.2007.106.4.710
35. del Valle RDA, Garnica SR, Aguilar E, Pérez-Pastenes M (2006) Radiocirurgia psiquiatrica con gammaknife. Salud mental 29(1):18–27
36. Jimenez-Ponce F, Soto-Abraham JE, Ramirez-Tapia Y, Velasco-Campos F, Carrillo-Ruiz JD, Gomez-Zenteno P (2011) Evaluation of bilateral cingulotomy and anterior capsulotomy for the treatment of aggressive behavior. Cir Cir 79(2):107–113
37. Baertschi B (2009) La neuroéthique ce que les neurosciences font à nos conceptions morales. Textes à l'appui Philosophie pratique. Éd. la Découverte, Paris
38. Franzini A, Marras C, Ferroli P, Bugiani O, Broggi G (2005) Stimulation of the posterior hypothalamus for medically intractable impulsive and violent behavior. Stereotact Funct Neurosurg 83(2–3):63–66. doi:10.1159/000086675. 86675 [pii]
39. Kuhn J, Lenartz D, Mai JK, Huff W, Klosterkoetter J, Sturm V (2008) Disappearance of self-aggressive behavior in a brain-injured patient after deep brain stimulation of the

hypothalamus: technical case report. Neurosurgery 62(5):E1182. doi:10.1227/01. neu.0000325889.84785.69. 00006123-200805000-00029 [pii]

40. Hernando V, Pastor J, Pedrosa M, Pena E, Sola RG (2008) Low-frequency bilateral hypothalamic stimulation for treatment of drug-resistant aggressiveness in a young man with mental retardation. Stereotact Funct Neurosurg 86(4):219–223. doi:10.1159/000131659 [pii]

41. Bottéro A (2001) Histoire de la psychiatrie—Révisionnisme psychochirurgical? Neuropsychiatrie: Tendances et Débats 14:21–22

42. Bottéro A (2009) Réserves sur la stimulation cérébrale profonde dans les troubles obsessionnels compulsifs. Neuropsychiatrie 37:9–12

43. Fins JJ, Schiff ND (2010) Conflicts of interest in deep brain stimulation research and the ethics of transparency. J Clin Ethics 21(2):125–132

44. Fraix V, Houeto JL, Lagrange C, Le Pen C, Krystkowiak P, Guehl D et al (2006) Clinical and economic results of bilateral subthalamic nucleus stimulation in Parkinson's disease. J Neurol Neurosurg Psychiatry 77(4):443–449. doi:10.1136/jnnp.2005.077677. 77/4/443 [pii]

45. Audry A, Ghislain JC (2009) Le dispositif médical. Presses universitaires de France

46. Erickson-Davis C (2011) Ethical concerns regarding commercialization of deep brain stimulation for obsessive compulsive disorder. Bioethics. doi:10.1111/j.1467-8519.2011.01886.x

47. Synofzik M, Schlaepfer TE (2011) Electrodes in the brain–ethical criteria for research and treatment with deep brain stimulation for neuropsychiatric disorders. Brain Stimul 4(1):7–16. doi:10.1016/j.brs.2010.03.002. S1935-861X(10)00020-3 [pii]

48. Finance USSCo (2006) FDA's approval process for the vagus nerve stimulation therapy system for treatment-resistant depression. Government Printing Office, Washington DC

49. Group O-DC (2002) Deep brain stimulation for psychiatric disorders. Neurosurgery 51 (2):519

50. Walkinshaw E (2012) Press that button again, please. CMAJ 184(5):E242–E243. doi:10.1503/cmaj.109-4112. cmaj.109-4112 [pii]

51. Fang J, Gu JW, Yang WT, Qin XY, Hu YH (2012) Clinical observation of physiological and psychological reactions to electric stimulation of the amygdaloid nucleus and the nucleus accumbens in heroin addicts after detoxification. Chin Med J (Engl) 125(1):63–66

52. Burn DJ, Troster AI (2004) Neuropsychiatric complications of medical and surgical therapies for Parkinson's disease. J Geriatr Psychiatry Neurol 17(3):172–180. doi:10.1177/0891988704267466

53. Aarsland D, Larsen JP, Lim NG, Janvin C, Karlsen K, Tandberg E et al (1999) Range of neuropsychiatric disturbances in patients with Parkinson's disease. J Neurol Neurosurg Psychiatry 67(4):492–496

54. Kulisevsky J, Berthier ML, Gironell A, Pascual-Sedano B, Molet J, Pares P (2002) Mania following deep brain stimulation for Parkinson's disease. Neurology 59(9):1421–1424

55. Krack P, Kumar R, Ardouin C, Dowsey PL, McVicker JM, Benabid AL et al (2001) Mirthful laughter induced by subthalamic nucleus stimulation. Mov Disord 16(5):867–875. 10.1002/mds.1174 [pii]

56. Daniele A, Albanese A, Contarino MF, Zinzi P, Barbier A, Gasparini F et al (2003) Cognitive and behavioural effects of chronic stimulation of the subthalamic nucleus in patients with Parkinson's disease. J Neurol Neurosurg Psychiatry 74(2):175–182

57. Chang CH, Chen SY, Hsiao YL, Tsai ST, Tsai HC (2010) Hypomania with hypersexuality following bilateral anterior limb stimulation in obsessive-compulsive disorder. J Neurosurg 112(6):1299–1300. doi:10.3171/2009.10.JNS09918

58. Romito LM, Raja M, Daniele A, Contarino MF, Bentivoglio AR, Barbier A et al (2002) Transient mania with hypersexuality after surgery for high frequency stimulation of the subthalamic nucleus in Parkinson's disease. Mov Disord 17(6):1371–1374. doi:10.1002/mds.10265

59. Witjas T, Baunez C, Henry JM, Delfini M, Regis J, Cherif AA et al (2005) Addiction in Parkinson's disease: impact of subthalamic nucleus deep brain stimulation. Mov Disord 20 (8):1052–1055. doi:10.1002/mds.20501

60. Morgan JC, diDonato CJ, Iyer SS, Jenkins PD, Smith JR, Sethi KD (2006) Self-stimulatory behavior associated with deep brain stimulation in Parkinson's disease. Mov Disord 21 (2):283–285. doi:10.1002/mds.20772

61. Moutaud B (2009) C'est un problème neurologique ou psychiatrique? Ethnologie de la stimulation cérébrale profonde appliquée au trouble obsessionnel compulsif. Université Paris Descartes, Paris

62. Portenoy RK, Jarden JO, Sidtis JJ, Lipton RB, Foley KM, Rottenberg DA (1986) Compulsive thalamic self-stimulation: a case with metabolic, electrophysiologic and behavioral correlates. Pain 27(3):277–290

63. Wise RA (1996) Addictive drugs and brain stimulation reward. Annu Rev Neurosci 19:319–340. doi:10.1146/annurev.ne.19.030196.001535

64. Fangerau H, Fegert J, Trapp T (2010) Implanted minds: the neuroethics of intracerebral stem cell transplantation and deep brain stimulation. Transcript Verlag, Bielefeld

65. Schermer M (2011) Ethical issues in deep brain stimulation. Front Integr Neurosci 5:17. doi:10.3389/fnint.2011.00017

66. Robert P, Rey A (2001) Le grand Robert de la langue française. Dictionnaires Le Robert

67. Kleiner-Fisman G, Herzog J, Fisman DN, Tamma F, Lyons KE, Pahwa R et al (2006) Subthalamic nucleus deep brain stimulation: summary and meta-analysis of outcomes. Mov Disord 21(Suppl 14):S290–S304. doi:10.1002/mds.20962

68. Sensi M, Eleopra R, Cavallo MA, Sette E, Milani P, Quatrale R et al (2004) Explosive-aggressive behavior related to bilateral subthalamic stimulation. Parkinsonism Relat Disord 10(4):247–251. doi:10.1016/j.parkreldis.2004.01.007. S1353802004000240 [pii]

69. Bejjani BP, Houeto JL, Hariz M, Yelnik J, Mesnage V, Bonnet AM et al (2002) Aggressive behavior induced by intraoperative stimulation in the triangle of sano. Neurology 59 (9):1425–1427

70. Herzog J, Reiff J, Krack P, Witt K, Schrader B, Muller D et al (2003) Manic episode with psychotic symptoms induced by subthalamic nucleus stimulation in a patient with Parkinson's disease. Mov Disord 18(11):1382–1384. doi:10.1002/mds.10530

71. Houeto JL, Mesnage V, Mallet L, Pillon B, Gargiulo M, du Moncel ST et al (2002) Behavioural disorders, Parkinson's disease and subthalamic stimulation. J Neurol Neurosurg Psychiatry 72(6):701–707

72. Witt K, Krack P, Deuschl G (2006) Change in artistic expression related to subthalamic stimulation. J Neurol 253(7):955–956. doi:10.1007/s00415-006-0127-x

73. Schneider F, Habel U, Volkmann J, Regel S, Kornischka J, Sturm V et al (2003) Deep brain stimulation of the subthalamic nucleus enhances emotional processing in Parkinson disease. Arch Gen Psychiatry 60(3):296–302. yoa10144 [pii]

74. Witt K, Daniels C, Herzog J, Lorenz D, Volkmann J, Reiff J et al (2006) Differential effects of L-dopa and subthalamic stimulation on depressive symptoms and hedonic tone in Parkinson's disease. J Neuropsychiatry Clin Neurosci 18(3):397–401. doi:10.1176/appi.neuropsych.18.3.397 [pii]

75. Houeto JL, Mallet L, Mesnage V, Tezenas du Montcel S, Behar C, Gargiulo M et al (2006) Subthalamic stimulation in Parkinson disease: behavior and social adaptation. Arch Neurol 63(8):1090–1095. doi:10.1001/archneur.63.8.1090 [pii]

76. Berney A, Vingerhoets F, Perrin A, Guex P, Villemure JG, Burkhard PR et al (2002) Effect on mood of subthalamic DBS for Parkinson's disease: a consecutive series of 24 patients. Neurology 59(9):1427–1429

77. Funkiewiez A, Ardouin C, Caputo E, Krack P, Fraix V, Klinger H et al (2004) Long term effects of bilateral subthalamic nucleus stimulation on cognitive function, mood, and behaviour in Parkinson's disease. J Neurol Neurosurg Psychiatry 75(6):834–839

78. Temel Y, Blokland A, Ackermans L, Boon P, van Kranen-Mastenbroek VH, Beuls EA et al (2006) Differential effects of subthalamic nucleus stimulation in advanced Parkinson disease on reaction time performance. Exp Brain Res 169(3):389–399. doi:10.1007/s00221-005-0151-6

79. Burkhard PR, Vingerhoets FJ, Berney A, Bogousslavsky J, Villemure JG, Ghika J (2004) Suicide after successful deep brain stimulation for movement disorders. Neurology 63 (11):2170–2172. 63/11/2170 [pii]

80. Soulas T, Gurruchaga JM, Palfi S, Cesaro P, Nguyen JP, Fenelon G (2008) Attempted and completed suicides after subthalamic nucleus stimulation for Parkinson's disease. J Neurol Neurosurg Psychiatry 79(8):952–954. doi:10.1136/jnnp.2007.130583 [pii]

81. Witt K, Daniels C, Reiff J, Krack P, Volkmann J, Pinsker MO et al (2008) Neuropsychological and psychiatric changes after deep brain stimulation for Parkinson's disease: a randomised, multicentre study. Lancet Neurol 7(7):605–614. doi:10.1016/S1474-4422(08)70114-5. S1474-4422(08)70114-5 [pii]

82. Smeding HM, Speelman JD, Koning-Haanstra M, Schuurman PR, Nijssen P, van Laar T et al (2006) Neuropsychological effects of bilateral STN stimulation in Parkinson disease: a controlled study. Neurology 66(12):1830–1836. doi:10.1212/01.wnl.0000234881.77830.66. 66/12/1830 [pii]

83. Schupbach M, Gargiulo M, Welter ML, Mallet L, Behar C, Houeto JL et al (2006) Neurosurgery in Parkinson disease: a distressed mind in a repaired body? Neurology 66 (12):1811–1816. doi:10.1212/01.wnl.0000234880.51322.16. 66/12/1811 [pii]

84. Gisquet E (2008) Cerebral implants and Parkinson's disease: a unique form of biographical disruption? Soc Sci Med 67(11):1847–1851. doi:10.1016/j.socscimed.2008.09.026. S0277-9536(08)00480-2 [pii]

85. Perozzo P, Rizzone M, Bergamasco B, Castelli L, Lanotte M, Tavella A et al (2001) Deep brain stimulation of subthalamic nucleus: behavioural modifications and familiar relations. Neurol Sci 22(1):81–82

86. Agid Y, Schupbach M, Gargiulo M, Mallet L, Houeto JL, Behar C et al (2006) Neurosurgery in Parkinson's disease: the doctor is happy, the patient less so? J Neural Transm Suppl 70:409–414

87. Bell E, Mathieu G, Racine E (2009) Preparing the ethical future of deep brain stimulation. Surg Neurol 72(6):577–586. doi:10.1016/j.surneu.2009.03.029. S0090-3019(09)00285-7 [pii] (discussion 86)

88. Fins JJ, Rezai AR, Greenberg BD (2006) Psychosurgery: avoiding an ethical redux while advancing a therapeutic future. Neurosurgery 59(4):713–716. doi:10.1227/01. NEU.0000243605.89270.6C. 00006123-200610000-00001 [pii]

89. Appleby BSR, Rabins PV (2009) Ethical considerations in psychiatric surgery. In: Lozano A (ed) Textbook of stereotactic and functional neurosurgery, 2nd edn. Springer, New York, pp 2856

90. Hariz M (2012) Twenty-five years of deep brain stimulation: celebrations and apprehensions. Mov Disord 27(7):930–933. doi:10.1002/mds.25007

91. Fins JJ, Mayberg HS, Nuttin B, Kubu CS, Galert T, Sturm V et al (2011) Misuse of the FDA's humanitarian device exemption in deep brain stimulation for obsessive-compulsive disorder. Health Aff (Millwood) 30(2):302–311. doi:10.1377/hlthaff.2010.0157

92. Vandewalle V, van der Linden C, Groenewegen HJ, Caemaert J (1999) Stereotactic treatment of Gilles de la tourette syndrome by high frequency stimulation of thalamus. Lancet 353 (9154):724. S0140673698059649 [pii]

93. Nuttin B, Cosyns P, Demeulemeester H, Gybels J, Meyerson B (1999) Electrical stimulation in anterior limbs of internal capsules in patients with obsessive-compulsive disorder. Lancet 354(9189):1526. doi:10.1016/S0140-6736(99)02376-4. S0140-6736(99)02376-4 [pii]

94. Fins JJ (2003) From psychosurgery to neuromodulation and palliation: history's lessons for the ethical conduct and regulation of neuropsychiatric research. Neurosurg Clin N Am 14 (2):303–319

95. Fins JJ (2000) A proposed ethical framework for interventional cognitive neuroscience: a consideration of deep brain stimulation in impaired consciousness. Neurol Res 22(3):273–278

96. Benabid AL, Pollak P, Louveau A, Henry S, de Rougemont J (1987) Combined (thalamotomy and stimulation) stereotactic surgery of the VIM thalamic nucleus for bilateral Parkinson disease. Appl Neurophysiol 50(1–6):344–346
97. Kuhn J, Gaebel W, Klosterkoetter J, Woopen C (2009) Deep brain stimulation as a new therapeutic approach in therapy-resistant mental disorders: ethical aspects of investigational treatment. Eur Arch Psychiatry Clin Neurosci 259(Suppl 2):S135–S141. doi:10.1007/s00406-009-0055-8
98. Kringelbach ML, Aziz TZ (2009) Deep brain stimulation: avoiding the errors of psychosurgery JAMA 301(16):1705–1707. doi:10.1001/jama.2009.551. 301/16/1705 [pii]
99. Ramamurthi B (2000) Stereotactic surgery in India: the past, present and the future. Neurol India 48:1–7

Chapter 6
What Is Next?

Abstract Due to its reversible nature, deep brain stimulation allows for the exploration of a greater number of anatomical structures and can therefore increase the number of psychiatric pathologies that can be ameliorated with psychosurgical intervention. It is probable that the progress seen in nanotechnology, biology, information technology, and cognitive sciences will lead to a paradigm shift for the treatments of certain mental illnesses that are currently at a therapeutic impasse. This progress may in turn lead to attempts not only to heal patients, but augment healthy individuals as well.

Some Questions

The Influence of Treatments on the Classification of Clinical Entities

A recurring criticism of the American Diagnostic Statistical Manual, the DSM [1], which is integral to the current psychiatric culture, is its tendency to emphasize the objective symptoms as opposed to the subjective ones. M. Corcos, a psychiatrist and psychoanalyst, claims that the *DSM is marked by a compartmentalist and biological view which denies the hypothesis of the unconscious, and is therefore a document accepting only one type of symptom which is in fact two superimposed symptoms (the conscious and unconscious) covering an internal conflict that is attempting to make itself known. It attempts to be a purely descriptive approach to mental pathologies, only accepting a purely physicalist view of patient symptomology, with no psychological components* [2]. Certain psychiatrists criticize the DSM by saying that it attempts to identify mental "disorders" in order to have them correspond to a pharmacological category and molecule. In fact, collusion between the pharmaceutical industry and the authors of the DSM is regularly decried [3]. Despite the debates surrounding this classification system, the DSM has enabled the

M. Lévêque, *Psychosurgery*, DOI: 10.1007/978-3-319-01144-8_6,
© Springer International Publishing Switzerland 2014

creation of a universal clinical language, leading to large epidemiological studies and clinical evaluation of the efficacy of a number of psychotropic drugs. It is also probable that genetics will begin to play a part in posological classifications. Why are some patients suffering from bipolar disorder treated with lithium while others are not? Why are certain patients resistant to antidepressants? The progress of pharmacogenetics, by predicting the response of the cellular metabolism for each molecule, will refine the taxonomy of these psychiatric pathologies. Genetics will become the future of clinical psychiatry as was predicted in the *American Journal of Psychiatry* [4] in 2006. One can also be sure that functional brain imagery will also influence the categorization of psychiatric illnesses. We will then be able to distinguish between a patient suffering from severe depression resistant to treatment with hyperactivity in the subgenual cortex from one without hyperactivity using functional imagery. In the former's case, for example, the illness may be treatable with deep brain stimulation of the subgenual cortex whereas the other patient will be treated using other methods. As the American psychiatrist H. Mayberg, states, *During the last 20 years of neuroscience research, we have witnessed a fundamental shift in the conceptualization of psychiatric disorders, with the dominant psychological and neurochemical theories of the past now complemented by a growing emphasis on developmental, genetic, molecular, and brain circuit models. Facilitating this evolving paradigm shift has been the growing contribution of functional neuroimaging, which provides a versatile platform to characterize brain circuit dysfunction underlying specific syndromes as well as changes associated with their successful treatment* [5]. In addition to sociological knowledge, the psychiatrist will soon have results from genetic and functional imagery examinations to aid him in adapting psychotherapeutic or pharmacological treatments to his patient. These new methods are exciting and promising but also raise new questions and fears. Is there not a risk that the human qualities of understanding and listening that a psychiatrist possesses may be substituted for the scientific ability to code symptoms and interpret complementary data?

Lesion or Stimulation?

The revival of psychosurgery is due in large part to the advent of deep brain stimulation. The reversible and adjustable character of this technique allows for greater exploration of anatomical structures and, therefore, the discovery if new psychiatric pathologies which can also be treated by psychosurgery. However, today, certain neurosurgeons question the superiority of this technique over lesional techniques. Recently, the London team of Hariz sought to compare the efficacy of capsulotomies with that of deep brain stimulation of the internal capsule or the nucleus accumbens[1] for treating OCD [6]. His conclusions favored

---

[1] Cf. p. 294.

Table 6.1 Respective advantages and disadvantages of stimulation and lesional techniques of the anterior portion of the internal capsule for the treatment of OCD

	DBS of ALIC	Gamma-capsulotomy
Efficacy	Good	Excellent
Surgical complications	Moderate	Low
Neuropsychological complications	Reversible	Irreversible
Cost	High	Low
Possibility for double blind studies	Yes	
Hospitalization period	5–10 days	1–3 days

lesional techniques. With regard to the potential complications from either technique results have also been mixed. Stimulation offers the advantage of reducing the risk of neuropsychological complications: if a problem arises, chances are that it can be fixed by adjusting the parameters of the stimulation. Nonetheless, when compared to radiosurgery, deep brain stimulation has an augmented risk of infection or hemorrhage, in addition to the vulnerability of the implanted materials. There is still insufficient data to compare the efficacy and the risk of complication of stimulation and lesion therapies. This controversy can only truly be resolved once prospective, randomized studies are conducted. As stimulation techniques evolve, so do lesional procedures, thus limiting the disadvantages and complications from these types of "ablative" surgery (Table 6.1).

One of the handicaps of radiosurgery is creating lesions lasting only a couple of months after the GammaKnife radiosurgery procedure is performed. The nature of this lesion makes it impossible to perform a clinical evaluation during the procedure. If clinical evaluation were possible, it would enable physicians to control the size of the lesion as a function of the clinical efficacy or the appearance of complications. The development of High Intensity Focalized Ultrasounds (HIFU) in neurosurgery allows us to envision new treatment modalities in psychosurgery.

Ultrasounds

Similar in principle to GammaKnife radiosurgery, HIFU replaces gamma waves with high-intensity focalized ultrasounds which cause coagulation at their points of convergence through a very controlled and localized temperature increase. The targeted tissue reaches 57–60 °C (Fig. 3.11, p. 128). This technique which is already used to perform thalamotomies in order to control neuropathic pain [7] is now being experimentally used to treat essential tremors [8]. During this procedure, the abnormal movements of the patient are measured in real-time by the neurologist while the temperature is progressively raised in a specific region of the thalamus (Vim). The physician is therefore able to measure the effect on the symptoms as the size of the lesion changes. If the physician follows proper protocols, the procedure can be stopped in time to prevent complications [9]. This technique needs further research to become a part of the psychosurgical therapeutic arsenal, but it is already promising.

Advances

New Targets

In 1999, the anterior limb of the internal capsule was the first anatomical region to be targeted by deep brain stimulation in order to treat OCD[2] [10]. This target was chosen by Nuttin's team as a result of the knowledge learned through ablative surgeries carried out in the 1950s.[3] In contrast, the subthalamic nucleus, which was the second structure to be targeted by stimulation to treat OCD, was chosen following observations made by Mallet and Fontaine of patients with Parkinson's disease and OCD [11, 12]. The unintended beneficial effects on the obsessive and compulsive symptoms of Parkinson's patients during stimulation of the subthalamic nucleus opened a new treatment path [13]. The first deep brain stimulation targets were thus discovered both by chance [14–16] and knowledge gained from surgical lesional treatments. New targets to treat resistant forms of depression,[4] such as the subgenual area, were later found using functional imaging. In 1997, this region was noticed due to its hyperactivity in patients suffering from major depressive disorders [17]. A few years later, the team of H. Mayberg and A. Lozano successfully treated patients suffering from this pathology by targeting the subgenual cortex [18]. In the future, it will probably be discoveries made by functional imagery that will lead new targets to be included in research protocols. Within the next decade, the improved spatial resolution of functional magnetic resonance imaging should unveil new anatomical regions implicated in psychiatric pathologies [19–21]. The high prevalence of comorbidities in psychiatric disorders, such as anorexia nervosa, OCD [22] and depression [23], and depression and addiction[5] [24], make it likely that new experimental targets found to be effective for one pathology will, in fact, be effective in the treatment of a comorbidity. Thanks to the diminishing size of electrodes, and the potential of nanotechnologies and the resulting ability to track electrode data with reduced invasiveness, our understanding of cerebral activity for various mental pathologies will certainly increase.

NBIC Convergence

Nanotechnology will refine neuromodulation. Soon, this stimulation will be able to target groups of neurons [25, 26] instead of a certain number of cubic millimeters surrounding the electrode. The quality of the electrode–neuron interaction should also progress due, in particular, to carbon nanotubes [27, 28]. *Nanotechnologies are extremely promising for the brain–computer interface domain*, states the neuroethics

----

[2] Cf. p. 271.
[3] Cf. p. 51.
[4] Cf. p. 221.
[5] Cf. p. 358.

specialist N. Kopp. *Thus, the interface between electronics and biology: neuroelectronics, is progressing quickly. We are starting to be able to communicate in an effective manner between the transistor, the base unit of the integrated system, with the base unit of the brain; the neuron. An electrical signal, sent through the integrated circuit, generates an action potential in the neuron; in return, an action potential in the neuron can prompt a modification of the electrical properties of the transistor* [29]. This next stage in nanotechnologies will allow for the recording of the electrical activity of neurons. This possibility, coupled with progress in the analysis of this signal, will lead to "personalized" [27] neuromodulation. The computational power needed to deal with this colossal quantity of information is prodigious, but the exponential reduction in the size of electronic chips and the increases in their speed suggest that these resources will be available soon. In fact, Moore's law[6] should allow us to predict the exact date when they will be available! The simultaneous progress occurring in *Nanotechnology, Biotechnology, Information technology*, neurosciences, and, more generally, *Cognition* is leading toward an important *NBIC convergence*. The concept highlights the convergence of the infinitely small, the study of the brain, and human and information technology. According to theorists of this multidisciplinary science, findings in each of these different domains aid and supplement one another. The brain–machine interface incarnates one of these hybridizations—that of the natural and the artificial. Deep brain stimulation, cortical stimulation, and vagus nerve stimulation are a part of these new interfaces and should benefit considerably from the progress being made. It is possible to imagine that neuromodulation as we know it today, meaning of a structure reached by descending an electrode through the cranium and tissue, may be replaced by "endovascular" techniques—techniques using the cerebral vascular system (Fig. 6.1).

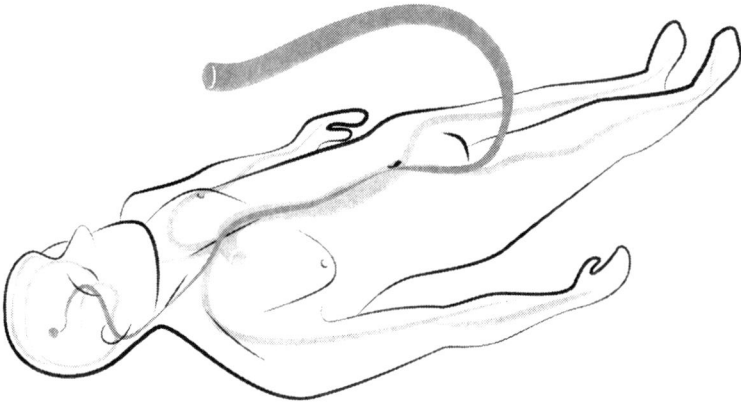

Fig. 6.1 Will we soon have endovascular "nano-electrodes?"

---

[6] In 1975, an engineer named Gordon Moore demonstrated that the density of microprocessors on silicon chips doubles every 2 years and that the cost is halved over the same period. This empirical law has held true as transistor density has doubled every 1.96 years.

This noninvasive technique, which spares the cerebral parenchyma and avoids the need for a craniotomy, have been extensively tested in the last 20 years to the point of becoming the norm in the treatment of intracranial aneurisms. The 25 m of capillaries offer access to any region of the brain. These vessels, with a diameter of only a couple of dozen microns, can be used by submicronic *ultra-micro-electrodes* capable of recording as well as stimulating [30]. A group of *ultra-micro-electrodes* will be able to record and, in response to the monitoring, mediate an extremely specific region of the brain [31, 32]. It is also plausible that such a group of carbon microtubules, measuring only 5 μ in diameter could measure in real-time, neuromediator concentrations in an extremely circumscribed region of the brain [27].

In-situ diffusion of synthetic molecules is another area of research. One of the greatest challenges for neuropharmacological treatments presently is the inability to observe the anatomical regions where incorrect levels of neurotransmitters are produced. Today, it is becoming possible thanks to carbon ultra-microelectrodes to measure the transmission of dopamine in the striatum even when concentrations are as low as 100 nmol [31, 33, 34]. In conjunction with electrical neuromodulation, a biochemical modulation will complete the therapeutic arsenal of the future.

Optogenetics

Several years ago, only electrical currents and neuromediators were able to modify neuronal activity. But today, thanks to optogenetics we are beginning to be able to use light to interact with nerve tissue (Fig. 6.2). At the intersection of optics and genetics, optogenetics is a technique able to mediate activity of genetically modified cells using light. A carrier virus introduces genes coding for opsin proteins into neurons in the brain, thus creating photosensitive ion channels which will open or close depending solely on whether light is present or not. Opening and closing of these channels modulates neuronal activity. Light is brought in through an optical fiber which is implanted under the surface of the cranium near the zone to be stimulated. Light of different wavelengths, each of which activates one particular type of opsin, is transmitted through this fiber. Thus, neurons carrying genes for rhodopsin 2 or halorhodopsin can be turned on or off, meaning they have an electrical activity or not, by being exposed to blue or yellow light, respectively [35].

Currently, optogenetics is only applicable in animals. Researchers are able to control an event in a genetically chosen cellular target in an intact system. This is a powerful investigative tool which should lead to advances allowing us to better understand mental pathologies [36]. Current research is attempting to understand the link between depression and neurobiology and find new targets for therapy [37]. In a speech at the French Senate, the researcher P. Vernier stated that *this simple, and only slightly invasive method is mostly used as an alternative to stimulation by electrodes. But the transfer of this type of treatment to humans,* via

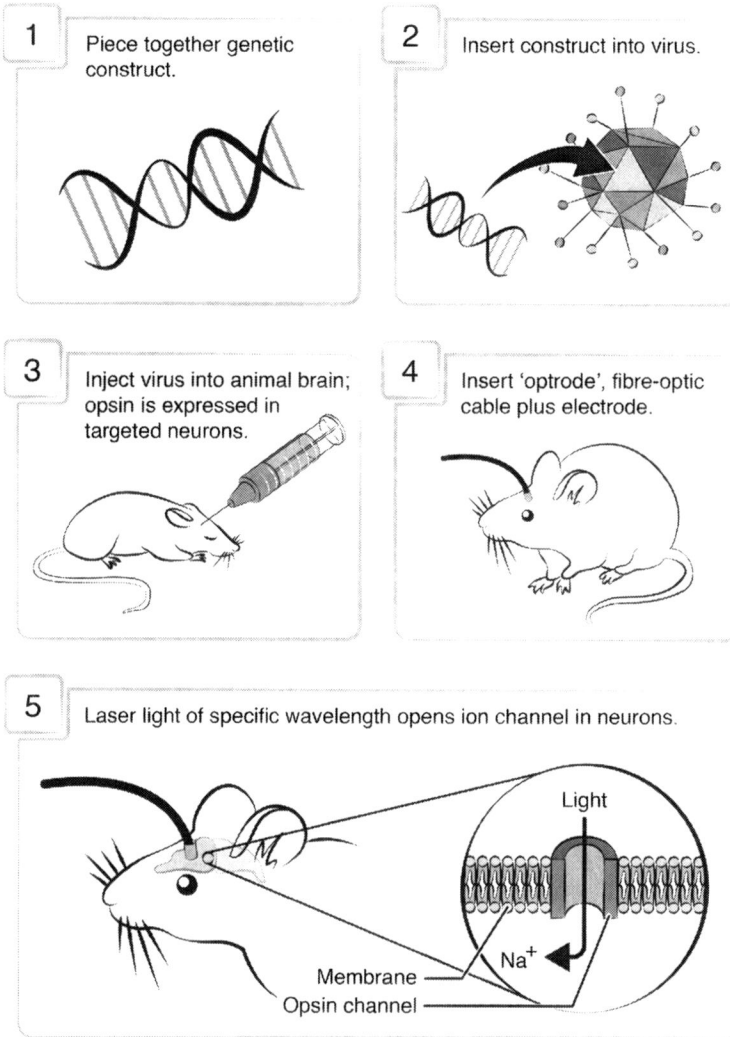

Fig. 6.2 Optogenetic principle

cells which we can be grafted and integrated into the neuronal circuit, is not impossible. And there are currently researchers in centers around the world, including France, who have begun to explore this possibility [38]. As with nanotechnologies, the question is not whether this technique is applicable to humans but when will it be offered to patients. This *kaleidoscope of opportunity,* [25] to quote Apuzzo in an editorial in *Neurosurgery* in 2008, now becoming available to *surgery of mood and mind,* [39, 40] will complicate our approach to mental illnesses and will probably lead to a paradigm shift [41].

Toward an Augmented Human?

Unknown only 5 years ago, optogenetics is gaining momentum [42] and promises to revolutionize modern biology. This effervescent field in bio-nanotechnology still holds many surprises. Thanks to Moore's law, we can be sure that the spread of information technology tools will continue. The computer, for instance, made sequencing of the human genome possible. It is possible to predict that by 2020 the decoding of genes will cost less than 50 euros,[7] or that by 2050 there will be artificial intelligences (AI) able to capture the essence of what it is to be human.[8] These projections suggest that, at one point or another, progress in the field of psychosurgery will be used to not only fix pathologies, but also to improve normal humans. We will thus shift from notions of *fixing people to augmenting them*. The recent work on augmenting the memory of humans [47, 48] or erasing selected painful memories in animals [49] tells us that this practice of *neuroenhancement* is not far off. Many will argue, citing *cosmetic psychopharmacology,* a term which appeared in the 1980s at about the same time as Prozac[®], that we are already there. It is true that we no longer count the number of molecules which can be used to drug our mental faculties or to augment our senses. For instance, medications which are prescribed for dementia (donepezil), depression (fluoxetine), attention deficits (methylphenidate), or narcolepsy (modafinil) are sometimes used for reasons other than their primary indications [50]. Beyond the issue of doping with any of these drugs, what would an *augmented human* with a brain–machine interface be like? As mentioned in a previous chapter, in 2008 a patient with Alzheimer's [51] saw improved performance after stimulation of his hypothalamus [47] opening new possibilities for a treatment for Alzheimer disease. More recently, the stimulation of the entorhinal cortex in seven patients as they undertook tasks encoding memory led to significantly improved spatial memorization. A 67 % reduction in the length of the subject's route, compared to an ideal route, was recorded in six of the seven patients. Despite these perspectives, and although it was unimaginable 10 years ago, deep brain stimulation is likely to enable *memory enhancement* through *brain chips* or even *neuromorphic* chips [52]. Current research focuses on the plasticity of these implants, meaning their ability to be tolerated by the cerebral environment and their capacity to establish functional connections with neurons. The efficacy of the cellular connections is one of the most important *frontiers* in biotechnology and is one of the keys for the

---

[7] Around 1,000 euros today compared with almost two million euros in 2007. Even more astounding, the first full genetic sequencing ever accomplished cost three billion dollars and required hundreds of researchers working for 13 years!

[8] Specialists predict that zetaflop, one thousand billion billion operations a second, processing should allow the connections among the one hundred billion neurons in our brain to be modeled. An American project called "Connectome" is attempting just that [43–45]. The leaders of this ambitious research program to map the almost infinity connections, which are "the product of our genes and our intellectual experiences," believe that the required computational power will be available in the next 10–20 years [46].

success of the brain–machine field. *Carbon nanotubes*, [53] *nanowires*, [54] *nanoscale coating*, [55] and *labs-on-a-chip*, [53, 56] are being used to explore this frontier. If the problem of plasticity is solved, the brain–machine interface may tie humans' evolution to Moore's Law... If that is the case, the application of implants will surpass simple memory augmentation: humans—*cyborgs* linguists may say—will be *directly* connected to a vast network of information. Currently, we access information through our five senses. Brain–machine interfaces, however, will lead us into a *pervasively networked* era in which information bypasses our sense to affect us directly, thus ushering us into *Transhumanity*.[9] A future world populated by humans full of bionic devices will certainly cause great controversy and debate between "bio-conservatives" and "bio-progressives," as well as raise a great number of grave new ethical questions.

References

1. American Psychiatric Association (2000) American Psychiatric Association. Task force on DSM-IV. Diagnostic and statistical manual of mental disorders: DSM-IV-TR, 4th edn. American Psychiatric Association, Washington
2. Corcos M (2011) L'homme selon DSM: Le nouvel ordre psychiatrique. Editions Albin Michel
3. Cosgrove L, Krimsky S (2012) A comparison of DSM-IV and DSM-5 panel members' financial associations with industry: a pernicious problem persists. PLoS Med 9(3):e1001190. doi:10.1371/journal.pmed.1001190 PMEDICINE-D-11-03049 [pii]
4. Hariri AR, Lewis DA (2006) Genetics and the future of clinical psychiatry. Am J Psychiatry 163(10):1676–1678. doi:10.1176/appi.ajp.163.10.1676 [pii]
5. Mayberg HS (2009) Targeted electrode-based modulation of neural circuits for depression. J Clin Invest 119(4):717–725. doi:10.1172/JCI38454 [pii]
6. Pepper J, Hariz M (2012) Anterior capsulotomy versus dbs for obsessive compulsive disorder: a review of the literature. XXth congress of the European society for stereotactic and functional neurosurgery, Cascais, Portugal
7. Martin E, Jeanmonod D, Morel A, Zadicario E, Werner B (2009) High-intensity focused ultrasound for noninvasive functional neurosurgery. Ann Neurol 66(6):858–861. doi:10.1002/ana.21801
8. Lozano A (2012) Functional neurosurgery—an illustrious past, an exciting future. XXth congress of the European society for stereotactic and functional neurosurgery, Cascais, Portugal
9. Medel R, Monteith SJ, Elias WJ, Eames M, Snell J, Sheehan JP et al (2012) Magnetic resonance-guided focused ultrasound surgery: part 2: a review of current and future applications. Neurosurgery 71(4):755–763. doi:10.1227/NEU.0b013e3182672ac9
10. Nuttin B, Cosyns P, Demeulemeester H, Gybels J, Meyerson B (1999) Electrical stimulation in anterior limbs of internal capsules in patients with obsessive-compulsive disorder. Lancet 354(9189):1526. doi:10.1016/S0140-6736(99)02376-4 [pii]

---

[9] For more on the subject, read *Bienvenue en Transhumanie* (Welcome to Transhumania), by Geneviève Ferone and Jean-Didier Vincent (Grasset, 290 p.). A captivating work on *technology forcing* and its ethical and political implications.

11. Mallet L, Mesnage V, Houeto JL, Pelissolo A, Yelnik J, Behar C et al (2002) Compulsions, Parkinson's disease, and stimulation. Lancet 360(9342):1302–1304. doi:10.1016/S0140-6736(02)11339-0 [pii]

12. Fontaine D, Mattei V, Borg M, von Langsdorff D, Magnie MN, Chanalet S et al (2004) Effect of subthalamic nucleus stimulation on obsessive-compulsive disorder in a patient with Parkinson disease. Case report. J Neurosurg 100(6):1084–1086. doi:10.3171/jns.2004.100.6.1084

13. Mallet L, Polosan M, Jaafari N, Baup N, Welter ML, Fontaine D et al (2008) Subthalamic nucleus stimulation in severe obsessive-compulsive disorder. N Engl J Med 359(20):2121–2134. doi:10.1056/NEJMoa0708514 359/20/2121 [pii]

14. Baumeister AA (2006) Serendipity and the cerebral localization of pleasure. J Hist Neurosci 15(2):92–98. doi:10.1080/09647040500274879 Q68T775847306678 [pii]

15. Benabid AL, Torres N (2012) New targets for DBS. Parkinsonism Relat Disord 8(Suppl 1):S21–S23. doi:10.1016/S1353-8020(11)70009-8 S1353-8020(11)70009-8 [pii]

16. Benabid AL (2006) Attention, la psychochirurgie est de retour. Revue de neurologie 162(8):797–799

17. Drevets WC, Price JL, Simpson JR, Todd RD, Reich T, Vannier M et al (1997) Subgenual prefrontal cortex abnormalities in mood disorders. Nature 386(6627):824–827. doi:10.1038/386824a0

18. Mayberg HS, Lozano AM, Voon V, McNeely HE, Seminowicz D, Hamani C et al (2005) Deep brain stimulation for treatment-resistant depression. Neuron 45(5):651–660. doi:10.1016/j.neuron.2005.02.014

19. Abosch A, Yacoub E, Ugurbil K, Harel N (2010) An assessment of current brain targets for deep brain stimulation surgery with susceptibility-weighted imaging at 7 tesla. Neurosurgery 67(6):1745–1756, discussion 56. doi:10.1227/NEU.0b013e3181f74105 00006123-20101 2000-00041 [pii]

20. Metzger CD, Eckert U, Steiner J, Sartorius A, Buchmann JE, Stadler J et al (2010) High field FMRI reveals thalamocortical integration of segregated cognitive and emotional processing in mediodorsal and intralaminar thalamic nuclei. Front Neuroanat 4:138. doi:10.3389/fnana.2010.00138

21. Lenglet C, Abosch A, Yacoub E, de Martino F, Sapiro G, Harel N (2012) Comprehensive in vivo mapping of the human basal ganglia and thalamic connectome in individuals using 7T MRI. PLoS One 7(1):e29153. doi:10.1371/journal.pone.0029153 PONE-D-11-12474 [pii]

22. Halmi KA, Tozzi F, Thornton LM, Crow S, Fichter MM, Kaplan AS et al (2005) The relation among perfectionism, obsessive-compulsive personality disorder and obsessive-compulsive disorder in individuals with eating disorders. Int J Eat Disord 38(4):371–374. doi:10.1002/eat.20190

23. Milanfranchi A, Marazziti D, Pfanner C, Presta S, Lensi P, Ravagli S et al (1995) Comorbidity in obsessive-compulsive disorder: focus on depression. Eur Psychiatry 10(8):379–382. doi:10.1016/0924-9338(96)80341-5 0924-9338(96)80341-5 [pii]

24. Thimann J, Gauthier JW (1959) The management of depression in alcoholism and drug addiction. J Clin Exp Psychopathol Q Rev Psychiatry Neurol 20:320–325

25. Elder JB, Hoh DJ, Oh BC, Heller AC, Liu CY, Apuzzo ML (2008) The future of cerebral surgery: a kaleidoscope of opportunities. Neurosurgery 62(6 Suppl 3):1555–1579; discussion 79–82. doi:10.1227/01.neu.0000333820.33143.0d 00006123-200806001-00062 [pii]

26. Elder JB, Liu CY, Apuzzo ML (2008) Neurosurgery in the realm of 10(-9), part 2: applications of nanotechnology to neurosurgery-present and future. Neurosurgery 62(2):269–284; discussion 84–5. doi:10.1227/01.neu.0000315995.73269.c3 00006123-200802000-00009 [pii]

27. Li J, Andrews RJ (2007) Trimodal nanoelectrode array for precise deep brain stimulation: prospects of a new technology based on carbon nanofiber arrays. Acta Neurochir Suppl 97(Pt 2):537–545

28. Mazzatenta A, Giugliano M, Campidelli S, Gambazzi L, Businaro L, Markram H et al (2007) Interfacing neurons with carbon nanotubes: electrical signal transfer and synaptic stimulation

in cultured brain circuits. J Neurosci 27(26):6931–6936. doi:10.1523/JNEUROSCI.1051-07. 2007 27/26/6931 [pii]

29. Kopp N. Neuroéthique et nanotechnologies (2007) In: Hervé C (ed) La nanomédecine: Enjeux éthiques, juridiques et normatifs. Dalloz, Paris, pp 142–156

30. Llina R, Walton K, Hunter M, Nakao I, Anquetil P (2005) Neuro-vascular central nervous recording/stimulating system: using nanotechnology probes. J Nanopart Res 7:111–127

31. Andrews RJ (2010) Neuromodulation: advances in the next decade. Ann N Y Acad Sci 1199:212–220. doi:10.1111/j.1749-6632.2009.05380.x NYAS5380 [pii]

32. Roco MC, Bainbridge WS (2003) Converging technologies for improving human performance: nanotechnology, biotechnology, information technology and cognitive science. Kluwer Academic Publishers, Dordrecht

33. Venton BJ, Zhang H, Garris PA, Phillips PE, Sulzer D, Wightman RM (2003) Real-time decoding of dopamine concentration changes in the caudate-putamen during tonic and phasic firing. J Neurochem 87(5):1284–1295. doi:2109 [pii]

34. Robinson DL, Venton BJ, Heien ML, Wightman RM (2003) Detecting subsecond dopamine release with fast-scan cyclic voltammetry in vivo. Clin Chem 49(10):1763–1773

35. Gradinaru V, Thompson KR, Zhang F, Mogri M, Kay K, Schneider MB et al (2007) Targeting and readout strategies for fast optical neural control in vitro and in vivo. J Neurosci 27(52):14231–14238. doi:10.1523/JNEUROSCI.3578-07.2007 27/52/14231 [pii]

36. Han MH, Friedman AK (2012) Virogenetic and optogenetic mechanisms to define potential therapeutic targets in psychiatric disorders. Neuropharmacology 62(1):89–100. doi:10.1016/j.neuropharm.2011.09.009

37. Lobo MK, Nestler EJ (2012) Covington HE, III. Potential utility of optogenetics in the study of depression. Biol Psychiatry 71(12):1068–1074. doi:10.1016/j.biopsych.2011.12.026

38. Vernier P (2011) L'impact et les enjeux des nouvelles technologies d'exploration et de thérapie du cerveau (Rapport). In: Rapports d'office parlementaire Apdj, editor. Sénat, République Française

39. Heller AC, Amar AP, Liu CY, Apuzzo ML (2006) Surgery of the mind and mood: a mosaic of issues in time and evolution. Neurosurgery 59(4):720–733; discussion 33–9 doi:10.1227/01.NEU.0000240227.72514.27 00006123-200610000-00003 [pii]

40. Robison RA, Taghva A, Liu CY, Apuzzo ML (2012) Surgery of the mind, mood, and conscious state: an idea in evolution. World Neurosurg doi:10.1016/j.wneu.2012.03.005 S1878-8750(12)00345-2 [pii]

41. Deisseroth K (2012) Optogenetics and psychiatry: applications, challenges, and opportunities. Biol Psychiatry 71(12):1030–1032. doi:10.1016/j.biopsych.2011.12.021

42. Minet P (2012) L'optogénétique gagne tous les organes. La recherche (460)

43. Axer M, Amunts K, Grassel D, Palm C, Dammers J, Axer H, Pietrzyk U, Zilles K (2011) A novel approach to the human connectome: ultra-high resolution mapping of fiber tracts in the brain. Neuroimage 54:1091–1101

44. Cammoun L, Gigandet X, Meskaldji D, Thiran JP, Sporns O, Do KQ, Maeder P, Meuli R, Hagmann P (2012) Mapping the human connectome at multiple scales with diffusion spectrum MRI. J Neurosci Methods 203:386–397

45. Toga AW, Clark KA, Thompson PM, Shattuck DW, Van Horn JD (2012) Mapping the human connectome. Neurosurgery 71:1–5

46. Vance A (2010) In pursuit of a mind map slice by slice. New York Times, New York

47. Hamani C, McAndrews MP, Cohn M, Oh M, Zumsteg D, Shapiro CM et al (2008) Memory enhancement induced by hypothalamic/fornix deep brain stimulation. Ann Neurol 63(1):119–123. doi:10.1002/ana.21295

48. Suthana N, Haneef Z, Stern J, Mukamel R, Behnke E, Knowlton B et al (2012) Memory enhancement and deep-brain stimulation of the entorhinal area. N Engl J Med 366(6):502–510. doi:10.1056/NEJMoa1107212

49. Han JH, Kushner SA, Yiu AP, Hsiang HL, Buch T, Waisman A et al (2009) Selective erasure of a fear memory. Science 323(5920):1492–1496. doi:10.1126/science.1164139 323/5920/1492 [pii]

50. Gross D (2010) Traditional vs. modern neuroenhancement: notes from a medico-ethical and societal perspective. In: Fangerau H, Fegert J, Trapp T (eds) Implanted minds: the neuroethics of intracerebral stem cell transplantation and deep brain stimulation. Transcript Verlag, London, pp 291–311
51. Laxton AW, Tang-Wai DF, McAndrews MP, Zumsteg D, Wennberg R, Keren R et al (2010) A phase I trial of deep brain stimulation of memory circuits in Alzheimer's disease. Ann Neurol 68(4):521–534. doi:10.1002/ana.22089
52. Neuner I, Podoll K, Janouschek H, Michel TM, Sheldrick AJ, Schneider F (2009) From psychosurgery to neuromodulation: deep brain stimulation for intractable Tourette syndrome. World J Biol Psychiatry 10(4 Pt 2):366–376. doi:10.1080/15622970802513317 905440831 [pii]
53. Nguyen-Vu TD, Chen H, Cassell AM, Andrews R, Meyyappan M, Li J (2006) Vertically aligned carbon nanofiber arrays: an advance toward electrical-neural interfaces. Small 2(1):89–94. doi:10.1002/smll.200500175
54. Green JE, Choi JW, Boukai A, Bunimovich Y, Johnston-Halperin E, DeIonno E et al (2007) A 160-kilobit molecular electronic memory patterned at 10(11) bits per square centimetre. Nature 445(7126):414–417. doi:10.1038/nature05462 nature05462 [pii]
55. He W, Bellamkonda RV (2005) Nanoscale neuro-integrative coatings for neural implants. Biomaterials 26(16):2983–2990. doi:10.1016/j.biomaterials.2004.08.021 S0142-9612(04)00770-7 [pii]
56. He W, McConnell GC, Bellamkonda RV (2006) Nanoscale laminin coating modulates cortical scarring response around implanted silicon microelectrode arrays. J Neural Eng 3(4):316–326. doi:10.1088/1741-2560/3/4/009 S1741-2560(06)31677-1 [pii]

Conclusion

In a 2006 article,[1] provocatively entitled, "Beware, Psychosurgery is back!" the father of deep brain stimulation, Alim-Louis Benabid, addressed all those "who will have the grave responsibility of redeveloping therapeutic methods able to bring certain relief to patients suffering from diseases which lead to their exclusion from society, their family and their own dignity." The celebrated neurosurgeon from Genoble warned that, "the renaissance of psychosurgery gives us, patients as well as physicians and scientists, a second chance, and it is our duty to use it as best we can and to positive effect. We will be responsible if once again because of our errors and lack of judgement we let it fail and give rise to a new era of darkness." The path forward for psychosurgery will not be easy. It is burdened with a history of past controversies that are hard to escape. Some authors have therefore suggested renaming psychosurgery "neuromodulation" but such a semantic trick is of little value. Quite the contrary, it invalidates efforts to educate the public about the difference between lobotomies practiced in the 1950s and current interventions, which are no longer synonymous with mutilations of patients' personality. Going forward, there is a risk of abuses if this intervention is practiced without heeding fundamental ethical principles. The future of psychosurgery, caught between past errors and the threat of being condemned for ideological reasons or because of technophobia, is uncertain. Nonetheless, this discipline seems the offer a way to improve the lives of tens of thousands of patients who today face a lack of treatments and are condemned to suffer from mental illness. In order for it to flourish, the future of psychosurgery must be strictly supervised. It therefore seems essential to end this book with a reminder of the safeguards without which the continued development of "deep brain stimulation for psychiatric pathologies may be doomed[2]" as Marwan Hariz warns.

First, these techniques must be used exclusively for patients suffering from serious debilitating disorders for whom less invasive therapies have failed.

---

[1] Benabid, A. L. 2006. "Beware psychosurgery is back" (Attention, la psychochirurgie est de retour). Revue de neurologie 162:797–799.

[2] Hariz MI, and Hariz GM (2012) Hyping deep brain stimulation in psychiatry could lead to its demise. BMJ 345: e5447.

M. Lévêque, *Psychosurgery*, DOI: 10.1007/978-3-319-01144-8,
© Springer International Publishing Switzerland 2014

Secondly, these treatments must be discussed by multidisciplinary teams with the proper authority and the indications approved in a collegial manner.

Thirdly, independent ethics bodies must ensure that fundamental principles of bioethics are respected. The issues of free and informed consent and conflicts of interest require the utmost vigilance.

Only democracies are capable of guaranteeing the requisite independence of these ethics bodies. Psychosurgery is inseparable from the political order.[3] For example, the press can be both a tool for emancipation in democracies as well as a tool for manipulation in dictatorships. Psychosurgery can likewise be used for good or evil: as a treatment or a tool for control. To counter this danger our societies must be kept informed, with utmost transparency, of the advances being made in this field and of its applications throughout the world.

---

[3] Breggin, P. R. 1975. Psychosurgery for political purposes. Duquesne Law Rev 13:841–862 et Delgado, J. M. R. 1969. Physical control of the mind; toward a psychocivilized society, 1st edn. Harper & Row, New York.

Afterword

We are at the beginning of an era of renewed interest in neurosurgery for psychiatric illness. The keyword of this new era of psychosurgery is "neuromodulation," as opposed to the neuro-ablation of the past. Neuromodulation makes use of a surgical technique called Deep Brain Stimulation (DBS). This new technique is promoted, and perceived, as being non-destructive, adaptable, and especially "reversible." Psychosurgery, including stereotactic psychosurgical ablative procedures—which had been thrown out through the door, sometimes reminding of the idiomatic expression of throwing the baby with the bath water—is now re-entering through the window of "neuromodulation," a disguise meant to reassure the public of the innocuity and leniency of this "modern" procedure.

The great contribution of this book by neurosurgeon Marc Lévêque is to put this new emerging era of non-ablative surgery into a historical, scientific, and ethical context. Reading this book is like reading an anthology, or rather an encyclopaedia of the field of psychiatric surgery, spanning more than a century. This is a work with an unprecedented degree of erudition and knowledge, and the subject is presented in a didactic, scholar, and scientific manner, and is extensively referenced and illustrated. If only one book is to be read by anybody interested in this field, regardless of specialty, this is The Book to read.

Where is the field now going? One may reflect upon the fact that, as described in the book, modern DBS for psychiatric illness was pioneered already in 1999 with DBS for obsessive compulsive disorder (OCD) and DBS for Tourette syndrome. A few years later, DBS for major depression was introduced. Today, there are about eight published brain targets for DBS in OCD, ten published brain targets for DBS in Tourette, and nine published brain targets for DBS in depression. Some of these brain targets overlap each other, and none of the brain targets and indeed none of the psychiatric indications for DBS is yet "established," despite the plethora of scientific papers published in the last 14 years of activity in the field. Despite this lack of consensus about DBS in these three major psychiatric illnesses, DBS is now trialled or advertised as a potential treatment for drug addiction, anorexia nervosa, post-traumatic stress disorder, and dementias. Lately, an alarming qualitative jump has occurred in that DBS is being considered as a tool, not for diseases and illnesses, but for enhancement of

M. Lévêque, *Psychosurgery*, DOI: 10.1007/978-3-319-01144-8,
© Springer International Publishing Switzerland 2014

cognition in *normal* people. Finally, that alarming jump has now approached an abyss as illustrated in a recent article published in the prestigious Journal BRAIN, in which "scientists" suggested the theoretical use of DBS to treat "antisocial behaviour" and to improve "morality"!

All this shows that the prophecy of Dr. Joseph H. Friedman from Rhode Island in 2004 is being confirmed. Friedman wrote then: "Now that DBS means that psychosurgery is reversible, we no longer have to worry about permanent harm. On the other hand, now that psychosurgery could be readily available, potentially for a large number of conditions, we have a lot more to worry about."

Indeed if the field continues in this direction we will have a lot more to worry about, and we may witness then another setback for surgery for psychiatric illness. The tragedy of the past is well illustrated in this book in relation to old times DBS as practiced in Tulane University in the 1950s through the 1970s, and that had been condemned by Beaumeister in 2000 as being unethical *"by yesterdays standards"*). This tragedy of the past may well become the farce of the future.

Neuromodulation should not be allowed to become neuro-manipulation, and the DBS technique as such is neither always "reversible," nor is it per se necessarily more "ethical" than well-performed stereotactic lesions such as anterior capsulotomy or cingulotomy, in the treatment of refractory psychiatric illness. The "second chance" of psychosurgery—as Benabid put it in 2006—and that is permitted by DBS, should not be allowed to degenerate into a farce. One should bear in mind the famous quote attributed to the Great Swedish neurosurgeon Lars Leksell: "a fool with a tool is still a fool." This book of Marc Lévêque will invite those who read it to a profound reflection about the field of psychiatric surgery, and about the moral and ethical guardrails (garde-fous) needed, if real severely ill patients who suffer from real diseases of the mind that are refractory to all other non-surgical treatments, are to benefit from a justified, well-performed, well-evaluated stereotactic procedure, be it stereotactic DBS surgery, or stereotactic ablative surgery.

November 2013

Professor Marwan Hariz
Chair of Functional Neurosurgery,
UCL Institute of Neurology,
Queen Square, London, UK
Adjunct Professor of Stereotactic Surgery,
Umeå University, Umeå, Sweden
London and Umeå

Thanks

This book is the product of a reflection on psychiatry, neurosurgery, and ethics. I would like to thank Monique Carton, who through her humanity and talent taught me to love psychiatry. My thanks to Patrice Simon, who guided me during my internship at the Charles Perrens Hospital and showed me the richness of psychoanalytic discourse. Jean Guérin, Dominique Liguoro in Bordeaux and Thierry Gustin and Claude Gilliard at the UCL helped me with their generosity and talents take my first steps in surgery of the nervous system. Thank you. My two years as a fellow in Montreal alongside Michel Bojanowski were incredibly fruitful. He is an exceptional neurosurgeon and a peerless teacher. Our discussions on neuroanatomy, ethics... the French language nourished me as much as the smoked-meat sandwiches at Schwartz's we would eat after those interminable interventions. My thanks to Danielle Laudy at the Université de Montréal who awakened me to the field of medical ethics and then made it possible for me to teach alongside her. With all their talent, Jean-Claude Péragut and Jean Régis at the Timone trained me in functional neurosurgery. I am grateful to them and to Jean-Philippe Azulay who encouraged me to learn more about the fascinating and promising field of psychosurgery. My thanks to Marwan Hariz and Bart Nuttin, two eminent specialists in psychosurgery, who welcomed me into their department and took the time to answer my numerous questions.

This book would not have been possible without the astute comments and eye for detail of Emmanuel Ly-Batallan, Fabrice Bartholomei, Michel W. Bojanowski, Romain Carron, Monique Carton, C. Rees Cosgrove, Edgar Durand, Alexandre Eusebio, Denys Fontaine, Anne Jilger, Marie-Pierre Fournier-Gosselin, Björn Meyerson, Grégoire Moutel, Mircea Polosan, Raphaëlle Richieri, Napoléon Torres, who all generously contributed their time to rereading parts or the whole of this text. I am indebted to Philippe Cornu, who agreed to preface this work. I thank from the bottom of my heart my friend, Laurent Alexandre, for his advice and our fascinating conversations about technomedecine. I had the privilege of being immediately understood by Nathalie L'Horset-Poulain, who welcomed my book into her collection. I express my immense gratitude as a young author. I thank Charlotte Porcheron, whose brush strokes reflected my thoughts perfectly. This book would never have seen the light of day without the encouragement of Philippe and the tender support of Sophie. I dedicate it to our daughter, Marie.

Bibliography

History

El-Hai J (2005) The lobotomist: a maverick medical genius and his tragic quest to rid the world of mental illness. Wiley & Hoboken

Freeman W (1942) Psychosurgery. Charles C. Thomas, Baltimore

Fulton JF (1951) Frontal Lobotomy and affective behavior: a neurophysiological analysis. Norton

Le Beau JC, Gaches M, Rosier J (1954) Psycho-chirurgie et fonctions mentales: techniques—resultats applications physiologiques. Masson, Paris

Mark VH, Ervin FR (1970) Violence and the brain. Medical Department., Harper & Row. New York

Pressman JD (2002) Last resort: psychosurgery and the limits of medicine. Cambridge University Press, Cambridge

Puech P, Guilly P, Lairy-Bounes GC (1950) Introduction à la psychochirurgie. Masson

Valenstein ES (1974) Brain control. Wiley, New York

Valenstein ES (1986) Great and desperate cures: the rise and decline of psychosurgery and other radical treatments for mental illness. Basic Books, New York

Techniques

Denys D, Feenstra M, Schuurman R (2012) Deep brain stimulation: a new frontier in psychiatry. Springer, Berlin

Higgins ES, George MS (2008) Brain stimulation therapies for clinicians. American Psychiatric Pub

Kellner CH (2012) Brain stimulation in psychiatry: ECT, DBS. Cambridge University Press, TMS and Other Modalities

Lisanby SH (2004) Brain Stimulation in psychiatric treatment. American Psychiatric Pub

Lozano AM, Gildenberg PL, Tasker RR (2009) Textbook of stereotactic and functional neurosurgery. Springer, Berlin

Winn HR, Youmans JR (2011) Youmans' neurological surgery, 6th edn. Saunders, Philadelphia

Ethics

Fangerau H, Fegert JM, Trapp T (2010) Implanted minds: the neuroethics of intracerebral stem cell transplantation and deep brain stimulation. Transcript Verlag, Roswitha Gost, Sigrid Nokel

Kleinig J (1985) Ethical issues in psychosurgery. Allen & Unwin, London

M. Lévêque, *Psychosurgery*, DOI: 10.1007/978-3-319-01144-8,
© Springer International Publishing Switzerland 2014

About the Author

Marc Lévêque is a neursosurgeon at the Pitié-Salpêtrière hospital in Paris, France. After beginning his residency in psychiatry, he was appointed physician at the French Embassy in China before joining neurosurgery. Trained at the University of Leuven and the Université de Montréal, he is a former fellow of the functional neurosurgery and stereotaxy department at the Timone hospital in Marseille. Marc Lévêque has contributed to several research protocols in deep brain stimulation for the treatment of OCD and has participated in the elaboration of a study on cortical stimulation for the treatment of treatment-refractory depression.

The latest scientific findings, testimonies, public domain elements of the bibliography as well as illustrations and videos on psychosurgery are available on the author's blog:

www.psychochirurgie.info

M. Lévêque, *Psychosurgery*, DOI: 10.1007/978-3-319-01144-8,
© Springer International Publishing Switzerland 2014

Blurb

With a controversial past, psychosurgery, or the surgical treatment of mental disorders, has undergone a spectacular revival over the past 10 years as new brain stimulation techniques have become available. Neuromodulation offers new possibilities for the treatment of psychiatric disorders such as depression, obsessive-compulsive disorders (OCD), addiction, and eating disorders. This work presents the history of this singular specialty and investigates current techniques and ethical challenges. With a wealth of illustrations and accessible anatomical diagrams, this book aims to inform and entertain medical practitioners as well as anyone interested in the fascinating advances being made in neuroscience today.

M. Lévêque, *Psychosurgery*, DOI: 10.1007/978-3-319-01144-8,
© Springer International Publishing Switzerland 2014

Name Index

M. Lévêque, *Psychosurgery*, DOI: 10.1007/978-3-319-01144-8,
© Springer International Publishing Switzerland 2014

Index

M. Lévêque, *Psychosurgery*, DOI: 10.1007/978-3-319-01144-8,
© Springer International Publishing Switzerland 2014

CPSIA information can be obtained at www.ICGtesting.com
Printed in the USA
LVOW12*2157130814

398980LV00009B/108/P